D1568411

PATHOLOGY OF ASBESTOS-ASSOCIATED DISEASES

PATHOLOGY OF ASBESTOS-ASSOCIATED DISEASES

VICTOR L. ROGGLI, M.D.
Associate Professor of Pathology, Duke University School of Medicine;
Staff Pathologist, Veterans Administration Hospital,
Durham, North Carolina

S. DONALD GREENBERG, M.D.
Professor of Pathology, Baylor College of Medicine; Attending Physician,
Ben Taub General Hospital, Houston, Texas

PHILIP C. PRATT, M.D.
Professor Emeritus of Pathology,
Duke University School of Medicine,
Durham, North Carolina

LITTLE, BROWN and COMPANY
Boston/Toronto/London

Library of Congress Cataloging-in-Publication Data
Roggli, Victor L.
    Pathology of asbestos-associated diseases / Victor L. Roggli, S.
Donald Greenberg, Philip C. Pratt
        p.   cm.
    Includes bibliographical references and index.
    ISBN 0-316-75423-4
    1. Asbestosis—Pathophysiology.   2. Mesothelioma—Pathophysiology.
3. Lungs—Cancer—Etiology.   I. Greenberg, S. Donald, 1930–
II. Pratt, Philip C.   III. Title.
    [DNLM: 1. Asbestosis—pathology.   2. Lung Neoplasms—pathology.
3. Mesothelioma—pathology.   4. Pleural Diseases—pathology.   WF
654 R733p]
RC775.A8R64   1992
616.2′44—dc20
DNLM/DLC
for Library of Congress   92-13417
                                                            CIP

Printed in the United States of America
HAL

Contents

PREFACE

The purpose of *Pathology of Asbestos-Associated Diseases* is to give a detailed description of the pathologic abnormalities associated with exposure to asbestos fibers. The past decade has witnessed substantial advances in our understanding of the pathology of asbestos-associated diseases, as a result of observations using both human and animal tissue samples. A book with this information summarized in a single volume is a valuable resource for pathologists, pulmonologists, radiologists, occupational medicine practitioners, industrial hygienists, and others with an interest in this subject.

Knowledge of asbestos-associated diseases has been derived primarily from three lines of investigation: (1) observations and detailed descriptions of pathologic changes in tissues of individuals exposed through their occupations to airborne asbestos fibers, including quantification of asbestos content; (2) reproduction of these diseases in animals exposed to asbestos fibers under controlled conditions; and (3) epidemiologic observations made of asbestos workers examined as part of either cross-sectional or longitudinal studies. Because these latter two lines of investigation have contributed to knowledge of the pathology of asbestos-associated diseases, they are also summarized in this volume. The chapters dealing with specific diseases include a review of pertinent epidemiologic studies. One entire chapter is devoted to a review of the contributions of experimental animal studies to knowledge of asbestos-associated diseases.

The book is organized into thirteen chapters, each dealing with a specific aspect of asbestos-associated diseases. The first chapter is designed to tell the reader what asbestos is and includes a simplified description of asbestos mineralogy, its sources, and the methods used to detect and identify asbestos fibers. The second chapter describes how individuals are exposed to asbestos, both in the workplace and in the home environment. Chapter 3 gives a detailed description of asbestos bodies, how they are formed, and how they can be distinguished from ferruginous bodies lacking an asbestos core.

The first three chapters give the background for the chapter on asbestosis, a form of pneumoconiosis that has been recognized since the early decades of this century. This is followed by a chapter dealing with the pathologic features of malignant mesothelioma, a signal neoplasm occurring with alarming regularity in populations exposed to asbestos. An explosion of information regarding the specific features of this neoplasm has greatly increased the reliability of the pathologist's diagnostic armamentarium for distinguishing mesothelioma from other malignancies with which it may be confused. The sixth chapter is devoted to the non-neoplastic alterations in the pleura that may occur in individuals exposed to asbestos.

Chapter 7 is a review of the pathologic and epidemiologic features of carcinoma of the lung related to asbestos exposure. This is a particularly difficult and controversial area, mainly due to the strong and confounding association of the various lung carcinomas with cigarette smoking. Other asbestos-related neoplasms are the topic of the following chapter, an area of investigation that is badly in need of more detailed studies. Chapter 9 reviews the contributions of cytopathology to the diagnosis of asbestos-associated diseases, a source of valuable information often neglected in the past.

A book on the pathology of asbestos-associated diseases would be incomplete without a discussion of the contributions of experimental animal studies. Chapter 10 shows how these models of asbestos-related disease have greatly expanded our understanding of the interactions of asbestos with the respiratory system and the resulting changes that ultimately lead to disease. In addition, they have in a more general sense increased our knowledge of pulmonary pathobiology. With the current rapid progress in molecular biology research, the coming decade should witness even greater progress in understanding the mechanisms at the molecular level, whereby asbestos is able to induce pulmonary fibrosis or effect neoplastic transformation of cells of the lung and pleura.

A great deal of information has also been gained in the past decade with regard to the tissue asbestos levels associated with various asbestos-induced diseases. Although these analytic and quantitative techniques have yet to be standardized, the information provided by different laboratories has been surprisingly consistent. This information is summarized in Chapter 11, including a considerable amount of previously unpublished data from the authors' own laboratories.

The medicolegal repercussions of asbestos-related diseases have affected a large segment of our population through asbestos litigation, and Chapters 12 and 13 deal with the pathologic aspects of asbestos-associated diseases from an attorney's perspective. Both the plaintiff's and the defendant's points of view are presented by prominent attorneys with extensive experience in this litigation.

Each of the chapters also contains a brief historic review to place the discussion in proper perspective. The information in these reviews is largely derived from a few excellent and detailed sources on the historic perspective of asbestos and asbestos-related diseases.

Due to increasing public awareness of asbestos and its effects on health, as well as increasing concern of public health officials on the prevention of future disease, it is important that pathologists have a working knowledge of the various manifestations of asbestos-related tissue injury. It is hoped that this volume will provide pathologists and other health-care workers with this necessary information.

V. L. R.
S. D. G.
P. C. P.

CONTRIBUTING AUTHORS

Arnold R. Brody, Ph.D.
Group Leader, Laboratory of Pulmonary Pathobiology, National Institute of Environmental Health Sciences, Research Triangle Park, North Carolina

Patrick Coin, Ph.D.
Research Technician, Department of Pathology, Duke University Medical Center; Research Physiologist, General Medical Research, Veterans Administration Hospital, Durham, North Carolina

Dennis J. Darcey, Ph.D.
Assistant Clinical Professor of Occupational Medicine, Duke University School of Medicine, Durham, North Carolina

Henry G. Garrard, III, J.D.
Attorney, Blasingame, Burch, Garrard & Bryant, P.C., Athens, Georgia

Gary N. Greenberg, M.D.
Assistant Clinical Professor of Occupational and Environmental Medicine, Duke University School of Medicine; Associate in General Internal Medicine, Duke University Hospital, Durham, North Carolina

S. Donald Greenberg, M.D.
Professor of Pathology, Baylor College of Medicine; Attending Physician, Ben Taub General Hospital, Houston, Texas

Ivan A. Gustafson, J.D.
Attorney, Blasingame, Burch, Garrard & Bryant, P.C., Athens, Georgia

Ronald L. Motley, J.D.
Attorney, Ness, Motley, Loadholt, Richardson, and Poole, P.A., Charleston, South Carolina

Charles W. Patrick, Jr., J.D.
Attorney, Ness, Motley, Loadholt, Richardson, and Poole, P.A., Charleston, South Carolina

Philip C. Pratt, M.D.
Professor Emeritus of Pathology, Duke University School of Medicine, Durham, North Carolina

Victor L. Roggli, M.D.
Associate Professor of Pathology, Duke University School of Medicine; Staff Pathologist, Veterans Administration Hospital, Durham, North Carolina

Fred Sanfilippo, M.D., Ph.D.
Professor of Pathology, Duke University School of Medicine; Director, Immunopathology Lab, Duke University Medical Center, Durham, North Carolina

John D. Shelburne, M.D., Ph.D.
Professor of Pathology, Duke University School of Medicine; Chief, Laboratory Service, Veterans Administration Hospital, Durham, North Carolina

Merry Reetz Stovall
Legal Assistant, Blasingame, Burch, Garrard & Bryant, P.C., Athens, Georgia

PATHOLOGY OF ASBESTOS-ASSOCIATED DISEASES

1. Mineralogy of Asbestos

Victor L. Roggli and Patrick Coin

The term *asbestos* refers to a group of mineral fibers that share properties of thermal and chemical resistance, flexibility, and high tensile strength. The word derives from the Greek σασβεστοσ, signifying "inextinguishable" or "indestructible."[1] Asbestos is actually a commercial term rather than a mineralogic one. Because of its many useful properties, asbestos has been incorporated into some 3000 different products in our industrialized society.[2] Indeed, it has been referred to as the "magic mineral," and, for many applications, substitutes having similar properties and equally as cheap are extremely difficult to find.[3] This chapter describes what asbestos is, where it is found, and what analytical techniques are available for its identification and characterization. (A description of how one might be exposed to asbestos in the workplace, at home, or in the environment is given in Chap. 2, and techniques for analyzing asbestos in tissue samples are presented in Chap. 11.)

HISTORICAL BACKGROUND

The use of asbestos dates back to at least 2500 B.C., when it was employed in the manufacture of Finnish pottery. One of the earliest historical accounts of asbestos describes its incorporation into the wick of a gold lamp for the goddess Athena in the fourth to fifth century B.C. Records from this same period note the use of asbestos cloth for retaining the ashes of the dead during cremation, and Pliny, in the first century A.D., refers to asbestos cloth as the funeral dress of kings.[1] Both the Chinese and the Egyptians wove asbestos into mats.[4] The Emperor Charlemagne is said to have displayed a tablecloth, around 800 A.D., made from asbestos. After a great feast, the cloth and its contents would be thrown into a fire and the cloth then removed unharmed, to the amazement of his guests. Marco Polo, in his travels around 1250 A.D., also referred to a cloth in one of the northern provinces of the Great Khan with the property of being unconsumed and even purified by fire.[1,3]

The discovery of substantial deposits of asbestos in the Ural Mountains around 1720 led to the establishment of the first factory for making asbestos products, including textiles, socks, gloves, and handbags. This factory operated for about 50 years, beginning during the reign of Peter the Great, but eventually closed due to lack of demand.[1,4] Chevalier Aldini constructed an asbestos suit for protection against fire; this was exhibited in the Royal Institution of London in 1829.[3] Chrysotile asbestos was discovered in Quebec, Canada, in 1860, a specimen of which was exhibited in London in 1862.[1,3,4] Mining of Quebec chrysotile deposits was started in 1878, with 50 tons being produced during the first year of operation. Crocidolite asbestos was discovered in South Africa in 1815,[4] but mining of substantial amounts did not begin until 1910.[1] Amosite was discovered in the central Transvaal in 1907, with mining operations commencing about 1916.[4] Thus, with the institution of mining operations in the latter half of the nineteenth century and the early decades of the twentieth century and the advent of the Industrial Revolution, the stage was set for the widespread exploitation of asbestos. (The industrial application of asbestos in the manufacture of various products is recounted in greater detail in Chap. 2.)

GEOLOGICAL CHARACTERISTICS OF ASBESTOS

Asbestos is a naturally occurring mineral and is conventionally divided into two mineralogic groups: amphiboles and serpentines. The *amphiboles* include crocidolite (blue asbestos), amosite (brown asbestos), tremolite, anthophyllite, and actinolite. Among the amphiboles, only crocidolite and amosite have had widespread commercial utilization. The noncommercial amphiboles (tremolite, anthophyllite, and actinolite) are the most commonly occurring amphibole asbestos minerals and are widely distributed,[4] but their primary importance is as contaminants of other minerals, such as chrysotile, vermiculite, and talc.[5] The other group of asbestos minerals is the *serpentine* group, of which chrysotile (white) asbestos is the sole variety. Chrysotile accounts for 90–95% of the asbestos used commercially in the United States.[2]

Asbestos deposits occur in four types of rocks: (I) alpine-type ultramafic rocks, including ophiolites (chrysotile, anthophyllite, and tremolite); (II) stratiform ultramafic intrusions (chrysotile and tremolite); (III) serpentinized limestone (chrysotile); and (IV) banded ironstones (amosite and crocidolite). Type I deposits are by far the most important, with the best-known commercial deposits located in Quebec and what was formerly the Soviet Union. Types II and III deposits, found mostly in South Africa, are of limited commercial importance. Type IV deposits are found only in the Precambrian banded ironstones of the Transvaal and Cape Province regions of South Africa and the Wittenoom Gorge area of Western Australia. Only the South African deposits are still actively mined. Geologic evidence indicates that asbestos deposits form where there is a favorable stress environment, such as where folding or faulting occurs.

The amphibole and serpentine minerals occur both as asbestiform (fibrous) varieties (Fig. 1-1) and as nonasbestiform (massive) varieties of identical chemical composition. The nonasbestiform counterpart of crocidolite is known as riebeckite, and the nonasbestiform counterpart of amosite is cummingtonite-grunerite. The nonasbestiform counterparts of tremolite, anthophyllite, and actinolite have the same names as their asbestiform varieties. Nonasbestiform serpentines include antigorite and lizardite. Amphibole crystallization is believed to occur initially as the massive form under conditions of

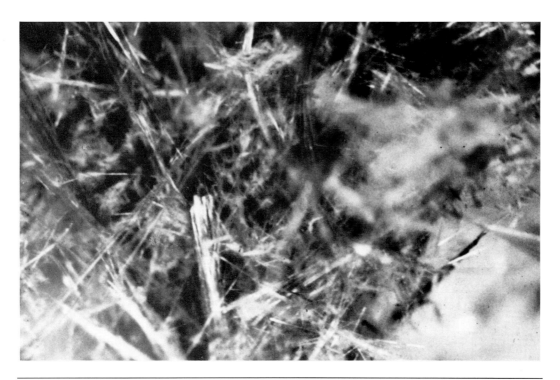

FIGURE 1-1. Crude chrysotile asbestos from Quebec. Note the fibrous character of the mineral. Reprinted from Greenberg SD: Asbestos-Associated Pulmonary Diseases, Medcom, Inc., 1981, with permission.

moderate temperature and pressure, and transformation to the fibrous form occurs when the unstable massive form is submitted to rock stresses. Similarly, serpentine minerals first crystallize as the massive form, and chrysotile is formed subsequently by recrystallization.[4] The best-known geographic locations of the various asbestiform minerals are summarized in Table 1-1.

PHYSICOCHEMICAL PROPERTIES OF ASBESTOS

Chrysotile is a hydrated magnesium silicate with the chemical composition indicated in Table 1-2. Individual fibrils of chrysotile have diameters of 20–40 nm (0.02–0.04 µm).[4] Crushing of chrysotile ore produces fiber bundles consisting of varying numbers of aggregated individual fibrils. These fibers have varying lengths but may exceed 100 µm. Typically, chrysotile fibers have a curved, curly, or wavy morphology that is particularly apparent in fiber bundles exceeding 10 µm in length (Fig. 1-2). In addition, the ends of chrysotile fiber bundles often have a splayed appearance due to the separation of the individual fibrillar units. This curly morphology influences the interceptive deposition of chrysotile fibers, which in turn affects the depth of penetration into the lower respiratory tract[6,7] (see Chap. 10).

TABLE 1-1. Geographic locations of best-known deposits of asbestiform minerals

Asbestos variety	Geographic locations
Chrysotile	Quebec (Canada), Rhodesia, Russia (Ural Mountains), China, Italy, United States (California, Vermont)
Crocidolite	South Africa (northwestern Cape Province, Transvaal), western Australia, Bolivia, northern Rhodesia
Amosite	South Africa (Transvaal), India
Tremolite	Turkey, Cyprus, Greece, Italy, Pakistan, South Korea
Anthophyllite	Finland, United States
Actinolite	South Africa (Cape Province), India

SOURCE: Adapted from Refs. 1, 4.

However, inhalational studies in rats have shown that substantial numbers of chrysotile fibers 5 μm or greater in length can penetrate into the lung periphery.[6,8] The diameter of chrysotile fibers tends to increase with increasing fiber length; however, some very long chrysotile fibers may be extremely thin.

The amphiboles are a group of hydrated silicates with a wide range of cation substitutions within the silicate backbone of the crystal structure. The idealized chemical formulas of the asbestiform varieties of amphibole minerals are summarized in Table 1-2. The diameters of individual fibers vary considerably, with substantial overlap among the members of the amphibole group. Crocidolite generally has the finest fiber diameters, especially dust obtained from the northwestern Cape Province in South Africa or the Wittenoom Gorge in Western Australia. Amosite fibers are on average somewhat thicker, and the noncommercial amphiboles (tremolite, anthophyllite, and actinolite) tend to have the coarsest fibers. Fiber diameters may vary considerably, depending on the source. For example, tremolite fibers from South Korea and the Metsovo region of Greece may be very fine with high aspect (length-to-diameter) ratios. The amphibole fibers have varying lengths, but the authors have observed amosite fibers with diameter less than one micron and length in excess of 200 μm. The amphiboles have typically straight fibers with parallel sides, and often have readily identified longitudinal grooves (see Fig. 1-2). They do not have splayed ends or the tendency

TABLE 1-2. Chemical composition of asbestiform minerals

Asbestos variety	Chemical formula
Chrysotile	$Mg_3 Si_2 O_5 (OH)_4$
Crocidolite	$Na_2 Fe_3^{++} Fe_2^{+++} Si_8 O_{22}(OH)_2$
Amosite	$(Fe-Mg)_7 Si_8 O_{22} (OH)_2 \quad Fe > 5$
Tremolite	$Ca_2 Mg_5 Si_8 O_{22} (OH)_2$
Anthophyllite	$(Mg-Fe)_7 Si_8 O_{22} (OH)_2 \quad Mg > 6$
Actinolite	$Ca_2 Mg Fe_5 Si_8 O_{22} (OH)_2$

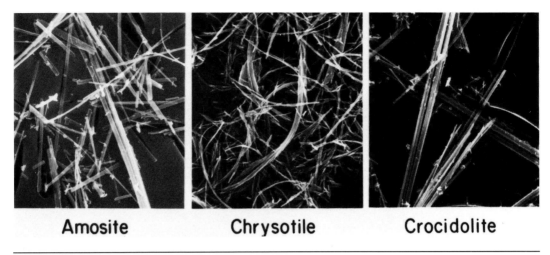

Amosite   Chrysotile   Crocidolite

FIGURE 1-2. Scanning electron micrographs contrast the curved fibers of chrysotile asbestos (*center*) with the straight fibers of amosite asbestos (*left*) and crocidolite asbestos (*right*). Magnified ×2000. Reprinted from Greenberg SD:
Environmentally Induced Pulmonary Disease, Medcom, Inc., 1987, with
permission.

toward longitudinal splitting typically observed with chrysotile. The
diameters of amphibole fibers generally tend to increase with increasing fiber length.

CRYSTALLOGRAPHIC STRUCTURE

SERPENTINE ASBESTOS

Chrysotile is a phyllosilicate, or sheet silicate, in which a silica layer
is joined to a brucite ($Mg[OH]_2$) layer. The silica layer consists of a
pseudohexagonal network of linked silica tetrahedra. There is considerable mismatching between the silica and brucite layers, resulting in
considerable strain in the crystal lattice and curvature of the sheet
structure. This is due to the fact that the brucite layer is slightly larger
than the silica layer. When viewed end on, chrysotile fibers have the
appearance of a sheet rolled up into a scroll. The scroll or tubule of an
individual chrysotile fibril thus has a central capillary with a diameter of 2–4.5 nm (Fig. 1-3). Selected area electron diffraction (SAED)
patterns obtained from chrysotile fibers have a characteristic appearance consisting of smearing of the dot patterns along the layer lines
and a layer line spacing of 5.3 Å (Fig. 1-4). A schematic diagram of
the crystal structure of chrysotile is given in Fig. 1-5.[9,10] Chrysotile
occurs as three distinct polymorphs referred to as clinochrysotile, or-
thochrysotile, and parachrysotile. Of these three polymorphs, clinochrysotile is by far the most common.[4]

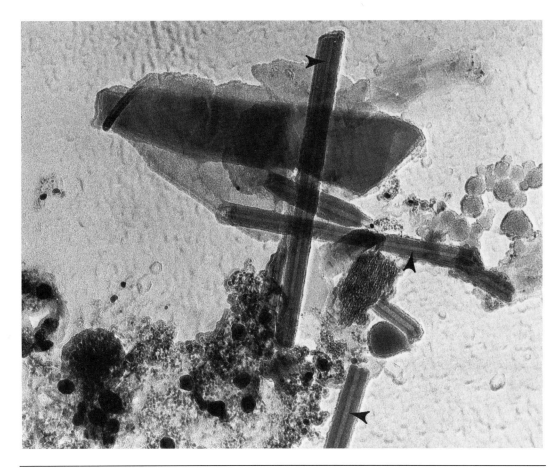

FIGURE 1-3. Transmission electron micrograph of individual chrysotile fibrils in longitudinal section showing the distinct central capillary (arrowheads) characteristic of chrysotile. Magnified ×60,000. Courtesy Mr. Frank D'Ovidio, Manville Sales Corp., Denver, CO.

AMPHIBOLE ASBESTOSES

The amphiboles are inosilicates, or chain silicates,[11] in which the silica tetrahedra are arranged linearly and wrap around each other like the strands of a rope. The crystalline structure of the amphiboles displays a perfect prismatic cleavage. The structure of the amphiboles is in the monoclinic class, with the exception of anthophyllite, which is orthorhombic. Thus the diffraction patterns of the various amphibole asbestoses are indistinguishable, consisting of discrete dots along the layer lines and a layer line spacing of 5.3 Å (Fig. 1-6). End-on views of amphibole fibers reveal a rectangular or rhombic shape, with a ratio of width to thickness varying from 1:1 to 10:1.[12,13] This appearance is in contrast to the characteristic tubular morphology of chrysotile. A schematic diagram of the crystal structure of amphibole asbestos is presented in Fig. 1-7.[9,10]

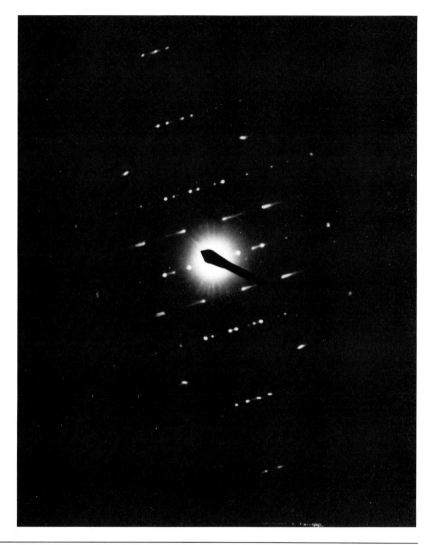

FIGURE 1-4. Selected area electron diffraction pattern of a chrysotile asbestos fiber showing the 5.3-Å interlayer line spacing. Note the very prominent "streaking" along the layer lines, a feature characteristic of chrysotile asbestos. Courtesy Dr. Neil Rowlands, JEOL USA Inc., Peabody, MA.

TECHNIQUES FOR IDENTIFICATION OF ASBESTOS

A variety of techniques has been devised for the identification of asbestos fibers,[14] taking advantage of the various features characterizing asbestos, including morphology, crystalline structure, and chemical composition. Each of these techniques has its advantages and its limitations (Table 1-3). A brief discussion of the more common techniques used for the identification of asbestos fibers is presented in the following sections.

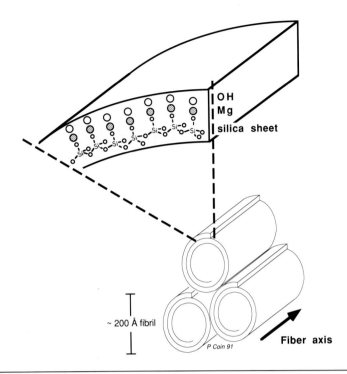

FIGURE 1-5. Schematic diagram of the crystalline structure of chrysotile asbestos. Modified from Refs. 9 and 10.

PHASE-CONTRAST MICROSCOPY

Phase-contrast light microscopy takes advantage of phase optics to increase the resolution and hence the sensitivity to the size of fibers that can be detected. Fibers with diameters as small as $0.2\,\mu m$ may be identified by means of this technique. Information obtainable with this approach is limited to morphologic features, such as size (length and diameter), shape, and aspect ratio (Fig. 1-8). However, information regarding specific fiber composition cannot be obtained, so one cannot readily distinguish among the various types of asbestos fiber. Nor can asbestos fibers be distinguished from nonasbestos mineral fibers. Furthermore, fibers with diameters less than $0.2\,\mu m$ are beyond the resolution of phase-contrast light microscopy and therefore cannot be detected with this technique. Today, phase contrast is seldom used for the detection or identification of asbestos in environmental or tissue samples.[14,15]

POLARIZING MICROSCOPY WITH DISPERSION STAINING

Polarizing microscopy takes advantage of the property of rotation of polarized light by anisotropic (i.e., crystalline) substances. This technique thus provides information on the relative crystallinity of a fibrous particle and, if immersion oils are also used, on its index of refraction. The latter procedure is referred to as *dispersion staining;* by

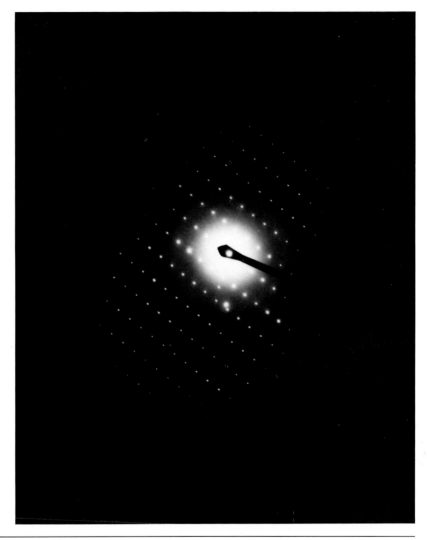

FIGURE 1-6. Selected area electron diffraction pattern of a crocidolite asbestos fiber showing the 5.3-Å interlayer line spacing. Note the discrete localization of the dots (representing diffraction maxima) along the layer lines (compare with Fig. 1-4). Courtesy Dr. Neil Rowlands, JEOL USA Inc., Peabody, MA.

careful selection of immersion oils, it can be used to distinguish among the various asbestos fiber types as well as distinguishing between asbestos and nonasbestos mineral fibers.[14,15] For example, asbestos fibers are birefringent when viewed with polarizing microscopy due to their crystalline nature, whereas fibrous glass (which is amorphous) is nonrefringent. According to some authorities, polarizing microscopy with dispersion staining is the method of choice for the identification of asbestos fibers in bulk samples, and may also be

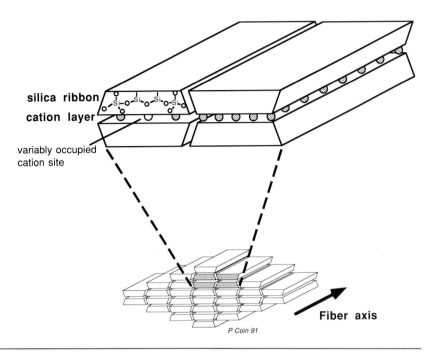

FIGURE 1-7. Schematic diagram of the crystalline structure of amphibole asbestos. Modified from Refs. 9 and 10.

useful in the analysis of air samples.[16,17] Its advantages include low cost, minimal sample preparation, simplicity of the analytical procedure, and reproducibility of results. Disadvantages include limitations of light microscopy for detection of the finest-diameter fibers and some inaccuracies in the determination of specific mineral types based on indices of refraction due to overlapping values for the bulk of the asbestos mineral types.[15]

INFRARED SPECTROSCOPY
Asbestos minerals produce characteristic spectra when examined by means of infrared spectrophotometry (IR).[14,15,18] IR is a bulk analytical technique and thus cannot be used for the identification of individual fibers. The advantages of this procedure include its relatively low cost and simple operation. Disadvantages include inaccuracies in the presence of a mixed particulate population (e.g., chrysotile mixed with clay minerals or talc) and interferences from organic debris. This technique is seldom used for the detection or identification of asbestos in environmental or tissue samples.

MAGNETIC ALIGNMENT AND LIGHT SCATTERING (MALS)
The MALS method of estimating asbestos content in a sample involves the use of a magnetic field to achieve alignment of fibers in a thin transparent film that is then examined by light scattering. The

TABLE 1-3. Techniques for identification of asbestos

Analytical technique	Specificity	Limitations	Advantages	Disadvantages
Phase-contrast microscopy	Nonspecific	Fiber detection only	Inexpensive; ease of sample preparation	Resolution limited to fibers ≥ 0.2 μm in diameter
Polarizing microscopy with dispersion staining	Relatively specific	Bulk samples	Inexpensive; minimal sample preparation; reproducible	Resolution limited; inaccurate, especially for biological samples
Infrared spectroscopy	Relatively specific	Bulk samples	Relatively inexpensive; simple operation	Inaccurate in presence of mixed particle population; interference from organic residues
Magnetic alignment and light scattering	Nonspecific	Bulk samples	Rapid; simple; relatively inexpensive	Does not allow for determination of specific mineral fiber types
X-ray diffraction	Highly specific	Bulk samples	Rapid, simple	Relatively insensitive
Selected area electron diffraction (SAED)	Specific for chrysotile	Individual fiber analysis	Crystallographic information regarding individual fiber	Tedious; time-consuming; expensive
Transmission electron microscopy with EDS	Highly specific	Individual fiber analysis	Specific identification of individual fibers by EDS/SAED; superior resolution	More complex sample preparation; tedious; expensive
Scanning electron microscopy with EDS	Highly specific	Individual fiber analysis	Specific identification of individual fibers; minimal sample preparation	Tedious; time-consuming; expensive

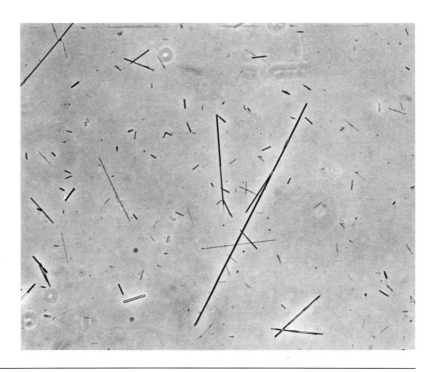

FIGURE 1-8. Phase-contrast light micrograph of U.I.C.C. amosite asbestos fibers. Magnified ×375.

fibers are suspended in an agar solution within a shallow brass ring mounted on a glass slide, which is supported in the air gap of an electromagnet. When such a film is illuminated orthogonally with a parallel beam of white light, scattering by the fibers produces a distinctive bright band that when measured photometrically provides information on fiber mass, fiber number, and median fiber length and diameter.[19,20] Fiber surface area can also be estimated with this technique. The MALS method has been used to measure the fiber content of lung tissue and to compare various fiber parameters with severity of fibrosis among patients with asbestosis. Comparison of individuals exposed to a wide variety of asbestos fiber types showed that the fibrosis score estimated by light microscopy correlated best with the relative fiber surface area per unit weight of tissue.[21] The fibrosis score correlated less well with relative fiber number or mass per unit weight of tissue. The advantages of this technique are that it is rapid, simple, and relatively inexpensive. However, it is a bulk analytical technique and must be calibrated by means of transmission electron microscopy. It provides no information about the range of particle dimensions in a sample and does not allow determination of specific mineral fibers.

X-RAY AND ELECTRON DIFFRACTION

When x-rays or electrons pass through a crystalline material, they are diffracted by the regularly spaced atomic planes within the crystal, according to Bragg's law.[22] The diffraction pattern resulting from this interaction provides useful information with regard to the three-dimensional structure of the substance under consideration. For x-ray diffraction, the diffraction pattern can be recorded on x-ray–sensitive film or as peaks on a strip chart using an x-ray diffractometer. For electron diffraction, the pattern appears as a series of dots on the CRT of a transmission electron microscope and can be recorded on photographic film (see Figs. 1-4 and 1-6).

A bulk analytical technique, x-ray diffraction is suitable for the analysis of macroscopic samples. The diffraction pattern often appears as a series of concentric rings on the x-ray film, and the distance from any one ring to the center of the film is inversely proportional to the distance d between the planes of atoms in the crystal giving rise to that particular x-ray intensity maxima. The peaks of x-ray intensity maxima on a strip chart are presented as angular deviation 2θ from center, which in turn can be related to interplanar spacing d (given in angstrom units, Å). An x-ray diffraction tracing for amosite asbestos is shown in Fig. 1-9, with major peaks at 3.07 Å, 3.21 Å, and 8.33 Å. Although x-ray diffraction is generally considered a qualitative technique, methods have been devised by which x-ray diffraction can be used to measure quantitatively the amounts of asbestos present in a sample.[23] By comparing the integrated peaks of the x-ray tracing from known standards of chrysotile asbestos with those of unknown samples and correcting for x-ray absorption by the matrix and the filter, investigators have been able to measure chrysotile asbestos with detection limits as low as 3 µg/cm^2 of filter when chrysotile is present in small quantities (1% by weight of matrix material).

Whereas x-ray diffraction is a bulk analytical method, electron diffraction is a microanalytical technique capable of providing a diffraction pattern from a particle or area 1 µm or less in diameter.[24] Thus using this technique, often referred to as *selected area electron diffraction (SAED)*, one can obtain crystallographic data from an individual asbestos fiber. Some investigators consider electron diffraction to be the method of choice for separating the six asbestos minerals from most other nonasbestos minerals.[25] The diffraction pattern is formed by weakening the first projector lens in the transmission electron microscope, bringing the back focal plane of the objective lens into focus on the viewing screen.[22] This results in the imaging of the diffraction pattern as a series of dots on the CRT, and the distance R between the individual spots of the diffraction pattern and the central spot is inversely related to the interplanar spacing d of the planes of atoms in the crystal giving rise to that particular electron intensity maximum. As noted earlier, chrysotile has a characteristic diffraction

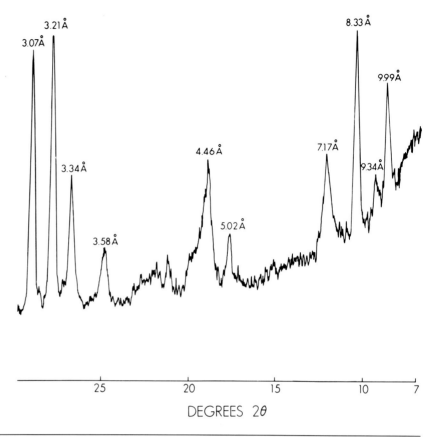

FIGURE 1-9. X-ray diffraction tracing of dust recovered from the lungs of an asbestos worker with asbestosis (same case as Fig. 4-5). The tracing shows several prominent peaks correlating with diffraction maxima for amosite asbestos (see text).

pattern (Fig. 1-4). However, diffraction patterns cannot be obtained from all fibers, and in practice the technique is tedious and time-consuming.

ANALYTICAL ELECTRON MICROSCOPY

Although there is a wide variety of techniques for identifying asbestos, most investigators prefer some form of analytical electron microscopy.[14,15] The analytical electron microscope has the ability to provide high-resolution images of the smallest of fibers, detailing their finest morphologic features, and spectral information regarding chemical composition by means of energy-dispersive spectrometry (EDS). The basic components of an analytical electron microscope are shown schematically in Fig. 1-10.

Perhaps the most widely used instrument for the detection and analysis of asbestos fibers is the analytical transmission electron microscope (TEM). This technique has the advantages of superior

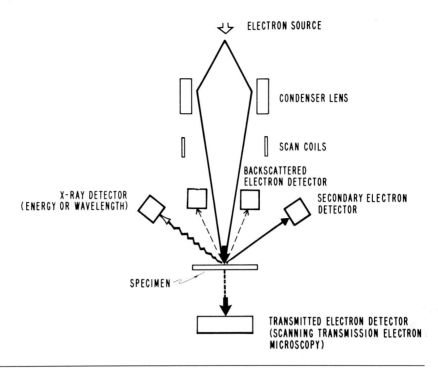

FIGURE 1-10. Basic components of the scanning electron microscope, equipped with back-scattered electron and x-ray detectors. Such an instrument is extremely valuable in the characterization of inorganic particulates such as asbestos fibers. Reprinted from Garner and Klintworth: Pathobiology of ocular disease, Marcel Dekker, Inc., NY, 1982.

resolution as well as the ability to obtain both crystallographic and elemental compositional data for an individual fiber by means of SAED (see earlier) and EDS, respectively.[26] The latter technique involves focusing the electron beam on an individual particle and observing the x-ray spectra produced by the interaction of the electrons of the primary beam with the atoms within the specimen. The resultant spectrum consists of peaks distributed according to the energy (KeV) of the x-rays generated, which is in turn related to the elements composing the particle (or fiber). The spectra generated can then be visually compared with known samples of asbestos (e.g., the U.I.C.C. standard asbestos samples) or can be subjected to discriminate function analysis. The latter is a more objective method that can differentiate among the various amphiboles with a high degree of confidence.[27] Analytical TEM has been used for at least two decades to analyze asbestos in dust recovered from human lung samples.[28,29] However, preparatory techniques for TEM are often complex, and the method is expensive and time-consuming.

Analytical scanning electron microscopy (SEM) has also been employed by various investigators for the detection and identification of asbestos.[27,30] This technique has the advantages of less complicated preparatory steps and larger sample size (e.g., an entire filter) as compared to TEM. Although it is generally acknowledged that TEM has superior resolution, state-of-the-art SEMs have resolutions approaching that of the TEM and are thus capable of resolving fine asbestos fibrils.[30] A potential disadvantage of the SEM is that electron diffraction cannot be readily performed with this technique. However, in the authors' experience, most fibers can be unequivocally identified based on their morphologic characteristics and energy-dispersive spectra.[30] A further advantage of analytical SEM is the potential for automation. Automated image x-ray analyzers are commercially available with capabilities of analyzing completely more than 1000 individual particles per hour under optimal conditions.[31] Although such systems have great potential for biological analyses, application has thus far been extremely limited. As is the case for analytical TEM, analytical SEM is an expensive and time-consuming technique.

REFERENCES

1. Lee DHK, Selikoff IJ: Historical background to the asbestos problem. *Environ Res* 18:300–314, 1979.
2. Craighead JE, Mossman BT: Pathogenesis of asbestos-associated diseases. *N Engl J Med* 306:1446–1455, 1982.
3. Murray R: Asbestos: A chronology of its origins and health effects. *Br J Ind Med* 47:361–365, 1990.
4. Pooley FD: Asbestos mineralogy, Ch. 1 In: *Asbestos-Related Malignancy* (Antman K, Aisner J, eds.), Orlando, FL: Grune & Stratton, 1987, pp. 3–27.
5. Addison J, Davies LST: Analysis of amphibole asbestos in chrysotile and other minerals. *Ann Occup Hyg* 34:159–175, 1990.
6. Brody AR, Hill LH, Adkins B, O'Connor RW: Chrysotile asbestos inhalation in rats: Deposition pattern and reaction of alveolar epithelium and pulmonary macrophages. *Am Rev Respir Dis* 123:670–679, 1981.
7. Lee KP: Lung response to particulates with emphasis on asbestos and other fibrous dusts. *CRC Crit Rev Toxicol* 14:33–86, 1985.
8. Roggli VL, Brody AR: Changes in numbers and dimensions of chrysotile asbestos fibers in lungs of rats following short-term exposure. *Expl Lung Res* 7:133–147, 1984.
9. Hodgson AA: Chemistry and physics of asbestos, In: *Asbestos: Properties, Applications, and Hazards* (Vol. 1) (Michaels L, Chissick SS, eds.), New York: Wiley, 1979, pp. 67–114.
10. Zussman J: The mineralogy of asbestos, In: *Asbestos: Properties, Applications, and Hazards* (Vol. 1) (Michael L, Chissick SS, eds.), New York: Wiley, 1979, pp. 45–65.
11. Roggli VL, Mastin JP, Shelburne JD, Roe MS, Brody AR: Inorganic particulates in human lung: Relationship to the inflammatory response, In: *Inflammatory Cells and Lung Disease* (Lynn WS, ed.), Boca Raton, FL: CRC Press, 1983, pp. 29–62.
12. Crawford D: Electron microscopy applied to studies of the biological significance of defects in crocidolite asbestos. *J Microscopy* 120:181–192, 1980.
13. Franco MA, Hutchison JL, Jefferson DA, Thomas JM: Structural imperfection and morphology of crocidolite (blue asbestos). *Nature* 266:520–521, 1977.

14. Langer AM, Ashley R, Baden V, Berkley C, Hammond EC, Mackler AD, Maggiore CJ, Nicholson WJ, Rohl AM, Rubin IB, Sastre A, Selikoff IJ: Identification of asbestos in human tissues. *J Occup Med* 15:287–295, 1973.

15. Berkley C, Langer AM, Baden V: Instrumental analysis of inspired fibrous pulmonary particulates. *NY Acad Sci Trans* 30:331–350, 1967.

16. McCrone WC: Asbestos monitoring. *Amer Lab* 17:20–28, 1985.

17. McCrone WC: Evaluation of asbestos in insulation. *Amer Lab* 11:19–31, 1979.

18. Coates JP: IR analysis of toxic dusts: Analysis of collected samples of quartz and asbestos. *Amer Lab* 9:105–111, 1977.

19. Timbrell V: Measurement of fibres in human lung tissue, In: *Biological Effects of Mineral Fibres*, Vol. 1 (Wagner JC, ed.), IARC Scientific Publications No. 30: Lyon, 1980, pp. 113–126.

20. Timbrell V: Deposition and retention of fibers in the human lung. *Ann Occup Hyg* 26:347–369, 1982.

21. Lippmann M: Asbestos exposure indices. *Environ Res* 46:86–106, 1988.

22. Roggli VL, Ingram P, Linton RW, Gutknecht WF, Mastin P, Shelburne JD: New techniques for imaging and analyzing lung tissue. *Environ Health Persp* 56:163–183, 1984.

23. Lange BA, Haartz JC: Determination of microgram quantities of asbestos by x-ray diffraction: Chrysotile in thin dust layers of matrix material. *Anal Chem* 51:520–525, 1979.

24. Geiss RH: Electron diffraction from submicron areas using STEM. *Scanning Electron Microsc* II:337–344, 1976.

25. Ruud CO, Barrett CS, Russell PA, Clark RL: Selected area electron diffraction and energy dispersive x-ray analysis for the identification of asbestos fibers, a comparison. *Micron* 7:115–132, 1976.

26. Churg A: Quantitative methods for analysis of disease induced by asbestos and other mineral particles using the transmission electron microscope, Ch. 4 In: *Microprobe Analysis in Medicine* (Ingram P, Shelburne JD, Roggli VL, eds.), New York: Hemisphere Publishing, 1989, pp. 79–95.

27. Millette JR, McFarren EF: EDS of waterborne asbestos fibers in TEM, SEM and STEM. *Scanning Electron Microsc.* III:451–460, 1976.

28. Langer AM, Rubin IB, Selikoff IJ: Chemical characterization of asbestos body cores by electron microprobe analysis. *J Histochem Cytochem* 20:723–734, 1972.

29. Langer AM, Rubin IB, Selikoff IJ, Pooley FD: Chemical characterization of uncoated asbestos fibers from the lungs of asbestos workers by electron microprobe analysis. *J Histochem Cytochem* 20:735–740, 1972.

30. Roggli VL: Scanning electron microscopic analysis of mineral fibers in human lungs, Ch. 5 In: *Microprobe Analysis in Medicine* (Ingram P, Shelburne JD, Roggli VL, eds.), New York: Hemisphere Publishing, 1989, pp. 97–110.

31. Johnson GG, White EW, Strickler D, Hoover R: Image analysis techniques, In: *Symposium on Electron Microscopy of Microfibers: Proceedings of the First FDA Office of Science Summer Symposium* (Asher IM, McGrath PP, eds.), Washington, DC: U.S. Government Printing Office, 1976, pp. 76–82.

2. Occupational and Environmental Exposure to Asbestos

GARY N. GREENBERG AND DENNIS J. DARCEY

Asbestos usefulness as an industrial material must be considered in order to understand the breadth of its consequent public health impact. Since its discovery as an indestructible material centuries ago, it has found countless applications, often because no identified substance rivals its engineering or commercial performance.

Asbestos applications result from its many unique physical attributes. Its high tensile strength stabilizes mixtures with concrete, asphalt, and plastic. Asbestos also offers a stable material for frictional use, that is, as a brake surface. Because of the length and pliability of its fibers, it has been incorporated into specially manufactured products, including gaskets, pads, fabric sheets, and asbestos paper with intrinsic properties of resistance and strength. Because it blocks heat transfer and is itself fireproof, it represents an ideal insulation material. Mixed into a slurry, it has been applied in economical fashion to building surfaces for fire protection and heat retention. In both its fabric and compacted-brick forms, it has been used to encase furnaces and kilns.

Economic advantages of asbestos must also be considered to explain its widespread application. As a natural (mined) rather than a manufactured substance, it was more available and its use not as closely evaluated by producers or consumers. Present in natural deposits on several continents, it has remained easily available for construction and industrial exploitation by all nations, both industrialized and developing. Its production cost, as a truly raw material, has always been far less than substitute agents, which require manufacture and even technology licensing.

HISTORICAL ORIGIN AND APPLICATIONS

PREINDUSTRIAL APPLICATIONS

Asbestos' first recorded use is as a wick material for oil lamps in ancient times. The material's name originates from the Greek for "inextinguishable" or "indestructible."[1] Woven into cloth, asbestos provided nearly miraculous resistance to fire, especially impressive for shrouds of deceased whose cremation was open to public display.

Combining asbestos with clay and other malleable materials is also cited as one of the earliest applications of the material. In Finland in 2500 B.C., asbestos was added to clay pots for greater strength. Asbestos as a fortifying additive remains its major present-day use—as a component of cement, concrete, paint, vinyl, and tar mixtures, accounting for 70% of current applications worldwide.

THE MODERN PERIOD
The past decades have witnessed a drastic change in America's patterns of asbestos use. Regulatory and health issues, rather than direct economic and engineering factors, now dominate. In the United States, regulatory concern regarding asbestos' use and continued presence has continually grown. Presently, the substance has been banned from commercial use, but there remains the critical issue of removal (abatement) from sites of previous use.

Dr. Irving J. Selikoff, whose scientific, clinical and public affairs careers are synonymous with asbestos and its effects, categorizes the societal impact of asbestos disease into three population "waves" of asbestos exposure and consequent clinical disease. Because of the well-documented latent interval for asbestos-related disease, the public health impact from each period of asbestos disease trails the period of exposure by 30–50 years.

The first wave of asbestos exposure comprises the workers whose activities actually generate asbestos for use, the miners and packagers who transformed an ore into an industrial material. This exposure period, involving relatively few workers, extends from the initial use of the mineral into the early twentieth century. These workers, in countries where asbestos was first processed, Canada and South Africa, prompted the initial recognition of the diseases that required a latent period of decades to manifest.[2]

The second wave of asbestos-induced disease represents the diagnostic impact of the manufacturing and construction use of the material. The most important peak in Western society's exposure to asbestos occurred during the period of rapid economic expansion surrounding World War II. Intense and high-volume ship construction, structural insulation, and the industrial fabrication of asbestos-containing products created a huge cohort of exposed workers during the mid-twentieth century. The ensuing period of public health impact is seen at present.

The third wave of asbestos exposure and disease generates the most controversy and conjecture regarding both its size and the intensity of its public health impact. This comprises the cohort of citizens exposed to asbestos already in place. This population is likely to be exposed during the disruption of preapplied asbestos insulation in homes and commercial buildings. Specific groups exposed to the highest dose of the mineral during this phase include building maintenance workers, construction workers, electricians, custodians, and the workforce employed specifically for asbestos abatement.

Worldwide use of asbestos remains sizable despite the increased recognition of its health consequences. Data provided by the Asbestos Institute[3] and the International Labour Organization[1] show very little change in either annual production or consumption during recent years (Figs. 2-1 and 2-2).

In the United States, use of asbestos had markedly diminished even before the outright ban regarding "the future manufacture, importation, processing, and distribution in commerce of asbestos in almost all products" was enacted by the U.S. Environmental Protection Agency (EPA) in July 1989. United States consumption of asbestos dropped from a 1984 total of 240,000 metric tons to less than 85,000 metric tons in 1987.[4]

OCCUPATIONAL EXPOSURE TO ASBESTOS

ASBESTOS PROCESSING

In the United States, for geological reasons, asbestos production has never been an important commercial enterprise. Even before restrictions for asbestos' use, the combined workforce involved in mining and milling were known to be less than 600.[5] Mining creates exposure levels that are surprisingly low when compared to those of materials manufactured, averaging 0.9 fibers/ml.[1] Because of the way the ore is handled, the fibers remain consolidated and have not yet become individualized. In contrast, the subsequent operation of mineral refining and milling (usually designed to "open" the bundles into individual fibers) generates worker exposure levels of 6.0–12.1 fibers/ml.[1]

Asbestos is shipped in bags, historically made of porous cloth but recently of paper and plastic. The handling of this material in secondary industries routinely began with cutting open these bags and manually emptying them into hoppers, e.g., for mixture with concrete. Since this material is both dry and nonaggregated, the likelihood of dispersal is then at its maximum. The waste packaging material constitutes a source of exposure separate from the intended construction or industrial application.

MANUFACTURE OF ASBESTOS-CONTAINING PRODUCTS

The exposures that occur during the manufacture of asbestos products are extremely variable. Additionally, the number of manufacturing workers exposed at any one time to the mineral's effects has been widely debated, with recent estimates ranging from 18,000–37,000.[6]

Production of asbestos textiles involved higher exposure than other products.[5] Carding and conventional spinning produced extreme air concentrations, resistant to environmental controls. Methods of manufacture utilizing liquid dispersion rather than dry asbestos are more successful at controlling potential exposure.

Work with material where the asbestos fibers were already entrapped, e.g., in roofing materials, floor tile, or cement pipe, do offer considerable exposure opportunities, but only when such products

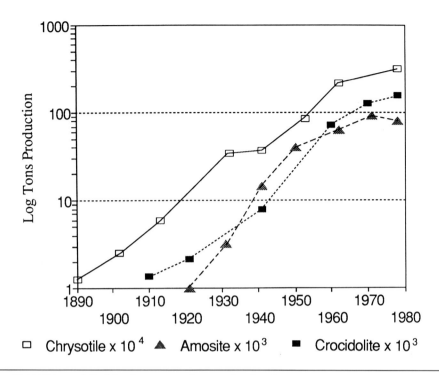

FIGURE 2-1. World asbestos production for the three major commercial types of asbestos, in tons produced annually, 1890–1980. Note logarithmic scale.

are broken, releasing respirable fibers. Information on job title provides some basis to assess actual exposure, but is often incomplete or misleading in estimating the degree of exposure. Certain jobs are more variable than others; for example, exposures for "inspectors" in manufacturing depend on the amount of loose asbestos dust remaining on the finished product. The exposures for this manufacturing step are cited as ranging from 0.1–8.0 fibers/ml.[5]

ASBESTOS INSULATION MATERIALS

During the 1940s and 1950s, covering boilers and furnaces with asbestos was universal and, before the health effects of the practice were recognized, considered a safety practice, preventing burns, heat release, and fire. Boiler makers and pipe coverers constitute the most important and widely evaluated cohort of exposed workers. Selikoff's 1964 study of New York insulation workers unionists[7] was one of the earliest reports of the health consequences of this work. Among 255 deaths evaluated in this mortality study, 18% were due to lung cancer, 11% to direct pulmonary damage from the dust, and 1.2% to mesothelioma. This staggering impact was an early demonstration of asbestos exposure risk.

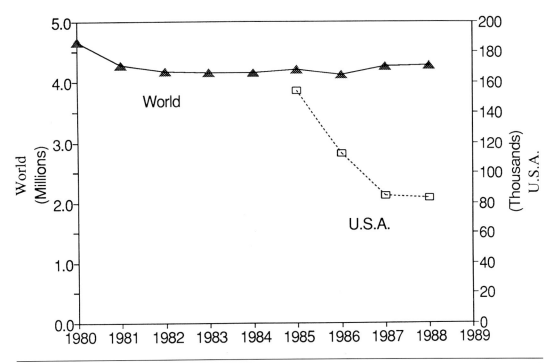

FIGURE 2-2. Annual asbestos use, in metric tons, for the U.S.A. compared to the rest of the world, 1980–1988. A sharp drop in U.S. importation is apparent from 1985–1988, whereas use by other nations has remained fairly constant.

Construction industry application of asbestos coating to structural steel beams increased immensely the societal breadth of this exposure. The spraying of asbestos-cement mixtures was initiated in 1935, and from 1958 through 1978 was widely employed for railway carriages, naval ships, and newly constructed buildings.[5] By one estimate, 1.2 billion square feet of asbestos-containing insulation (averaging 14% concentration) is present in 190,000 American buildings.[8] The process was actually employed more rather than less frequently in the final years of this period, until the practice was halted when health issues became widely known.

FRICTION MATERIALS

The use of asbestos for vehicular brakes takes advantage of its heat resistance and material strength. Asbestos concentrations in these materials are sizable, ranging from 30–80%. Because manufacture and repair of automotive wheels is geographically widely distributed, this application exposes individuals in a wide variety of trades and geography—the number of workers exposed as a consequence of asbestos brake and clutch work is estimated at 900,000. The practices of "blowing out" brake surfaces and beveling or grinding brake shoes produce high airborne fiber concentrations, for considerable periods of time and at distances extending many feet from the actual operation.[5]

The dispersion of asbestos dust particles from brake surfaces (even in situations of automotive traffic) remains a continuing concern. Airborne asbestos at a San Francisco bridge toll plaza was measured at 1400 fibers per cubic meter, nearly tripling from "ordinary" urban values for that area.[5]

CONSTRUCTION MATERIALS

In floor tile and in roof shingles and coatings, asbestos mixtures utilize the flexibility and strength of the mineral additive as an important stabilizing feature. Since these materials are popular for home improvement activities, this application provides additional opportunity for exposure to nonprofessional workers, who lack specific occupational monitoring or training. Ordinarily, exposures are quite low and require considerable disruption of the product's integrity to release respirable particles with asbestos content.

SHIPYARDS

Ship building makes unusually intense use of insulating materials because of the nature of the construction. Ships have greater vulnerability to fire because of their isolation and the confined spaces. Noise and heat from the immediate proximity of a shipboard power plant create an important need for effective thermal and acoustic insulation, which must also be fireproof. Additionally, preparing ships brings workers not necessarily directly involved with asbestos work (e.g., electricians, metal workers) into an asbestos-containing closed environment for the entire duration of the project. This closed-space exposure is, by its nature, difficult to control by the usual industrial measures, such as ventilation, wetting of the fiber sources, and containment.

Because workplace safety efforts were relaxed during the establishment of the war-time economy of the 1940s, the massive shipbuilding effort of that period put the largest segment of workers at risk for subsequent asbestos-related disease. The conditions of enclosed, poorly ventilated, and unmonitored assignments produced prolonged and heavy exposure to all interior shipworkers.

ASBESTOS REMOVAL

As a result of the regulatory recommendation[9] that asbestos must be removed from schools, industrial work sites, and residences, the most significant and identifiable current exposure to asbestos occurs during asbestos abatement. In the removal of pure asbestos lagging, potential exposures of 62–159 fibers/ml were reported.[5] This process often takes place in considerable disorder, because the surfaces are no longer easily accessible, and the work site is either in demand or in current use. Geographic isolation, soaking of the asbestos source, and personal containment represent the most important strategies for reduction of exposure.

The safety advantage in this process is that workers are required to be trained and to become aware of the nature of the task and its hazards. Current regulations for asbestos exposure provide for these workers detailed rules that contrast dramatically with the historically careless handling of the same material.

The administrative demands of asbestos worker protection are extensive. Currently, workers involved in asbestos abatement are required[10] to undergo a preemployment evaluation of their ability to work wearing a HEPA (high-efficiency-particulate air) filter respirator and impermeable (thus hot and humid) disposable clothing. Baseline and annual chest radiographs are taken, with measurement of pulmonary flows usually added. Before initiation of asbestos work, these individuals receive mandatory instruction regarding the health effects of asbestos-related disease and the means of dust and exposure control. Educational opportunities regarding the multiplicative effect of tobacco smoking on the risks from asbestos exposure are now a required component of asbestos worker training.

The area for asbestos removal is enclosed with a plastic barrier of specified 6-mil-thick polyethylene sheeting and by toxic-hazard warning signs. The site is kept at negative barometric pressure (relative to the surrounding area) by having fans blow air outward through HEPA filters. If possible asbestos-containing material is covered in plastic bags to encase escaping fragments. Additionally, workers wear intensive personal protective gear (mask, gown, and gloves, as in Fig. 2-3). Throughout removal, every effort is made to keep the material soaked so that respirable dust is minimized. Waste products are labeled and are handled with special care. Monitoring for airborne asbestos concentration is performed outside the confined asbestos-abatement area.

Following each work period, workers are required to discard all outer clothing and shower, to prevent secondary contamination from work clothes. Periodic medical monitoring is also required, although the decades-long latency of asbestos-related disease makes these sessions more appropriately an opportunity for discussions of health risk and for counseling on smoking cessation.

NONOCCUPATIONAL EXPOSURE TO ASBESTOS

Exposure to asbestos in the ambient indoor and outdoor environments results from many sources, both natural and man-made. Chrysotile asbestos, which accounts for over 90% of the asbestos used in the United States, has become a ubiquitous contaminant of ambient air. It has been noted that asbestos fibers can be found in

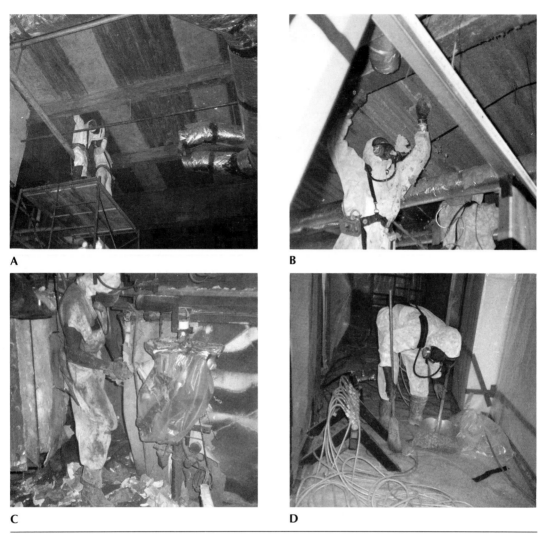

A

B

C

D

FIGURE 2-3. Workers in the North Carolina Asbestos Abatement Program. Asbestos removal occurs within confined spaces. Note the respiratory equipment and special protective clothing.

the lungs of almost everyone in the American population.[11] Natural sources of asbestos fiber release include weathering and erosion of asbestos-containing rock and of road surfaces composed of asbestos ores. If the primary areas of source rock are compared with high population density, the most critical areas for emissions from natural sources appear to be eastern Pennsylvania, southeastern New York, southwestern Connecticut, and greater Los Angeles and San Francisco.[5]

Man-made sources of exposure in the past have included off-site releases from mining, milling, and manufacture of asbestos products, exposing residents in nearby communities. Before occupational work practices improved in the 1970s, secondary contamination of homes occurred when employees brought home asbestos-laden work clothes. Weathering of asbestos cement wall and roofing materials is a relatively minor environmental source of exposure from man-made construction materials. However, off-site release from construction sites (primarily from sprayed-on asbestos fireproofing) have resulted in ambient asbestos levels 100 times background levels.[12]

Asbestos brake and clutch pads in automobiles contribute to the environmental load of asbestos. However, it is uncertain how much respirable fiber is released, because thermal degradation occurs at the high temperatures generated during braking. Waste disposal has become a growing source of potential exposure to asbestos fibers, and promises to continue as removal, abatement, and renovation occur in the existing building stock. Consumer products, water supplies, and food sources have been contaminated with asbestos-containing materials in the past. These man-made sources of exposure have been significantly reduced by regulatory activity over the past 20 years and will continue to decline as the 1989 EPA ban on the manufacture, importation, and processing of asbestos becomes fully implemented by 1996.

Currently, the most important source of nonoccupational exposure is the release of fibers from existing asbestos-containing surface materials in schools, residences, and public buildings or from sprayed asbestos-containing fireproofing in high-rise office buildings. The greatest potential for future exposure will be determined by the asbestos released during the maintenance, repair, and removal of these structures. The implementation of the Asbestos Hazard Emergency Response Act (AHERA), requiring inspection of the nation's public and private schools for asbestos, has resulted in an explosive commercial growth of the industry involved in asbestos identification and removal. Some have argued that removal itself presents more of an exposure hazard than leaving the materials undisturbed or encapsulated.[13]

MEASURING EXPOSURE

Different techniques have been developed for measuring the concentration of asbestos in ambient air and in the workplace. The phase-contrast light microscope for counting fibers in the workplace has been less useful in the ambient environment, where fiber identity and character are usually unknown, fibers are too small to be seen by light microscopy, and concentrations expressed as mass are usually hundreds or thousands of times lower than those in the workplace.

Fiber concentrations in the workplace have generally been measured as the number of fibers longer than 5 microns (Table 2-1). Ambient concentrations are now determined by transmission electron

TABLE 2-1. Exposure to airborne asbestos in selected asbestos product manufacturing industries

| | Asbestos concentrations (time-weighted average, in fibers/ml) | | | | | Employees affected | |
| | Most operations | | Operations with highest levels | | | | |
Industry	Typical	Range	Typical	Range	Name of operation	Production workers	Total
Friction products							
Primary	2	0.1–15.0	4	0.5–22.0	Forming or Rolling	4,900	7,300
Secondary		2.5–6.5					34,500
Asbestos paper							
Primary	1	0.75–2.7	2	0.3–2.8	Fiber Introduction	1,100	4,500
Secondary		1.0–3.5					198,000
Asbestos-reinforced plastics							
Primary	1	0.2–2.5	2	0.5–3.0	Fiber Introduction	900	2,600
Secondary		0.5–2.0					11,000
Cement pipe	1.5	0.25–3.5	2	0.6–4.5	Finishing	1,600	2,400
Cement sheet							
Primary	2	0.3–8.7	3	0.9–8.4	Dry Mixing, Sanding	600	1,300
Secondary		1.0–6.0					24,000
Floor tile	1	0.5–4.3	4	0.9–4.3	Fiber Introduction	2,900	6,700
Textile							
Primary	4	0.25–10.0	4	2.0–10.0	Carding	2,400	3,700
Secondary		2.0–6.0					7,500
Paints, Coatings, and Sealants	1	1.0–2.5	2.5	1.5–8.0	Fiber Introduction	350	3,000

SOURCE: From Ref. 5. Optical microscope visible fibers, 5 μm long or longer.

microscopy and usually are expressed as mass per unit volume (nanogram per cubic meter). Because of intrinsic variability in the unit weight of individual fibers, the conversion factors relating mass concentration to optical fiber concentration range from 5–150 $\mu g/m^3/f/ml$. Despite the uncertainty of these derived conversion factors, a factor of 30 $\mu g/m^3/f/ml$ has been adopted by the EPA[12] and other scientific bodies.

Measurements via transmission electron microscopy have established background concentrations of asbestos in urban ambient air at generally less than 1 nanogram per cubic meter (0.00003 fibers per ml) and rarely more than 10 nanograms per cubic meter (0.00033 fibers per ml).[14] Table 2-2 summarizes fiber concentration data from a variety of studies in both urban and rural areas over the period 1969–1983.

Asbestos concentrations in buildings, on the other hand, are more variable, revealing a three-fold variability among arithmetic mean concentrations.[14] Earlier studies often focused on buildings in which asbestos surface materials were visibly damaged and friable, which were not representative. In buildings with evidence of severe damage or deterioration, the probability of detecting excessive asbestos levels over background was high. If the asbestos-containing surface materials or thermal insulation was undamaged or encapsulated, lower air concentrations were observed.

Table 2-3 shows summary statistics for average airborne fiber concentrations near schools and buildings reflecting more recent sampling data. Levels are comparable to outdoor air and are several orders of magnitude lower than current workplace standards (OSHA permissible exposure level (PEL) of 0.20 fibers per ml).

Asbestos abatement work is a significant potential source of asbestos exposure, particularly in schools and public buildings. While abatement procedures already specified by the EPA should minimize

TABLE 2-2. Summary of asbestos exposure samples in different environments

Sample set	No. of samples	Measured concentration (ng/m³)		Equivalent concentration (fibers/cc)*	
		Median	90th Percentile	Median	90th Percentile
Air of 48 U.S. cities	187	1.6	6.8	0.00005	0.00023
Air in U.S. schoolrooms without asbestos	31	16.3	72.7	0.00054	0.00242
Air in Paris buildings with asbestos surfaces	135	1.8	32.2	0.00006	0.00107
Air in U.S. buildings with cementitious asbestos	28	7.9	19.1	0.00026	0.00064
Air in U.S. buildings with friable asbestos	54	19.2	96.2	0.00064	0.00321

SOURCE: Modified from Ref. 14. *Based on conversion factor of 30μg/m³ = 1 fiber/cc.

TABLE 2-3. Summary statistics for average airborne fiber concentrations in U.S. schools and buildings

			Public buildings		
Statistic	Schools (71)	Outdoor air (48)	Category 1 (6)	Category 2 (6)	Category 3 (37)
Median		0.00000	0.00010	0.00040	0.00058
Mean	0.00024*	0.00039	0.00099	0.00059	0.00073
Standard Deviation	0.00053	0.00096	0.00198	0.00052	0.00072

SOURCE: From Ref. 19, with permission.
* 80th percentile = 0.00045; 90th percentile = 0.00083.
The data used in the calculation of each statistic are the average concentrations (expressed as number of fibers greater than 5μm in length per cubic centimeter of air) in a building (for indoor samples) or the concentration outside each building (for outdoor samples). By visual inspection, category 1 buildings contained no asbestos-containing material (ACM), category 2 buildings contained ACM in primarily good condition, and buildings in category 3 showed at least one area of significantly damaged ACM. In the study on public buildings, 387 indoor and 48 outdoor air samples were evaluated. No asbestos fibers were detected in 83% of the 387 samples. The sample size is given in parentheses below each heading.

building contamination following renovation, removal, enclosure, or encapsulation of asbestos materials, these procedures may be violated.

The EPA has monitored the efficacy of the specified controls and cleanup procedures. Table 2-4 presents the results of one study of five schools where removal and encapsulation of asbestos-containing surfaces followed EPA procedures.[14] Although escape of asbestos fibers did occur during encapsulation and removal, there appeared to be a net reduction in fiber levels after encapsulation. Little improvement occurred in asbestos fiber levels following physical removal, with pre- and postabatement fiber levels being virtually the same. These results have brought into question both the health risk/benefit and the cost-benefit considerations of removal versus encapsulation. Currently, widespread removal of asbestos is not always recommended, and encapsulation is preferred in many situations.

REGULATORY ACTIVITY

Public health concern over the occupational and nonoccupational sources of asbestos exposure has created a vast array of governmental regulatory activity and the phasing out of asbestos production and its use in consumer products. Between 1900 and 1980 some 30 million tons of asbestos were used commercially in the United States,[12] most extensively from the end of World War II until the early 1970s, when its use began to decline. Asbestos use in this country has decreased dramatically in the last decade.[15] Currently, the largest categories of asbestos use are asbestos cement, pipe, and sheet products, and friction products, including brakes, coatings, and gaskets.

This marked reduction in use is the result of regulatory activities in the 1970s and 1980s, during which time five government agencies

TABLE 2-4. Geometric mean of chrysotile fiber and mass
concentrations before, during, and after asbestos abatement

Sampling Location	Concentration							
	Before abatement		During abatement*		Immediately after abatement		After school resumed	
	(f/l)[†]	(ng/m³)	(f/l)	(ng/m³)	(f/l)	(ng/m³)	(f/l)	(ng/m³)
Encapsulation								
Rooms with unpainted asbestos	1423.6	6.7	117.2	0.6	13.7	0.1	248.1	1.2
Rooms with painted asbestos	622.9	2.7	—	—	0.8	0.0	187.2	0.8
Asbestos-free rooms	250.6	1.2	0.5	0.0	9.3	0.0	30.7	0.2
Outdoors	3.5	0.0	0.0	0.0	6.5	0.0	2.8	0.0
Removal								
Rooms with asbestos	31.2	0.2	1736.0	14.4	5.6	0.1	23.9	0.2
Asbestos-free rooms	6.1	0.1	12.0	0.1	1.6	0.0	18.1	0.1
Outdoors	12.6	0.1	1.3	0.0	20.0	0.1	7.9	0.0

SOURCE: Reprinted from Ref. 14, with permission.
*Measured outside work containment areas.
[†]Fibers of all lengths.

invoked statutory authority to regulate asbestos. The Occupational Safety and Health Administration (OSHA) regulates workplace exposure to asbestos and has set a PEL (an 8-hour time-weighted average for a 40-hour-per-week work shift) for occupational exposures. The PEL has been steadily lowered, as concern over health hazards and better monitoring methods have become established (Table 2-5).[5] The first permanent standard, set in 1972, was 5 fibers/ml. This was lowered in 1976 to 2 fibers/ml and in 1986 to the lowest level agreed to be technologically feasible, 0.2 fibers/ml. There is still great debate whether this provides adequate protection to prevent both lung cancer and mesothelioma in asbestos-exposed workers. The National Institute for Occupational Safety and Health (NIOSH) has recommended a PEL of 0.1 fibers/ml, and this was also proposed as a regulatory standard by OSHA in 1990.

The Mine Safety and Health Administration regulates the mining and milling of asbestos ore. The Food & Drug Administration (FDA) is responsible for regulating asbestos in food, drugs, and cosmetics. Consumer product bans on the use of asbestos in garments, dry-wall patching compounds, and fireplace emberizing materials have been implemented by the Consumer Product Safety Commission. Despite these selected events, most of the regulatory activity has emanated from the Environmental Protection Agency.

Through the National Emissions Standards for Hazardous Air Pollutants (NESHAP) program, the EPA regulates external emissions from asbestos mills and from manufacturing and fabricating operations. The EPA also regulates the use of asbestos in roadway surfacing and

TABLE 2-5. Regulatory activities regarding permissible exposure levels in the workplace

Date	U.K. Advisory Committee on Asbestos	British Occupational Hygiene Soc.	National Institute of Occupational Safety & Health	Occupational Safety & Health Admin. (proposed)	Occupational Safety & Health Admin. (regulation)	Environmental Protection Agency
1969		2 fibers/ml TWA chrysotile				
March, 1971						Asbestos listed as hazardous air pollutant
1972					5 fibers/ml STEL	
April, 1973						No visible emissions, milling and manufacturing Ban: Spray application of friable materials containing more than 1% asbestos
Oct. 1975				0.5 fibers/ml TWA		
July, 1976					2 fibers/ml TWA 10 fibers/ml STEL	
Dec, 1976			0.1 fibers/ml TWA			
1979	0.5 fibers/ml TWA chrysotile					

Date	Exposure limits	Actions
1983	0.5 fibers/ml TWA amosite 0.2 fibers/ml TWA crocidolite 0.5 fibers/ml TWA chrysotile	
June, 1986	0.2 fibers/ml TWA 1.0 fibers/ml STEL	
Sept. 1988		
July, 1990	0.1 fibers/ml TWA	Ban: cloth, felt, tile
July, 1993		Ban: gaskets, original equipment, brakes
July, 1996		Ban: after-market brakes, air conditioning, pipe, shingles, roof materials

SOURCE: Ref. 5.
NOTE: STEL = short term exposure limit
TWA = time weighted average

in insulation materials, and has banned most uses of sprayed-on asbestos materials and pipe wrapping. These standards also require specific work practices during demolition and renovation involving asbestos materials, and regulate the removal, transport, and disposal of asbestos-containing materials. The EPA has also established programs to evaluate and certify asbestos-removal contractors and established work rules to protect workers during asbestos-abatement activities.

Since 1982, when the EPA issued the Asbestos and Schools Identification and Notification Rule, the agency has required all local education agencies to inspect for friable asbestos materials; to notify parents and teachers if such materials are found; to place warning signs in schools where asbestos is found; and to keep accurate records of their actions eliminating this problem. With Congressional approval of the Asbestos School Hazards Abatement Act of 1984, the EPA was given responsibility for providing both financial and technical assistance to local education agencies.

In July 1989, the EPA banned almost all asbestos-containing products in the United States in a phase-out staged over seven years. The final rule, promulgated under the Toxic Substances Control Act (Section 6) bans the importation, processing, and manufacture of asbestos-containing products. When fully implemented, this rule will effectively remove over 94% of the new asbestos used in the United States. The primary factor in determining the elimination of each category of products is based on EPA's projection of the development and availability of a safe substitute with industrial qualities adequate to the asbestos it replaces.

For example, the rule bans asbestos use in automotive and other gaskets in 1993, automotive vehicle brakes beginning with the 1994 models, and asbestos-containing cement pipe and roof shingles by 1996. Certain products are exempt from the rule, because they do release insignificant amounts of asbestos over the life of the product. These were felt too costly to ban because of the unavailability of reasonable-cost substitutes. Examples include reinforced plastic, asbestos thread, asbestos diaphragms, and unique industrial applications. The rule does not affect existing asbestos materials in commercial products and buildings.

ASSESSING NONOCCUPATIONAL RISK

Asbestos-related disease resulting from nonoccupational exposure to asbestos has been recognized in published reports of mesothelioma among household contacts of asbestos workers and in residents living near asbestos mines and factories.[12] An increase in the prevalence of malignant mesothelioma and asbestos-related disease has been reported in nonoccupationally exposed populations in Turkey,[16] Cyprus[17] and Northeast Corsica.[18] These sites are associated with ambient exposures much higher than those observed in U.S. homes and public buildings.[19] The causal factor for at least some of the excess mesothelioma in Turkey may be due to the geologic presence of a nonasbestos mineral fiber, erionite (see Chap. 5).

No epidemiologic evidence is available to quantitatively link mesothelioma with general environmental, nonoccupational asbestos exposure in nonindustrialized countries. As a result, there is no directly observed quantitative risk estimate from observation of populations nonoccupationally exposed to asbestos.[20]

In an effort to assess the health risk of nonoccupational exposure to asbestos in buildings and schools, numerous international panels have been convened. In the absence of undisputed evidence, several mathematical models have been proposed to assess the lifetime risk of lung cancer and mesothelioma.[21–25] Underlying these varying risk assessment models are assumptions and uncertainties making the interpretation of these risk estimates inherently difficult.

The estimation of risk is based on extrapolation from high-dose workplace exposures in the past to low doses found in buildings and the ambient environment. Modern ambient exposures are orders of magnitude less than even today's OSHA permissible exposure level of 0.2 fibers per ml. Estimates of exposure assigned to these retrospective worker cohorts cannot be fully characterized, due in part to poor sampling and analytical methodology and the use of surrogate exposure categories based on job title. Mass-to-fiber conversions utilized in these models add substantial uncertainty. Models that include an assumption of a linear dose-response assume there is no exposure threshold for disease risk. This concept implies that exposure to one fiber of asbestos carries an inherent and finite risk for lung cancer and mesothelioma, and that the risk is cumulative for each fiber to which an individual is exposed. This hypothesis is still widely debated.

Differences between the carcinogenic potential of chrysotile and amphibole fiber types could not be fully considered because the fiber-specific exposure data are incomplete. Some recent reviews conclude that mesothelioma is the only asbestos-related disease likely to occur at relatively low nonoccupational exposures and that it is due overwhelmingly to amphibole asbestos.[19] This assumption is based on the finding that chrysotile fibers are more readily eliminated from the lung than the amphiboles. It is postulated that mesotheliomas attributed to chrysotile exposure in the past are instead the result of trace contaminants of amphibole asbestos.[26]

Examination of combined data from some of these published risk estimates shows that the risk of asbestos-related death (lung cancer and mesothelioma) due to exposure in schools is in the range of 0.005–0.093 deaths per year per million students for an average life expectancy of 75 years.[26] This estimate assumes an exposure of 0.00024 fibers per cubic centimeter of air for five school years beginning at age 10. These estimates are orders of magnitude lower than some commonplace risks from drowning, motor vehicle accidents, and household accidents.

Calculations of unit risk for asbestos at the low concentrations measured in the environment must also be viewed with great caution. The EPA's best estimate of the risk to the U.S. general population for a lifetime of continuous exposure to 0.0001 fibers/ml is 2.8 mesothelioma deaths and 0.5 excess lung cancer deaths per 100,000 females; and for males, 1.9 mesothelioma and 1.7 excess lung cancer deaths per 100,000. Excess gastrointestinal cancer mortality is estimated to be approximately 10–30% of the excess lung cancer mortality.[27] The World Health Organization proposes a range of cancer risks based on an exposure of 0.0005 fibers/ml. The predicted lifetime cancer risk per 100,000 (smokers and nonsmokers) for the general population is 1–10 for mesothelioma and 0.1–1 for lung cancer.[28]

Some studies of asbestos workers have observed an increased risk of cancer at other sites, including the gastrointestinal tract, larynx, esophagus, and kidney (see Chapter 8). However, these findings have not been consistent and there is still considerable controversy as to whether these cancers are associated with asbestos exposure. All reviews regarding asbestos risk considered nonmalignant disease, asbestosis, to be of no importance at levels now typical in the ambient environment and buildings.[12]

REFERENCES

1. Gilson JC: Asbestos, In: *Encyclopedia of Occupational Health and Safety* (Parmeggiani L, ed.), Geneva: International Labour Office, 1983, pp. 185–187.
2. Nicholson WJ, Selikoff IJ, Seidman H, Lilis R, Formby P: Long-term mortality of chrysotile miners and millers in the Thetford Mines, Quebec. *Ann NY Acad Sci* 330:11–21, 1979.
3. Prevost, M: Asbestos Institute, Montreal, Quebec, Canada, Personal communication, December 1989.
4. Asbestos: Manufacture, importation, processing and distribution in commerce prohibitions; final rule. 40 CFR 763. *Fed Reg* 54:29468.
5. U.S. Department of Health Education and Welfare, Public Health Service: Asbestos: an information resource (Levine RJ, ed.), 1978. DHEW Publication number 78–1681, pp. 41–60.
6. Dement JM: Asbestos, In: *Occupational Respiratory Diseases*, National Institute for Occupational Safety and Health, U.S. Department of Health and Human Services (Merchant JA, ed.), 1986, p. 288.
7. Selikoff IJ, Churg J, Hammond EC: Asbestos exposure and neoplasia. *JAMA* 188(1):142–146, 1964.
8. U.S. Environmental Protection Agency. Asbestos Fact Book, USEPA Office of Public Affairs (A-107), 1985, p. 5.
9. Report to the Congress, Study of Asbestos-Containing Materials in Public Buildings, U.S. EPA, February 1988, p. 5.
10. Code of Federal Regulations. Title 29, Chapter XVII, Subpart 1926.58, 1986.
11. Churg A: Current issues in the pathologic and mineralogic diagnosis of asbestos-induced disease. *Chest* 84(3):275–280, 1983.

12. Airborne Asbestos Health Assessment Update. U.S. Environmental Protection Agency, Office of Health and Environmental Assessment, EPA/600/8-84/003F, June 1986.
13. Corn M: Asbestos and disease: An industrial hygienist's perspective. *Am Indus Hyg Assoc J* 47(9):515–523, 1986.
14. Nicholson WJ: Airborne mineral fiber levels in the non-occupational environment, In: *Non-Occupational Exposure to Mineral Fibers* (Bignon J, Peto J, Saracci J, eds.), IARC Scientific Publication No. 90, Lyon, France, 1989, pp. 239–261.
15. Environmental News. EPA Announces Final Regulation to Ban New Asbestos Products. USEPA Washington, DC, July 6, 1989.
16. Simonato L, et al: Relation of environmental exposure to erionite fibers to risk of respiratory cancer, In: *Non-Occupational Exposure to Mineral Fibers* (Bignon J, Peto J, Saracci J, eds.), IARC Scientific Publication No. 90, Lyon, France, 1989, pp. 398–405.
17. McConnochie K, et al: Mesothelioma in Cyprus, In: *Non-Occupational Exposure to Mineral Fibers* (Bignon J, Peto J, Saracci J, eds.), IARC Scientific Publication No. 90, Lyon, France, 1989, pp. 411–419.
18. Boutin C, et al: Bilateral pleural plaques in Corsica: A marker for nonoccupational asbestos exposure, In: *Non-Occupational Exposure to Mineral Fibers* (Bignon J, Peto J, Saracci J, eds.), IARC Scientific Publication No. 90, Lyon, France, 1989, pp. 406–410.
19. Mossman BT, et al: Asbestos: Scientific developments and implications for public policy. *Science* 247(294):294–301, 1990.
20. Gardner MJ, Saracci R: Effects on health of nonoccupational exposure to airborne minerals, In: *Non-Occupational Exposure to Mineral Fibers* (Bignon J, Peto J, Saracci J, eds.), IARC Scientific Publication No. 90, Lyon, France, 1989, pp. 375–397.
21. Acheson ED, Gardner MJ: Asbestos: The control limit asbestos. Her Majesty's Stationery Office, London, 1983.
22. Report to the U.S. Consumer Product Safety Commission by the Chronic Hazard Advisory Panel on Asbestos. Consumer Product Safety Commission, Washington, DC, 1986.
23. Doll R, Peto J: Asbestos: Effects on health of exposure to asbestos. Her Majesty's Stationery Office, London, 1985.
24. Report on matters of health and safety arising from the use of asbestos in Ontario. Ontario Royal Commission, Ontario Ministry of the Attorney General, Toronto, 1984.
25. National Research Council, Committee on Nonoccupational Health Risks of Asbestiform Fibers: Nonoccupational Health Risks, Washington, DC: National Academy Press, 1984.
26. Mossman BT, Gee JB: Asbestos-related diseases, Medical Progress. *N Eng J Med* 320(26):1721–1730, 1989.
27. Evolution of the Potential Carcinogenicity of Asbestos. Carcinogen Assessment Group, Office of Health and Environmental Assessment, U.S. EPA, Washington, DC, 1988.
28. Air Quality Guidelines, World Health Organization, Copenhagen, 1987.

3. Asbestos Bodies and Nonasbestos Ferruginous Bodies

Victor L. Roggli

Asbestos bodies are the histologic hallmark of exposure to asbestos.[1–4] These structures are golden brown, beaded, or segmented, dumbbell-shaped objects with a characteristic microscopic appearance that is readily recognized by the pathologist. Their identification in histologic sections is an important component of the pathologic diagnosis of asbestosis (see Chap. 4), and their presence serves to alert the pathologist to exposure to air-borne asbestos fibers. This chapter discusses the structure and development of asbestos bodies, as well as their occurrence and distribution within human tissues. In addition, techniques for the quantification of asbestos bodies are reviewed, along with the relationship of asbestos-body formation to the various types of asbestos fibers. Finally, the distinction of asbestos bodies from other ferruginous bodies based on light microscopic and analytical electron microscopic observations is emphasized. (The identification and significance of asbestos bodies in cytologic specimens is discussed in Chap. 9, and the relationship between asbestos-body concentrations in pulmonary tissues and the various asbestos-associated diseases is reviewed in Chap. 11.)

HISTORICAL BACKGROUND

Asbestos bodies in the lung were first described by Marchand in 1906.[5] He called them peculiar "pigmented crystals" and did not recognize their relationship to asbestos fibers. Eight years later the German pathologist T. Fahr took note of peculiar crystals in the lungs of an asbestos worker with pulmonary interstitial fibrosis.[6] W. E. Cooke described these structures as "curious bodies,"[7] and by 1929 Stewart and Haddow had coined the term *asbestosis bodies*.[8] By this time Cooke[9] and Gloyne[10] recognized that these curious bodies had asbestos fibers at their core, although as late as 1930 in this country they were being confused with fungal hyphae.[11] The term *asbestosis body* was later changed to *asbestos body* when it was discovered that they also occurred in the lungs of workers who did not have asbestosis.[12,13] Experimental animal studies in the 1960s showed that structures resembling asbestos bodies were formed when a number of different types of fibrous dusts (fibrous aluminum silicate, silicon carbide whiskers, cosmetic talc, and fibrous glass) were instilled intratracheally into the lungs of hamsters.[14] As a result, it was suggested that the noncommittal term *ferruginous body* be used when the precise nature of the fibrous core was not known.[14,15] It then remained for Churg and Warnock[16,17] to show by means of energy-dispersive spectrometry and electron diffraction that ferruginous bodies isolated from human lungs and having a thin, translucent fibrous core were virtually always true asbestos bodies.

STRUCTURE AND DEVELOPMENT OF ASBESTOS BODIES

Asbestos bodies form when an asbestos fiber is inhaled and deposited in the distal regions of the lung parenchyma.[13] Here, the free alveolar macrophages phagocytose the fiber (Fig. 3-1). Subsequently, through a process that is still poorly understood, the fiber becomes covered with a layer of iron-protein-mucopolysaccharide material.[18-20] It has been proposed that this process is a means of host defense, since in vivo[21] as well as in vitro[22] studies have shown that asbestos bodies are nonfibrogenic and noncytotoxic in comparison to uncoated asbestos fibers. The coated asbestos fiber, or asbestos body, has a characteristic golden brown appearance, due to the iron component of the coating. These structures thus give a strong positive reaction with the Prussian blue stain. In histologic sections, asbestos bodies have a beaded, segmented, dumbbell or lancet shape, which is especially well appreciated in cytologic preparations (Fig. 3-2) and in Nuclepore filter preparations of lung tissue digests (Fig. 3-3). Branched forms, which result from the deposition of coating material on a splayed fiber, may also occur (Fig. 3-4). Curved or circular asbestos bodies may also be observed (Fig. 3-5), and usually have very thin core fibers (average core diameter of 0.2 μ).[17] Asbestos bodies are generally 20–50 μ in length,[20] with an average length of about 35 μ.[23] However, they may exceed 200 μ in length; some examples approaching 0.5 mm (500 μ) have been reported.[24] Asbestos bodies are usually 2–5 μ in diameter,[20] although, by scanning electron microscopy, the author has observed rare bodies only 0.5 μ in diameter.[13]

Only a small percentage of asbestos fibers found within the lung at any single time are coated. A number of factors exist that determine whether an individual fiber will become coated to form an asbestos body, including characteristics of the inhaled dust as well as characteristics pertaining to the host. Regarding the former, fiber dimensions are important factors in asbestos-body formation. Morgan and Holmes[25] found that, in humans, fibers less than 20 μ in length rarely become coated, while virtually all fibers 80 μ or greater in length are coated. Fiber diameter is also an important factor, with thicker fibers being more likely to become coated than thinner fibers.[26] Dodson et al.[27] suggested that fiber surface irregularities, such as etching, fracture, fraying, and multifibrillar composition, may also influence the coating process, with uncoated fibers having much smoother surface features. The type of fiber is also important (vide infra), with the vast majority of asbestos bodies isolated from human lungs possess-

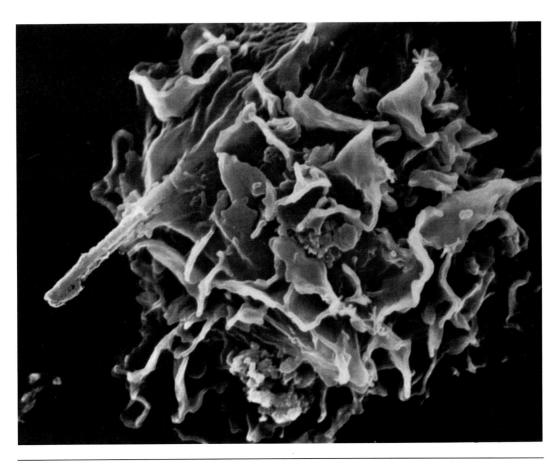

FIGURE 3-1. Scanning electron micrograph of a human free alveolar macrophage phagocytizing an amosite asbestos fiber. Magnified ×2000. Reprinted from Greenberg SD, Asbestos-Associated Pulmonary Diseases, Medcom, 1981, with permission.

ing an amphibole asbestos core.[13,16,17,20,26] The proportion of fibers 5 µ or more in length that are coated appears to increase as the tissue fiber burden increases (Fig. 3-6). The presence of other dusts in the lung may also influence the coating process. For example, the author has observed that welders, who have heavy burdens of iron oxide particles in their lungs, tend to have a high percentage of coated fibers (median value of 26% for nine welders, as compared to 10.8% for 254 other asbestos-exposed individuals).

With regard to host factors, coating efficiency depends on the animal species exposed to the asbestos fibers. Humans, hamsters, and guinea pigs form asbestos bodies efficiently, whereas cats, rabbits, and mice do so much less readily, and rats and dogs are poor asbestos-body formers.[21] There is also individual variability in coating efficiency, with some individuals appearing to be poor asbestos-body formers.[28,29] Considerable variation in coating efficiency has

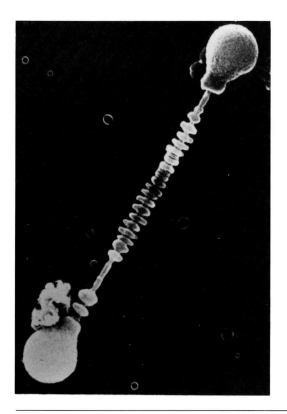 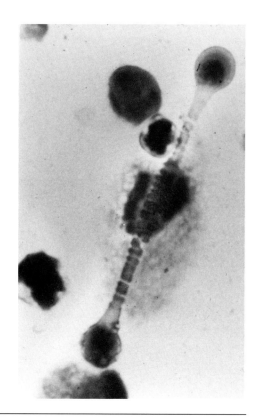

FIGURE 3-2. Side-by-side scanning electron micrograph of: (*left*) an asbestos body; (*right*) bronchoalveolar-lavage-recovered asbestos body and free alveolar macrophage. (SEM, magnified ×2000; Papanicolaou, magnified ×600). Reprinted from Ref. 2, with permission.

even been observed in different areas of the lung from a single individual.[26] In the author's laboratory, the percentage of fibers 5 μ or greater in length that are coated (as determined by scanning electron microscopy) has ranged from 0.002% to 72%, with a median value of 11.8%. This last value is very similar to the 11% coated fibers reported by Morgan and Holmes[26] using phase-contrast light microscopy. Finally, fiber clearance may be reduced in individuals with asbestosis, so that increased numbers of short fibers are retained and the proportion of fibers that become coated is greatly diminished.[26]

The mechanism of formation of asbestos bodies was studied in detail by Suzuki and Churg.[30] Asbestos fibers deposited in the distal regions of the lung parenchyma are phagocytosed by free alveolar macrophages. Those fibers that are approximately 20 μ or greater in length cannot be completely ingested by a single cell, and by poorly understood mechanisms this "frustrated phagocytosis" then triggers the coating process. Within 16 days of initial exposure, the iron micelles appear in the cytoplasm of the macrophages in close proximity to the ingested fibers, and by continuous accretion of these micelles

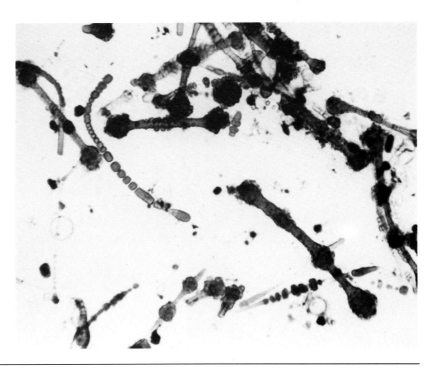

FIGURE 3-3. Asbestos bodies on a Nuclepore filter show the range of morphologic appearances, including dumbbell shapes, beaded structures, lancet forms, among others. Note the variable quantity of iron coating and the visible asbestos core fibers (arrowheads).

embedded in a homogeneous matrix material, the typical asbestos bodies recognizable by light microscopy are eventually formed.[30] The asbestos fiber is separated from the cytoplasm of the macrophage by a lysosomal limiting membrane. Recent evidence suggests that the process of asbestos-body formation occurs extracellularly and is analogous to the process of bone resorption by osteoclasts.[31] The source of the iron that coats the fiber is unknown, but it is probably derived from either hemoglobin or plasma transferrin. In experimental animals, asbestos bodies can be recognized by light microscopy within two or three months of exposure.[26] The finding of asbestos bodies in lung tissue digests of infants from three to twelve months of age[32] suggests that the time course for the formation of asbestos bodies is similar in man. It has been suggested that the peculiar segmentation of asbestos bodies is due to the fragmentation of the rigid, sheathlike coating, and that further "weathering" and dissolution of the coating eventually occurs.[33,34] This sequence of events has been supported by scanning electron microscopic observations of asbestos bodies isolated from human tissues[35] (Fig. 3-7). However, recent studies have shown that typical, segmented asbestos bodies can be formed in vitro in a mouse peritoneal macrophage culture system,[36] casting doubt on the "weathering" mechanism of asbestos-body segmentation.

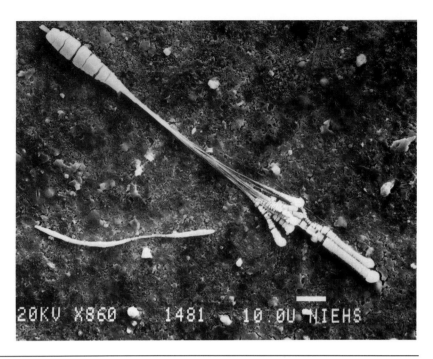

FIGURE 3-4. Scanning electron micrograph of an asbestos body with splaying of one end of the core fiber. Each splayed fiber has its own ferroprotein coating. Magnified ×860.

Not all asbestos bodies have a ferruginous coating. De Vuyst et al.[37] described a case in which amosite asbestos fibers coated with calcium oxalate crystals were recovered by bronchoalveolar lavage. Similar observations were reported by Le Bouffant et al.,[38] who described "enrobant" forms in which entire asbestos bodies are encased within an oxalate crystal. This author has observed two similar cases (Fig. 3-8), including one with long-standing renal failure. However, systemic disturbance in oxalate metabolism cannot be identified in some cases.[36,37] Coating of asbestos fibers with spherules of calcium phosphate has also been observed in humans and experimental animals[31,39] (Fig. 3-9). The formation of calcium phosphate salts in association with interstitial asbestos fibers appears to be a common reaction to injury in the white rat.[40] The calcium phosphate coatings are distinctive by virtue of their large size, spherical shape, and wide separation between deposits on an individual fiber. Intraalveolar calcium carbonate concretions (pulmonary "blue bodies") have also been reported in association with asbestos exposure[41] but have not been described as a coating material on asbestos fibers. It must be emphasized that calcium phosphate and calcium oxalate bodies are rare occurrences, and that ferruginized asbestos fibers are by far the most common form of asbestos body.

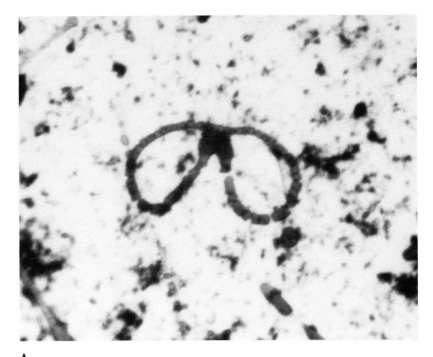

A

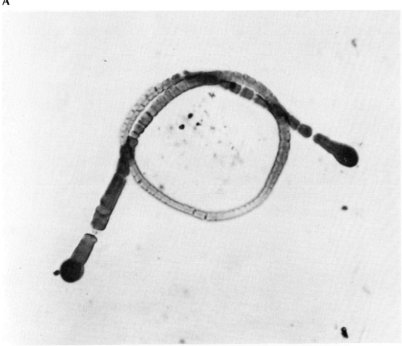

B

FIGURE 3-5. Examples of curved asbestos bodies with thin amphibole cores. (A) Pair of asbestos "spectacles." (B) This asbestos body, isolated from bronchoalveolar lavage fluid, appears to be tied in a knot.

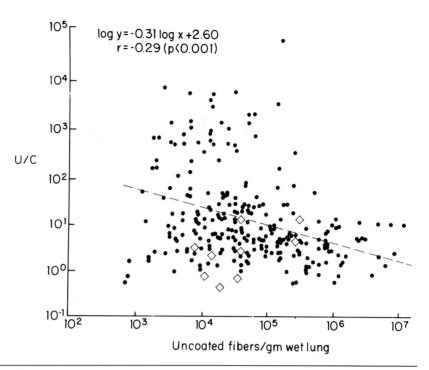

FIGURE 3-6. Graph showing the relationship between the pulmonary burden of uncoated fibers 5 μ or greater in length and the ratio of uncoated to coated fibers (U/C) isolated from the lung, as determined by scanning electron microscopy of 263 cases. The percentage of fibers that are coated increases significantly as the pulmonary asbestos burden increases. Welders (◇) tend to have especially low U/C ratios (i.e., high percentage of coated fibers).

OCCURRENCE AND DISTRIBUTION OF ASBESTOS BODIES

In 1963, Thomson et al.[42] reported that asbestos bodies could be found in scrapings of autopsy lungs in 24% of urban residents in South Africa. Since that time, a number of studies have demonstrated that when digestion-concentration techniques are employed to analyze sufficient quantities of lung tissue, some asbestos bodies can be recovered from the lungs of virtually all adults in industrialized nations.[1,43–51] The percentage of patients from a general autopsy adult population with asbestos bodies in their lungs has ranged from as low as 33% in Japan in a study using 0.5-gram samples of lung tissue[51] to as high as 100% in a study from the United States employing 5-gram samples.[44] The median value for the 10 cited studies is 92% (Table 3-1). Correlations with occupational data indicate that blue-collar men tend to have the highest counts,[48] reflecting some occupational exposure to asbestos for many of these individuals. Lower counts are often found in women as compared to men,[45,48,49] indicating that men are more likely to have jobs with some asbestos

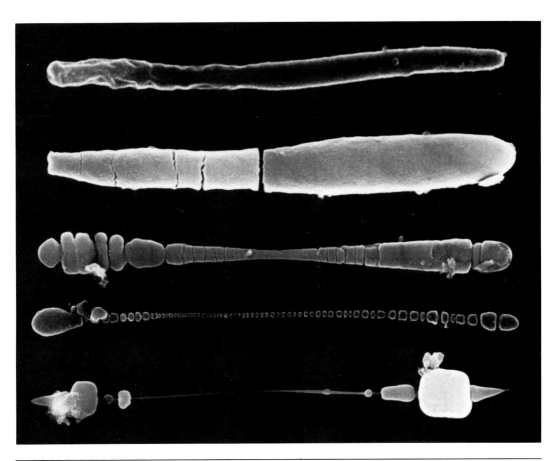

FIGURE 3-7. Composite scanning electron micrograph demonstrating the proposed sequence of events in asbestos-body segmentation. *From top:* (A) Membrane-limited smooth coating. (B) Partial cracks (small arrowheads) and complete cracks (large arrowheads) in a coated fiber. (C) Erosion of the sharp edges of cracked regions to form a smooth contour along an asbestos body. (D) Extensive beading along the axis of an asbestos body. (E) A bizarre form, with an extensive central uncoated fiber region capped by heavily eroded ends. Reprinted from Ref. 35, with permission.

exposure. In addition, smokers appear to have higher lung asbestos-body counts than nonsmokers.[48] Environmental asbestos contamination is not confined to urban areas, since rural dwellers are found to have asbestos bodies in their lungs just as often as urban dwellers (95% vs. 91%).[46] An increasing prevalence of asbestos bodies in autopsy lungs during the past several decades has also been reported, ranging from 41% in the 1940s to 91% of cases in 1970–72.[47] These investigators also found a significant increase with increasing age in the proportion of lungs containing asbestos bodies,[47] although others have found no increase in asbestos-body content with age.[45,48,49] Indeed, studies by Haque et al.,[32] who reported the isolation of

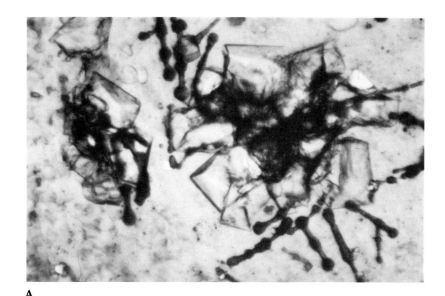

FIGURE 3-8. Calcium oxalate bodies. (A) Light micrograph of a cluster of asbestos bodies in sputum associated with numerous crystals of calcium oxalate dihydrate. (B) Scanning electron micrograph of asbestos fibers embedded in calcium oxalate crystals. Note the large bipyramidal form typical of caicium oxalate dihydrate. Courtesy of Dr. Robert Moore of the Richmond VA Medical Center and Dr. Mason Williams, Jr., of the University of Texas Health Center at Tyler.

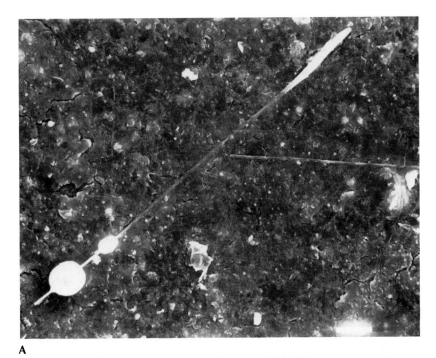

A

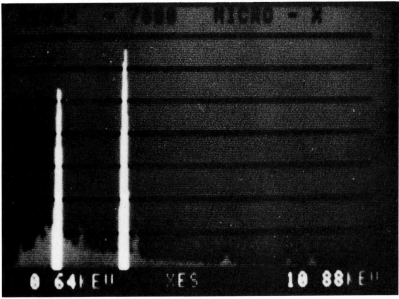

B

FIGURE 3-9. (A) Calcium-phosphate-coated asbestos fiber isolated from the lungs of a construction worker with asbestosis and squamous carcinoma of the lung. Note the uncoated fibers. Magnified ×1100. (B) Energy dispersive x-ray spectrum of the large spherical globule in part (A) shows peaks for calcium and phosphorus but not for iron. Reprinted from Ref. 39, with permission.

TABLE 3-1. Occurrence of asbestos bodies in the general population as determined by tissue digestion

Authors	Year	Country	No. cases	Percent*
Bignon et al.[43]	1970	France	100	100%
Smith and Naylor[44]	1972	United States	100	100
Rosen et al.[45]	1972	United States	86	90
Breedin and Buss[46]	1976	United States	124	93
Bhagavan and Koss[47]	1976	United States	145	91
Churg and Warnock[48]	1977	United States	252	96
Roggli et al.[1]	1980	United States	52	92
Steele and Thomson[49]	1982	United Kingdom	106	80
		New Zealand	248	75
Rogers[50]	1984	Australia	128	37
Kobayashi et al.[51]	1986	Japan	656	33

*Percent indicates the percentage of cases in which asbestos bodies were recovered from autopsy lung tissue by digestion.

asbestos bodies from the lungs of infants, indicate that exposure to asbestos in our industrialized society begins within the first year of life.

A few studies have examined the topographic distribution of asbestos bodies within the lung. Sebastien et al.[52] examined autopsy lung tissue from six patients with no known asbestos exposure, and found no consistent relationship between the concentration of asbestos bodies in the upper vs. lower lobes or central vs. peripheral lung parenchyma. Rosen et al.[45] reported on results from 14 cases in which lung tissue was analyzed for asbestos-body content from more than one site, and again found no consistent relationship between asbestos-body content in the upper vs. lower lobes or right vs. left lung. Gylseth and Baunan[53] described the asbestos-body content in two asbestos workers, and found considerable variation from site to site within the lungs. These observations are consistent with the data from this author's laboratory involving 41 cases for which tissue was available for digestion from two or more sites. The asbestos-body concentration in the upper lobe exceeded that in the lower lobe in 17 instances, whereas the reverse was true in 15 instances. Similarly, the asbestos-body concentration in the right lung exceeded that in the left lung in 24 cases, whereas the opposite was found in 17 cases. This variability in asbestos-body concentration from one site to another within the lung was dramatically demonstrated in the studies of Morgan and Holmes,[54,55] who extensively sampled lung tissue from one insulator and two Finnish anthophyllite mine workers. Their data show a five- to ten-fold variation in asbestos-body concentration in adjacent blocks of tissue. Experimental animal studies suggest that this site-to-site variability in asbestos content may be related to airway path lengths and branching patterns.[56]

QUANTIFICATION OF ASBESTOS BODIES

Since a few asbestos bodies can be found in the lungs of virtually everyone in industrialized nations, quantitative studies are required in order to draw inferences relative to exposure and various disease processes. A number of techniques have been devised for quantification of asbestos bodies in tissues, and these are reviewed in the following sections. They include quantification in histologic sections, lung tissue digests, lymph nodes, and extrapulmonary tissues.

HISTOLOGIC SECTIONS

Paraffin sections are routinely used by pathologists for diagnostic purposes, so it is only natural that histologic sections have played an important role with respect to identification and quantification of asbestos bodies in tissues. In early studies investigating the prevalence of asbestos bodies in the general population, 30-μ-thick paraffin sections were employed.[57] Selikoff and Hammond used basal smears and ashed tissue sections to study the prevalence of asbestos bodies in the lungs of New York City residents.[58] However, there was little attempt actually to quantify the numbers of asbestos bodies in histologic sections. A semiquantitative study was reported in 1980 by Roggli et al.,[1] who concluded that 5000 or more asbestos bodies per gram of wet lung tissue were required before bodies were likely to be encountered in 10 random high-power fields of iron-stained sections. Churg[59] observed in 1982 that roughly 500 asbestos bodies per gram of wet lung needed to be present before any bodies could be found in tissue sections. Then in 1983, Roggli and Pratt[23] reported a quantitative study relating the numbers of asbestos bodies observed in iron-stained tissue sections to asbestos-body counts in lung tissue digests. The observations in this study were validated using a more rigorous mathematical model,[60] and similar results have subsequently been reported by others.[29,51]

A key factor in the calculation of the numbers of asbestos bodies per gram of wet lung tissue from the number observed in a histologic section is the recognition that the same asbestos body may be observed in several serial sections.[23] This is because the average asbestos body is considerably longer than the average section is thick. Thus there is a finite probability that an asbestos body will be oriented in the block in such a way that it will appear on two or more adjacent sections. This concept is depicted schematically in Fig. 3-10. Once the orientation of the asbestos body in the paraffin block has been accounted for, it is a simple matter to calculate asbestos bodies per gram, using a conversion factor from volume of paraffin-embedded tissue to wet weight of lung. The relevant formulas are:[23]

$$N_g = \frac{N_c}{A_s \cdot t \cdot O_c \cdot R} \tag{1}$$

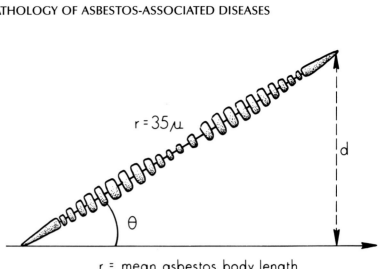

r = mean asbestos body length
θ = angle of orientation of asbestos
    body with respect to face of
    paraffin tissue block
d = r sin θ

FIGURE 3-10. Model for determining the orientation correction factor for counting asbestos bodies in tissue sections. Bodies are assumed to be rigid, straight structures with a mean length of 35 μm. The abscissa is parallel to the paraffin block face, θ is the angle between the asbestos body and the plane of the block face, which can range from 0°–90°, and d is the projection of the asbestos body (in μm) in a direction perpendicular to the plane of the tissue section. As d increases, so does the probability that the asbestos body will be observed in two or more serial sections. Reprinted from Ref. 23, with permission.

where

N_g = Number of asbestos bodies per gram of wet lung tissue
N_c = Number of asbestos bodies counted on iron-stained tissue section
A_s = Area of tissue section, in mm^2
t = Thickness of tissue section, in mm
O_c = Orientation correction factor (see Ref. 23 for details)
R = Ratio of wet weight of fixed lung tissue to volume of paraffin-embedded lung tissue

Typical values for these variables in our laboratory are:

t = 5 μm = 0.005 mm
O_c = 2.56 for an average asbestos body length of 35 μm
R = 2.1 gm/cm^3 (includes a factor for shrinkage of lung during paraffin embedding[23])

Therefore,

$$N_g = \frac{N_c}{A_s} \times 37{,}200 \text{ mm}^2/\text{gm} \tag{2}$$

Note Equation (2) is only applicable to sections cut at 5-μm thickness and an average asbestos-body length of 35 μm. Also, these formulas were derived using iron-stained sections examined at 200× magnification using a mechanical stage.[23] Since asbestos bodies are not necessarily distributed uniformly through tissue sections, the more sections and the more total area examined, the greater the accuracy of the estimated asbestos-body concentration. Similar results can be obtained by using the regression line in Fig. 3-11 [in lieu of Eq. (2)] to estimate the asbestos-body concentration per gram of wet lung from the numbers of asbestos bodies per mm^2 of tissue section.[23] Also, Table 3-2 shows the number of 400× microscopic fields that have to be examined, on the average, to find the first asbestos body for a given tissue asbestos-body concentration.[60] These calculations indicate that asbestos-body detection in tissue sections (i.e., one asbestos body per 4 cm^2 section area) requires 100 or more asbestos bodies per gram of wet lung tissue.[23,60]

LUNG TISSUE DIGESTS

A variety of techniques have been described for the extraction of asbestos bodies from lung tissue for subsequent quantification or identification.[14,20,26,43–51,61–67] Most of these techniques employ wet chemical digestion, although low-temperature plasma ashing techniques have been used as well.[53,66,67] The inorganic residue remaining after digestion is then suspended in ethanol and collected on an acetate or polycarbonate filter with an appropriate pore size (0.45 μm or less). If the intent of the study is to quantify asbestos bodies alone, then the filter can be examined by light microscopy at a magnification of 200–400×. However, scanning electron microscopy (SEM) can be used to count asbestos bodies just as well,[39,53] and there is an excellent correlation between asbestos-body concentrations determined by light microscopy and those determined by SEM (Fig. 3-12). Once the number of asbestos bodies on the filter has been determined, the asbestos-body concentration per gram of wet lung,[1,39,64] gram of dry lung,[20,29,62] or cm^3 of lung tissue[43,52] can be calculated. The relationship between these three ways of reporting results varies somewhat from case to case, but a useful rule of thumb for comparative purposes is

$$1 \text{ AB/gm wet wt.} \cong 1 \text{ AB/cm}^3 \cong 10 \text{ AB/gm dry wt.} \tag{3}$$

Digestion studies must be carefully performed, since there are a number of potential sources of error. Asbestos bodies (and fibers)

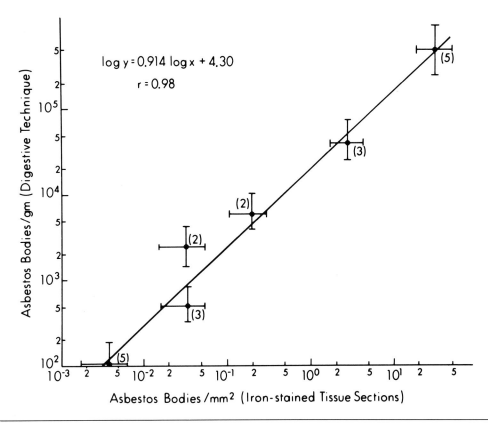

FIGURE 3-11. Relation (log-log scale) of the number of asbestos bodies seen in iron-stained sections (in units of bodies per mm^2) to the number measured by a tissue digestion technique (in units of asbestos bodies per gram of wet, formalin-fixed lung tissue). The number of sections evaluated per case is shown in parentheses, and each data point represents the mean result for one case, with error bars indicating one standard deviation. The least-squares fitted regression equation is shown at upper left, and the correlation coefficient is significant at the $P < 0.001$ level. Reprinted from Ref. 23, with permission.

may be lost during the extraction process through adhesion to glass surfaces, and this can result in substantial underestimation of the actual tissue concentration.[67] However, Corn et al.[68] have shown that, with their bleach digestion technique, the percentage error due to adherence of fibers or bodies to glass surfaces in cases with a heavy tissue asbestos burden is negligible. Whether this is true for low or moderate tissue asbestos burdens is unknown. Ashing of the specimen (especially in a muffle furnace at 400°–500°C) causes tissue shrinkage resulting in fracture of long fibers, which increases the asbestos-body count.[53,67] Morgan and Holmes[55] have also reported that dicing of the tissue sample prior to bleach digestion results in a decrease in median asbestos-body length and thus an apparent increase in asbestos-body concentration. However, this effect on

TABLE 3-2. Average number (N) of 400× microscopic fields examined to find first asbestos body for a given asbestos–body concentration (AB/gm)

N	AB/gm
1	181,000
5	36,200
10	18,100
18	10,000
25	7,240
36	5,000
50	3,620
100	1,810
181	1,000
362	500
1810	100

SOURCE: Modified from Ref. 60, with permission.

asbestos-body counts appears to be of the same order of magnitude as the coefficient of variation for counting different aliquots of the same sample (i.e., about 10%), and is substantially less than the five- to ten-fold variation that can occur from sampling different sites in the same lung.[54,55] This serves to emphasize the importance of sampling multiple sites for digestion whenever this is feasible.

The range of asbestos-body concentrations reported on lung samples from the general population as well as from individuals with various asbestos-related diseases (discussed in Chap. 11) spans at least nine orders of magnitude (from 0.1 to 10^7 AB's/gm wet lung tissue). It should be noted that while there is fairly good agreement in the determination of tissue asbestos-body concentrations among different laboratories employing different analytical techniques, the agreement is considerably worse for the determination of uncoated asbestos fiber concentrations.[69] However, there may be significant variation in tissue asbestos-body content from one region of the country to another.[1,20,39,48,64] Therefore, it is important for laboratories engaged in such determinations to calculate their own normal range of asbestos-body concentrations.

LYMPH NODES

Gloyne in 1933 described asbestos bodies in histologic sections of lymph nodes, and noted that, when present, they are usually found in areas of the node containing pigment.[70] Godwin and Jagatic reported asbestos bodies in the regional lymph nodes of six of seven patients with malignant mesothelioma.[71] Others have also mentioned the presence of asbestos bodies in histologic sections of lymph nodes,[20] but the author is not aware of any quantitative studies of asbestos bodies in pulmonary lymph nodes. The author has noted asbestos bodies in histologic sections in 20 cases from his consultation files[72] (Fig. 3-13). Seventeen of these patients had histologically

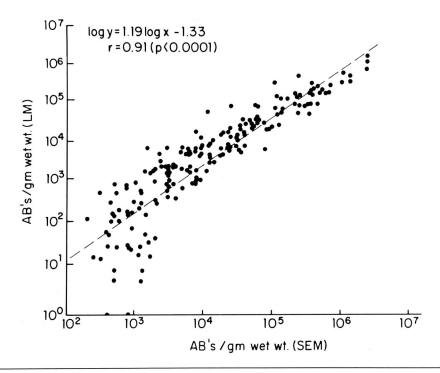

FIGURE 3-12. Correlation between asbestos-body counts by light microscopy and by scanning electron microscopy in 189 cases. Each dot represents one case. The linear regression line has a correlation coefficient of 0.91 ($p < 0.0001$). Note log-log scale.

confirmed asbestosis, and all were heavily exposed to asbestos for durations ranging from 4 to 40 years. The median asbestos-body concentration in the lung parenchyma as determined by light microscopy of lung tissue digests was more than 1000 times our upper limit of normal.[72] In four cases, lymph node tissue was also available for digestion, and the asbestos-body concentration in the lymph nodes ranged from 3000 to more than 300,000 asbestos bodies per gram of wet weight of lymph node. Asbestos bodies were not observed in iron-stained sections of lymph nodes in 14 autopsied controls, all of which had lung asbestos-body counts within our normal range of 0–20 AB's/gm. However, a few asbestos bodies were found in lymph node digests in 6 of 14 controls. The range of values for the lymph nodes was roughly the same as for normal lung parenchyma (0 to 17 AB's/gm of wet lymph node tissue).[72]

Considerations similar to those used for the determination of asbestos-body concentrations from asbestos-body counts in tissue sections of lung (see above) can be used to estimate the minimum asbestos-body concentration necessary in lymph node tissue for asbestos bodies to be observed in lymph node histologic sections. For an average lymph node measuring 1.0 by 0.5 cm, average asbestos-

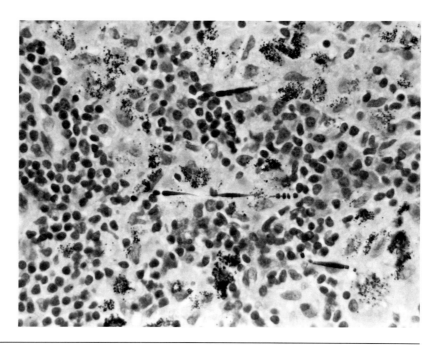

FIGURE 3-13. Asbestos bodies within a histologic section of a hilar lymph node from an insulator with asbestosis and squamous cell carcinoma of the right upper lobe. Hematoxylin and eosin, magnified ×520. Reprinted from Ref. 72, with permission.

body length of 35 μm, tissue section thickness of 6 μm, and lymph node density of 1 gm/cm^3, the finding of one asbestos body in an iron-stained section of lymph node is equivalent to approximately 1600 asbestos bodies per gram wet weight of lymph node[72] (Fig. 3-14). Several conclusions can be drawn from these observations. First, the finding of asbestos bodies in histologic sections of lymph nodes is indicative of a heavy asbestos-body burden within the node and is associated with considerably elevated lung asbestos-body burdens. Second, a few asbestos bodies can be found in digests of lymph nodes in many individuals with no known exposure to asbestos, indicating transport of some long fibers to the lymph nodes even at low tissue asbestos burdens. Finally, in some cases, the asbestos-body content of the hilar nodes exceeds that of the lung parenchyma at both low and high tissue asbestos burdens.

EXTRAPULMONARY TISSUES
As early as 1933, Gloyne had observed that asbestos bodies are readily transported from place to place on a scalpel or microtome blade, and can easily be carried over from one specimen jar to another.[70] It is common practice for pathologists to place portions of multiple organs in a single container of formalin. The author has recovered scores of asbestos bodies from one cc of formalin within a

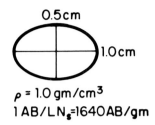

ρ = 1.0 gm/cm^3
1 AB/LN$_s$=1640AB/gm

FIGURE 3-14. Schematic diagram of a typical hilar lymph node section, measuring
1 × 0.5 cm and with approximate density (ρ) of 1.0 gm/cm^3. The finding of
one asbestos body in such a paraffin section is equivalent to roughly 1600
asbestos bodies per gram of wet fixed nodal tissue. Reprinted from Ref. 72,
with permission.

container in which lungs (and other organs) from an individual with
a heavy pulmonary asbestos burden had been placed. In addition,
asbestos bodies may adhere to glassware used in the digestion procedure, and thus potentially be carried over from one case to the
next.[67,73] All of these sources of contamination would have to be considered in studies of asbestos bodies in extrapulmonary tissues,
especially since the tissue concentrations would be so low that confirmation by means of histologic sections would be lacking.[23] Nevertheless, most investigators reporting asbestos bodies in extrapulmonary sites have failed to take these considerations into account.
Therefore, the reader should keep these confounding factors in mind
when considering the literature on this subject.

Extrapulmonary organs from which asbestos bodies have been
recovered are listed in Table 3-3. Auerbach et al.[74] reported the occurrence of asbestos bodies in extrapulmonary sites in 37 cases, including 19 with asbestosis and 18 with parietal pleural plaques. These
investigators recovered 20 mm^3 of tissue from paraffin blocks deparaffinized in xylene and digested in potassium hydroxide, with the
residue collected on an ashless paper filter and ashed on a glass slide
within a low-temperature plasma asher. Asbestos bodies were recovered from kidney, heart, liver, spleen, adrenals, pancreas, brain,
prostate, and thyroid. The authors concluded that, in individuals
with heavy pulmonary asbestos-body burdens, asbestos bodies are
likely to be present in other organs as well.[74] Kobayashi et al.[75] reported a similar study of 26 cases with varying levels of pulmonary
asbestos body burden. They used up to five grams of formalin-fixed
tissue that was digested with potassium hydroxide, with the residue
collected on a membrane filter. Asbestos bodies were found in esophagus, stomach, small and large intestine, spleen, pancreas, liver,
heart, kidney, urinary bladder, bone marrow, thyroid, and adrenals.
These investigators also noted that the incidence and the number
of asbestos bodies in extrapulmonary organs tend to increase as

TABLE 3-3. Extrapulmonary tissues from which
asbestos bodies have been recovered

Adrenal gland	Large intestine
Bone marrow	Small intestine
Brain	Stomach
Esophagus	Spleen
Heart	Pancreas
Kidney	Prostate
Larynx	Thyroid
Liver	Urinary bladder

SOURCE: From Refs. 74, 75, and 78.

the pulmonary asbestos burden increases.[75] However, this observation is also consistent with contamination of formalin by pulmonary asbestos bodies.

Ehrlich et al.[76] reported a case of an asbestos insulator with asbestosis who underwent a resection for carcinoma of the colon. Asbestos bodies were recovered from digests of 3–5 grams of tumor, adjacent normal bowel, mesentery, and serosal fat. In contrast, Rosen et al.[77] found no asbestos bodies in digests of colonic tissue from 21 cases of colon cancer from the general population. Roggli et al.[78] recovered asbestos bodies from digests of laryngeal mucosa in two of five asbestos workers but in none of 10 autopsy controls. The occurrence of asbestos bodies in the upper airway and the gastrointestinal tract is not unexpected, since asbestos bodies may be found in mucus from the lower respiratory tract, which is then coughed up and swallowed (see Chap. 9). Although asbestos bodies in other extrapulmonary sites may be artifactual (see earlier discussion), there are some data to indicate that vascular transport of dust from the lungs can occur.[79,80] Once an asbestos fiber gains access to the intravascular compartment, hematogenous transport to any of the organs listed in Table 3-3 could theoretically occur. However, one would then expect to find the largest numbers of asbestos bodies in the organs that receive the greatest percentage of systemic blood flow, i.e., the brain, the heart, and the kidneys. This has not been the case in the reported studies.[74,75]

ASBESTOS BODIES AND FIBER TYPE

The vast majority of asbestos bodies isolated from human lungs have been found to have an amphibole asbestos core.[13,16,17,20,28,64,81,82] Asbestos workers[39,64] and men from the general population[83] generally have the commercial amphiboles, amosite or crocidolite, forming the cores of asbestos bodies within their lungs. On the other hand, women from the general population are more likely to have one of the noncommercial amphiboles, tremolite or anthophyllite, as the core to asbestos bodies found in their lungs.[83] This latter finding may be related to contamination of commercial talcum powder with tremolite and anthophyllite.[84] The predominance of amphibole asbestos-body cores is somewhat curious, considering that the bulk of asbestos used commercially is chrysotile[85] (Fig. 3-15). Chrysotile asbestos bodies do occur, however (Fig. 3-16), and account for about 2% of all asbestos bodies that have been analyzed by our laboratory[39,86] and by others as well.[20,87] Moulin et al.[88] reported that chrysotile asbestos bodies accounted for 10% of bodies analyzed from asbestos-exposed workers but only 3% of bodies from members of the Belgian urban population. They are especially likely to occur in individuals exposed to long fibers of chrysotile, such as asbestos textile workers or chrysotile miners or millers. In the latter group of workers, most asbestos bodies isolated from lung tissue have chrysotile asbestos cores.[89] Thicker chrysotile bundles are more likely to become coated than thin chrysotile fibrils.[26] The rarity of chrysotile asbestos bodies apparently results from the ready fragmentation of chrysotile into shorter fibrils, and the fact that asbestos bodies tend to form only on fibers 20 µm or more in length.[25,26] As a result, asbestos bodies are generally a poor indicator of the pulmonary chrysotile asbestos burden.[20,29,62,63] On the other hand, the pulmonary asbestos-body content correlates very well with the burden of uncoated fibers 5 µm or greater in length (Fig. 3-17).[39,54,55,64] Among individuals exposed occupationally to asbestos, most fibers in this size range are commercial amphiboles.[39,64] An obvious exception to this is the relatively small percentage of asbestos workers exposed exclusively to chrysotile.

NONASBESTOS FERRUGINOUS BODIES

As noted in the earlier section on "Historical Background," fibrous dusts other than asbestos can become coated with iron, or ferruginized, so that one must be cautious in identifying asbestos bodies by light microscopy.[14,15] Fortunately, most of the nonasbestos ferruginous bodies, or pseudoasbestos bodies, can be distinguished from true asbestos bodies at the light microscopic level.[13,17,20,90] The author has observed nonasbestos ferruginous bodies in tissue digests from 97 of 406 cases (24%), but only rarely are they found in numbers approaching those of true asbestos bodies.[20] The morphologic features of the various types of nonasbestos ferruginous bodies are reviewed next.

SHEET SILICATES
These structures may form ferruginous bodies with a distinctive broad, yellow core. Churg et al.[17] described two patterns of ferruginous body formation with sheet silicate cores: (1) bodies with a

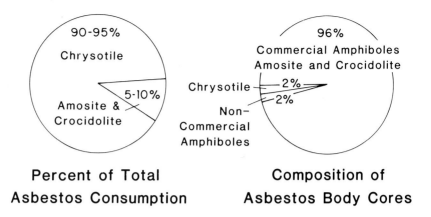

Percent of Total Asbestos Consumption

Composition of Asbestos Body Cores

FIGURE 3-15. Diagram showing the proportions of the various types of asbestos fibers consumed commercially (*left*) versus the composition of asbestos-body cores (*right*). Although chrysotile accounts for the great bulk (90–95%) of asbestos consumed commercially, asbestos bodies infrequently (approximately 2%) have a chrysotile core. Reprinted from Ref. 86, with permission.

highly irregular shape and platy structure with irregular, often sparse coating (Fig. 3-18), and (2) bodies with a rectangular shape, more uniform coating, and diameter only slightly greater than that of true asbestos bodies. The second pattern may be confused with true asbestos bodies; and when the core is particularly thin, this distinction may not be possible at the light-microscopic level. Electron diffraction shows a pseudohexagonal pattern, and energy-dispersive spectrometry shows that most of these bodies have cores of talc, mica, or kaolinite.[20] They are commonly found in the lungs of roofers and rubber factory workers, who are exposed to substantial amounts of talc,[20] and the author has observed them commonly in the lungs of shipyard welders. In the general population, they may contribute up to 20% of the total ferruginous body burden.[17]

CARBON FIBERS

Some ferruginous bodies have black cores, ranging from uniform, very thin black filaments to broader, more irregular platy forms. Gross et al. described ferruginous bodies of this type from human lungs and suggested that they had carbon cores.[91] The coating on these bodies is also variable, and may be segmented, sheathlike, or form right-angle branches.[17] Electron diffraction shows that these core fibers are amorphous, and energy-dispersive spectrometry indicates there are no elements with atomic number greater than or equal to that of sodium ($Z = 11$).[20] These observations are consistent with the carbonaceous nature of the cores. We have observed bodies of this type in the lungs of coal miners,[92] and recently in the lungs of a woman with an unusual exposure to woodstove dust[93] (Fig. 3-19). In

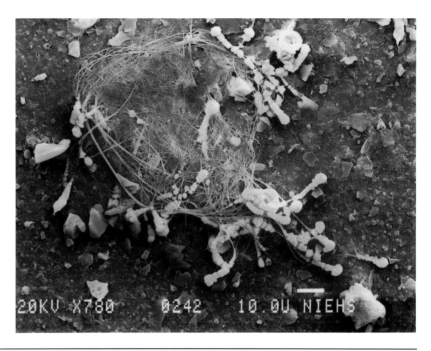

FIGURE 3-16. Cluster of chrysotile asbestos fibers on a Nuclepore filter isolated from the lungs of an asbestos textile worker with a pleural mesothelioma. The fiber ends appear to spin off the central mass like arms of a spiral galaxy, and have become coated to form numerous chrysotile asbestos bodies. Scanning electron microscopy, magnified ×850. Reprinted from Ref. 39, with permission.

the general population, they may contribute to as much as 90% of the total ferruginous body burden in some cases;[20] in our case with the unusual woodstove dust exposure, they accounted for 100% of the bodies recovered.[93]

METAL OXIDES

Fibrous forms of a variety of metal oxides can form ferruginous bodies with dark brown to black cores.[13] These structures usually have a core with a uniform diameter and segmented coating that, except for the color of the core, resemble typical asbestos bodies (Fig. 3-20). We have identified such ferruginous bodies with cores of titanium, iron, chromium, and aluminum, presumably in the form of the metal oxide. Titanium particles and fibers are commonly found in lung specimens;[39,92] when they reach a certain critical length,[25] they may then become coated to form a ferruginous body. Dodson et al.[94] described ferruginous bodies with iron-rich core fibers isolated from the lungs of a worker at an iron reclamation and manufacturing facility. We have observed ferruginous bodies with iron-rich cores and rarely with aluminum-rich cores from the lungs of shipyard welders. These individuals have large numbers of nonfibrous iron and aluminum oxide particles in their lungs. Finally, a unique case has been reported

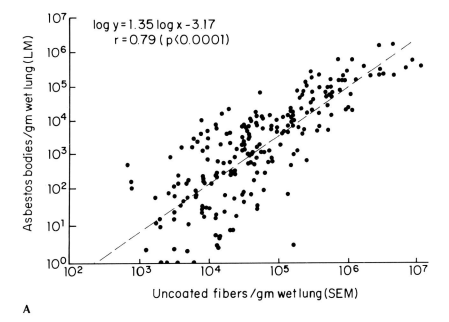

A

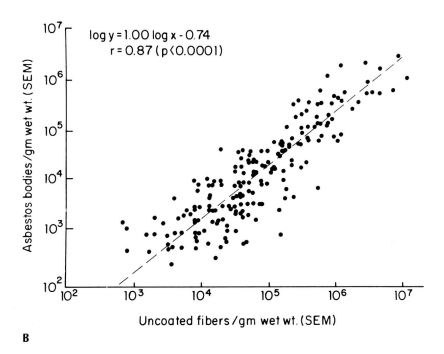

B

FIGURE 3-17. (A) Scattergram showing the relation between asbestos-body counts by light microscopy and uncoated fiber counts by scanning electron microscopy, for 223 cases. The correlation coefficient for the least-squares fitted linear regression line is 0.79 ($p < 0.0001$). (B) Correlation between asbestos-body and uncoated-fiber counts by scanning electron microscopy in 193 cases ($r = 0.87$, $p < 0.0001$). Note log-log scale.

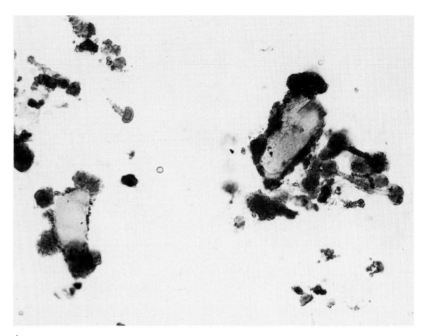

A

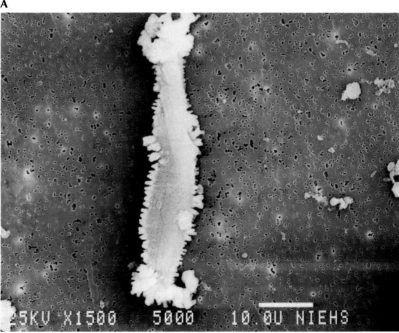

B

FIGURE 3-18. (A) Pseudoasbestos bodies of the sheet silicate type, isolated from the lungs of an insulator with asbestosis and small cell carcinoma of the lung, have broad, yellow cores (arrows). True asbestos bodies are also present (*right center and upper left*). Nuclepore filter preparation, ×520. (B) Scanning electron micrograph of a sheet silicate pseudoasbestos body. Note the heavy coating on the ends and the serrated edges. Magnified ×1500. Part (A) reprinted from Ref. 13, with permission.

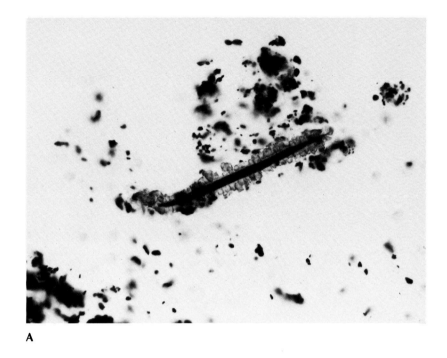

A

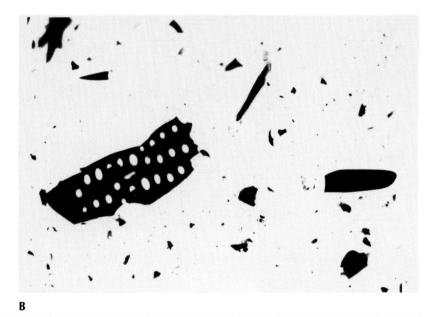

B

FIGURE 3-19. (A) Pseudoasbestos body isolated from the lungs of a coal worker has a black carbon core coated with segmented ferroprotein material. Magnified ×800. (B) Dust recovered from bronchoalveolar lavage fluid from a woman exposed to woodstove dust. Fiber in upper middle portion of field (arrow) is iron coated. Note gridlike structure left of center. Nuclepore filter preparation, magnified ×330. Part (A) reprinted from Ref. 92; part (B) reprinted from Ref. 95, with permission.

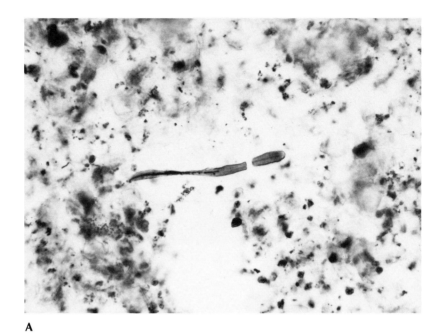

A

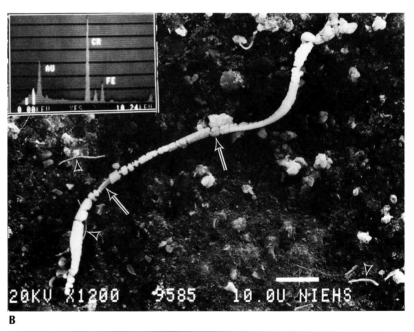

B

FIGURE 3-20. (A) Pseudoasbestos body with black core fiber recovered from lungs of a 76-year-old metal polisher. Magnified ×500. (B) Scanning electron micrograph of pseudoasbestos body, showing beaded iron coating as well as bare area revealing the core fiber (arrows). Additional uncoated fibers are present (arrowheads). *Inset:* EDXA spectrum from bare area of coated fiber, showing prominent peaks for chromium and a smaller peak for iron. Peak for gold is due to sputter-coating. Magnified ×1200. Reprinted from Ref. 95, with permission.

in which chromium-rich cores were identified in ferruginous bodies isolated from the lungs of a metal polisher.[95]

MAN-MADE MINERAL FIBERS

Man-made mineral fibers are commonly used in insulation materials and can form ferruginous bodies in experimental animals.[14] Therefore, it would not be unexpected to find such fibers at the cores of ferruginous bodies isolated from human lungs. Langer et al.[82] studied 50 ferruginous bodies isolated from the lungs of members of the general population of New York City, and concluded that the cores in most were either degraded chrysotile or fibrous glass. Roggli et al.[96] examined 90 ferruginous bodies isolated from the lungs of six individuals with malignant pleural mesothelioma and three with asbestosis, and found two with cores that had a chemical composition consistent with fibrous glass. Although fibrous glass may occasionally be found in samples of human lung tissue[92] (Fig. 3-21), it is uncommonly identified as the core of ferruginous bodies. This observation is most likely due to the brittleness of these fibers so that they tend to break transversely, producing shorter fibers,[97] and to the tendency for fibrous glass to dissolve in vivo.[98]

DIATOMACEOUS EARTH

Ferruginous bodies with cores of diatomaceous earth are infrequently encountered. By light microscopy, they are large, broad, segmented, and frequently serpiginous. They lack the clubbed ends so often observed in true asbestos bodies, and their color varies from golden yellow to deep orange-brown.[17] In some examples, the sievelike skeletal pattern of the diatom can be observed by electron microscopy[17,92] (Fig. 3-22). Since the diatom skeleton is composed of amorphous silica, the cores would appear silicon-rich with energy-dispersive spectrometry and show no pattern with electron diffraction. Some silica "fibers" encountered in the lung may be acicular cleavage fragments of quartz, and it is conceivable that such fragments, if of the proper dimension, might form the cores of ferruginous bodies and give a peak for silicon only with energy-dispersive spectrometry.

ZEOLITE BODIES

Zeolites are hydrated aluminum silicates that occur naturally, and some forms of zeolite, such as erionite, are fibrous. Erionite is found in volcanic tuff in Turkey, and has physical characteristics that closely resemble those of amphibole asbestos. Sebastien et al.[99] have isolated ferruginous bodies with erionite cores from the lungs of individuals from Turkish villages situated on volcanic tuff rich in erionite. By light microscopy, they are indistinguishable from typical asbestos bodies. The villagers in this region of Turkey have a high incidence of pleural mesothelioma (see Chap. 5) and pleural fibrosis and

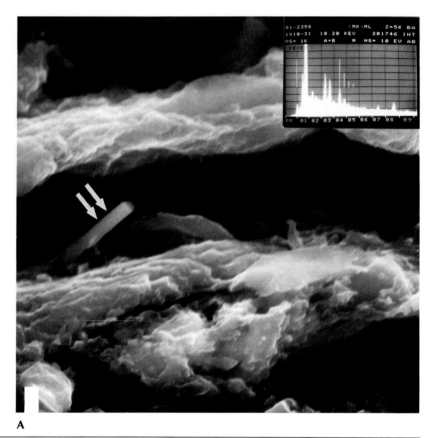

A

FIGURE 3-21. Lung tissue from a young woman with interstitial fibrosis. (A) Secondary electron image, showing a fiber protruding from an alveolar septum (double arrow). (B) Back-scattered electron image of the same field shown in part (A), demonstrating the fiber (double arrow) and an additional particle of talc (magnesium silicate) embedded in the tissue (single arrows). *Inset:* EDXA spectrum obtained from the fiber shown in parts (A) and (B), indicating a chemical composition of Na-Al-Si-K-Ca-Ba. This composition is consistent with fibrous glass. Parts (A) and (B) magnified ×3300. Reprinted from Ref. 92, with permission.

calcification (see Chap. 6). Zeolite bodies have thus far not been reported in lung tissue from individuals in North America.[13]

OTHERS
Silicon carbide whiskers can form ferruginous bodies in experimental animals,[14] and ferruginous bodies with black cores have been observed in the lung tissues of silicon carbide workers.[100,101] In addition, elastic fibers under certain conditions can undergo fragmentation and ferruginization, and hence form the cores of ferruginous bodies.[20] In consideration of the wide variety of nonasbestos mineral fibers that can be recovered from human lungs (see Chap. 11), it is

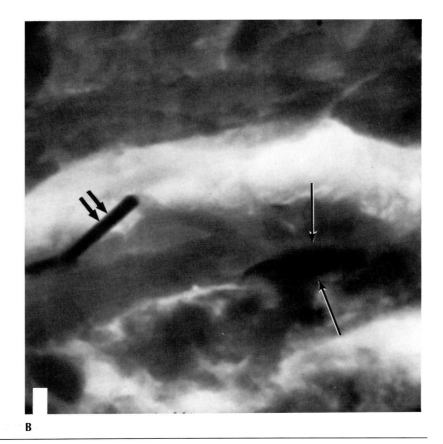

B

likely that nonasbestos ferruginous bodies of types other than those just described will be reported in the future.

REFERENCES

1. Roggli VL, Greenberg SD, Seitzman LH, McGavran MH, Hurst GA, Spivey CG, Nelson KG, Hieger LR: Pulmonary fibrosis, carcinoma, and ferruginous body counts in amosite asbestos workers: A study of six cases. *Am J Clin Pathol* 73:496–503, 1980.
2. Greenberg SD: Asbestos lung disease. *Sem Respir Med* 4:130–136, 1982.
3. Greenberg SD: Asbestos, Chapter 22, In: *Pulmonary Pathology* (Dail DH, Hammar SP, eds.), Springer-Verlag: New York, 1988, pp. 619–635.
4. Craighead JE, Abraham JL, Churg A, et al: The pathology of asbestos-associated diseases of the lungs and pleural cavities: Diagnostic criteria and proposed grading schema (Report of the Pneumoconiosis Committee of the College of American Pathologists and the National Institute for Occupational Safety and Health). *Arch Pathol Lab Med* 106:544–596, 1982.
5. Marchand F: Ueber eigentümliche Pigmentkristalle in den Lungen. *Verhandl d Deutsch path Gesellsch* 10:223–228, 1906.
6. Fahr T: Demonstrationen: Präparate und Microphotogrammes von einen Falle von Pneumokoniose. *Muench Med Woch* 11:625, 1914.

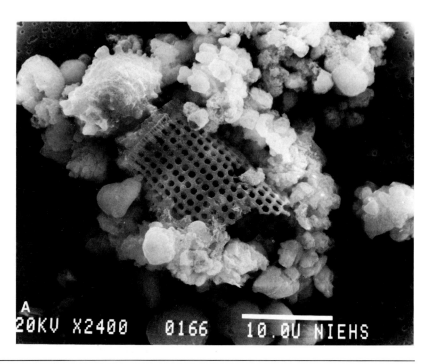

FIGURE 3-22. Diatomaceous earth pseudoasbestos body isolated from the lungs of an asbestos insulator in a shipyard. The diatom fragment with symmetrically aligned holes represents the silicon-containing diatom skeleton, which is surrounded by irregular granules of hemosiderin. Magnified ×2400. Reprinted from Ref. 92, with permission.

7. Cooke WE: Pulmonary asbestosis. *Br Med J* 2:1024–1025, 1927.
8. Stewart MJ, Haddow AC: Demonstration of the peculiar bodies of pulmonary asbestosis ("asbestosis bodies") in material obtained by lung puncture and in the sputum. *J Pathol Bact* 32:172, 1929.
9. Cooke WE: Asbestos dust and the curious bodies found in pulmonary asbestosis. *Br Med J* 2:578–580, 1929.
10. Gloyne SR: The presence of the asbestos fibre in the lesions of asbestos workers. *Tubercle* 10:404–407, 1929.
11. Craighead JE: Eyes for the epidemiologist: The pathologist's role in shaping our understanding of the asbestos-associated diseases. *Am J Clin Pathol* 89:281–287, 1988.
12. Castleman BI: *Asbestos: Medical and Legal Aspects*. New York: Harcourt Brace Jovanovich, 1984.
13. Roggli VL: Pathology of human asbestosis: A critical review. In: *Advances in Pathology*, vol. 2 (Fenoglio-Preiser, CM, ed.), Chicago: Yearbook Publishers, 1989, pp. 31–60.
14. Gross P, de Treville RTP, Cralley LJ, Davis JMG: Pulmonary ferruginous bodies: Development in response to filamentous dusts and a method of isolation and concentration. *Arch Pathol* 85:539–546, 1968.
15. Gaensler EA, Addington WW: Asbestos or ferruginous bodies. *N Engl J Med* 280:488–492, 1969.
16. Churg A, Warnock ML: Analysis of the cores of ferruginous (asbestos) bodies from the general population. I: Patients with and without lung cancer. *Lab Invest* 37:280–286, 1977.

17. Churg A, Warnock ML, Green N: Analysis of the cores of ferruginous (asbestos) bodies from the general population. II. True asbestos bodies and pseudoasbestos bodies. *Lab Invest* 40:31–38, 1979.

18. Davis JMG: Further observations on the ultrastructure and chemistry of the formation of asbestos bodies. *Exp Mol Pathol* 13:346–358, 1970.

19. Governa M, Rosanda C: A histochemical study of the asbestos body coating. *Br J Ind Med* 29:154–159, 1972.

20. Churg AM, Warnock ML: Asbestos and other ferruginous bodies: Their formation and clinical significance. *Am J Pathol* 102:447–456, 1981.

21. Vorwald AJ, Durkan TM, Pratt PC: Experimental studies of asbestosis. *Arch Ind Hyg Occup Med* 3:1–43, 1951.

22. McLemore TL, Mace ML, Roggli V, Marshall MV, Lawrence EC, Wilson RK, Martin RR, Brinkley BR, Greenberg SD: Asbestos body phagocytosis by human free alveolar macrophages. *Cancer Letts* 9:85–93, 1980.

23. Roggli VL, Pratt PC: Numbers of asbestos bodies on iron-stained tissue sections in relation to asbestos body counts in lung tissue digests. *Hum Pathol* 14:355–361, 1983.

24. Farley ML, Greenberg SD, Shuford EH, Jr., Hurst GA, Spivey CG, Christianson CS: Ferruginous bodies in sputa of former asbestos workers. *Acta Cytologica* 27:693–700, 1977.

25. Morgan A, Holmes A: Concentrations and dimensions of coated and uncoated asbestos fibres in the human lung. *Br J Ind Med* 37:25–32, 1980.

26. Morgan A, Holmes A: The enigmatic asbestos body: Its formation and significance in asbestos-related disease. *Environ Res* 38:283–292, 1985.

27. Dodson RF, O'Sullivan MF, Williams MG, Jr., Hurst GA: Analysis of cores of ferruginous bodies from former asbestos workers. *Environ Res* 28:171–178, 1982.

28. Dodson RF, Williams MG, O'Sullivan MF, Corn CJ, Greenberg SD, Hurst GA: A comparison of the ferruginous body and uncoated fiber content in the lungs of former asbestos workers. *Am Rev Respir Dis* 132:143–147, 1985.

29. Warnock ML, Wolery G: Asbestos bodies or fibers and the diagnosis of asbestosis. *Environ Res* 44:29–44, 1987.

30. Suzuki Y, Churg J: Structure and development of the asbestos body. *Am J Pathol* 55:79–107, 1969.

31. Koerten HK, Hazekamp J, Kroon M, Daems WTh: Asbestos body formation and iron accumulation in mouse peritoneal granulomas after the introduction of crocidolite asbestos fibers. *Am J Pathol* 136:141–157, 1990.

32. Haque AK, Kanz MF: Asbestos bodies in children's lungs: An association with sudden infant death syndrome and bronchopulmonary dysplasia. *Arch Pathol Lab Med* 112:514–518, 1988.

33. Gloyne SR: The formation of the asbestosis body in the lung. *Tubercle* 12:399–401, 1931.

34. Botham SK, Holt PF: Development of asbestos bodies on amosite, chrysotile, and crocidolite fibres in guinea-pig lungs. *J Pathol* 105:159–167, 1971.

35. Mace ML, McLemore TL, Roggli V, Brinkley BR, Greenberg SD: Scanning electron microscopic examination of human asbestos bodies. *Cancer Letts* 9:95–104, 1980.

36. Koerten HK, de Bruijn JD, Daems W Th: The formation of asbestos bodies by mouse peritoneal macrophages: An in vitro study. *Am J Pathol* 137:121–134, 1990.

37. DeVuyst P, Jedwab J, Robience Y, Yernault J-C: "Oxalate bodies," another reaction of the human lung to asbestos inhalation? *Eur J Respir Dis* 63:543–549, 1982.

38. Le Bouffant L, Bruyère S, Martin JC, Tichoux G, Normand C: Quelques observations sur les fibres d'amiante et les formations minérales diverses

rencontrèes dans les poumons asbestosiques. *Rev Fr Mal Respir* 4:121–140, 1976.

39. Roggli VL: Scanning electron microscopic analysis of mineral fibers in human lungs. Ch. 5, In: *Microprobe Analysis in Medicine* (Ingram P, Shelburne JD, Roggli VL, eds.), Washington, DC: Hemisphere Publishing, 1989, pp. 97–110.

40. Brody AR, Hill LH: Interstitial accumulation of inhaled chrysotile asbestos fibers and consequent formation of microcalcifications. *Am J Pathol* 109:107–114, 1982.

41. Koss MN, Johnson FB, Hochholzer L: Pulmonary blue bodies. *Hum Pathol* 12:258–266, 1981.

42. Thomson JG, Kaschula ROC, MacDonald RR: Asbestos as a modern urban hazard. *S Afr Med J* 37:77–81, 1963.

43. Bignon J, Goni J, Bonnaud G, Jaurand MC, Dufour G, Pinchon MC: Incidence of pulmonary ferruginous bodies in France. *Environ Res* 3:430–442, 1970.

44. Smith MJ, Naylor B: A method of extracting ferruginous bodies from sputum and pulmonary tissues. *Am J Clin Pathol* 58:250–254, 1972.

45. Rosen P, Melamed M, Savino A: The "ferruginous body" content of lung tissue: A quantitative study of eighty-six patients. *Acta Cytologica* 16:207–211, 1972.

46. Breedin PH, Buss DH: Ferruginous (asbestos) bodies in the lungs of rural dwellers, urban dwellers and patients with pulmonary neoplasms. *South Med J* 69:401–404, 1976.

47. Bhagavan BS, Koss LG: Secular trends in presence and concentration of pulmonary asbestos bodies—1940 to 1972. *Arch Pathol* 100:539–541, 1976.

48. Churg A, Warnock ML: Correlation of quantitative asbestos body counts and occupation in urban patients. *Arch Pathol Lab Med* 101:629–634, 1977.

49. Steele RH, Thomson KJ: Asbestos bodies in the lung: Southampton (UK) and Wellington (New Zealand). *Br J Ind Med* 39:349–354, 1982.

50. Rogers AJ: Determination of mineral fibre in human lung tissue by light microscopy and transmission electron microscopy. *Ann Occup Hyg* 28:1–12, 1984.

51. Kobayashi H, Watanabe H, Zhang WM, Ohnishi Y: A quantitative and histological study on pulmonary effects of asbestos exposure in general autopsied lungs. *Acta Pathol Jpn* 36:1781–1791, 1986.

52. Sebastien P, Fondimare A, Bignon J, Monchaux G, Desbordes J, Bonnaud G: Topographic distribution of asbestos fibres in human lung in relation to occupational and nonoccupational exposure. In: *Inhaled Particles*, vol. IV (Walton WH, ed.), Oxford: Pergamon Press, 1977, pp. 435–446.

53. Gylseth B, Baunan R: Topographic and size distribution of asbestos bodies in exposed human lungs. *Scand j Work Environ Health* 7:190–195, 1981.

54. Morgan A, Holmes A: Distribution and characteristics of amphibole asbestos fibres, measured with the light microscope, in the left lung of an insulation worker. *Br J Ind Med* 40:45–50, 1983.

55. Morgan A, Holmes A: The distribution and characteristics of asbestos fibers in the lungs of Finnish anthophyllite mine-workers. *Environ Res* 33:62–75, 1984.

56. Pinkerton KE, Plopper CG, Mercer RR, Roggli VL, Patra AL, Brody AR, Crapo JD: Airway branching patterns influence asbestos fiber location and the extent of tissue injury in the pulmonary parenchyma. *Lab Invest* 55:688–695, 1986.

57. Um CH: Study of the secular trend in asbestos bodies in lungs in London, 1936–1966. *Br Med J* 2:248–252, 1971.

58. Selikoff IJ, Hammond EC: Asbestos bodies in the New York City population in two periods of time, Pneumoconiosis: Proceedings of the Inter-

national Conference, Johannesburg, 1969 (Shapiro HA, ed.), Capetown: Oxford University Press, 1970, pp. 99–105.

59. Churg A: Fiber counting and analysis in the diagnosis of asbestos-related disease. *Hum Pathol* 13:381–392, 1982.

60. Vollmer RT, Roggli VL: Asbestos body concentrations in human lung: Predictions from asbestos body counts in tissue sections with a mathematical model. *Hum Pathol* 16:713–718, 1985.

61. Williams MG Jr., Dodson RF, Corn C, Hurst GA: A procedure for the isolation of amosite asbestos and ferruginous bodies from lung tissue and sputum. *J Toxicol Environ Health* 10:627–638, 1982.

62. Warnock ML, Prescott BT, Kuwahara TJ: Correlation of asbestos bodies and fibers in lungs of subjects with and without asbestosis. *Scanning Electron Microsc* II:845–857, 1982.

63. Warnock ML, Kuwahara TJ, Wolery G: The relation of asbestos burden to asbestosis and lung cancer. *Pathol Annu* 18(2):109–145, 1983.

64. Roggli VL, Pratt PC, Brody AR: Asbestos content of lung tissue in asbestos-associated diseases: A study of 110 cases. *Br J Ind Med* 43:18–28, 1986.

65. Ehrlich A, Suzuki Y: A rapid and simple method of extracting asbestos bodies from lung tissue by cytocentrifugation. *Am J Ind Med* 11:109–116, 1987.

66. Manke J, Rödelsperger K, Brückel B, Woitowitz H-J: Evaluation and application of a plasma ashing method for STEM fiber analysis in human lung tissue. *Am Ind Hyg Assoc J* 48:730–738, 1987.

67. Gylseth B, Baunan RH, Overaae L: Analysis of fibres in human lung tissue. *Br J Ind Med* 39:191–195, 1982.

68. Corn CJ, Williams MG Jr, Dodson RF: Electron microscopic analysis of residual asbestos remaining in preparative vials following bleach digestion. *J Electron Microsc Tech* 6:1–6, 1987.

69. Gylseth B, Churg A, Davis JMG, Johnson N, Morgan A, Mowe G, Rogers A, Roggli V: Analysis of asbestos fibers and asbestos bodies in tissue samples from human lung: An international interlaboratory trial. *Scand J Work Environ Health* 11:107–110, 1985.

70. Gloyne SR: The morbid anatomy and histology of asbestosis. *Tubercle* 14:550–558, 1933.

71. Godwin MC, Jagatic J: Asbestos and mesotheliomas. *Environ Res* 3:391–416, 1970.

72. Roggli VL, Benning TL: Asbestos bodies in pulmonary hilar lymph nodes. *Mod Pathol* 3:513–517, 1990.

73. Roggli VL, Piantadosi CA, Bell DY: Asbestos bodies in bronchoalveolar lavage fluid: A study of 20 asbestos-exposed individuals and comparison to patients with other chronic interstitial lung diseases. *Acta Cytolog* 30:470–476, 1986.

74. Auerbach O, Conston AS, Garfinkel L, Parks VR, Kaslow HD, Hammond EC: Presence of asbestos bodies in organs other than the lung. *Chest* 77:133–137, 1980.

75. Kobayashi H, Ming ZW, Watanabe H, Ohnishi Y: A quantitative study on the distribution of asbestos bodies in extrapulmonary organs. *Acta Pathol Jpn* 37:375–383, 1987.

76. Ehrlich A, Rohl AN, Holstein EC: Asbestos bodies in carcinoma of colon in an insulation worker with asbestosis. *JAMA* 254:2932–2933, 1985.

77. Rosen P, Savino A, Melamed M: Ferruginous (asbestos) bodies and primary cancer of the colon. *Am J Clin Pathol* 61:135–138, 1974.

78. Roggli VL, Greenberg SD, McLarty JL, Hurst GA, Spivey CG, Hieger LR: Asbestos body content of the larynx in asbestos workers. *Arch Otolaryngol* 106:553–555, 1980.

79. Holt PF: Transport of inhaled dust to extrapulmonary sites. *J Pathol* 133:123–129, 1981.
80. Lee KP, Barras CE, Griffith FD, Waritz RS, Lapin CA: Comparative pulmonary responses to inhaled inorganic fibers with asbestos and fiberglass. *Environ Res* 24:167–191, 1981.
81. Pooley FD: Asbestos bodies, their formation, composition and character. *Environ Res* 5:363–379, 1972.
82. Langer AM, Rubin IB, Selikoff IJ: Chemical characterization of asbestos body cores by electron microprobe analysis. *J Histochem Cytochem* 20:723–734, 1972.
83. Churg AM, Warnock ML: Analysis of the cores of ferruginous (asbestos) bodies from the general population: III. Patients with environmental exposure. *Lab Invest* 40:622–626, 1979.
84. Miller A, Teirstein AS, Bader MD, Bader RA, Selikoff IJ: Talc pneumoconiosis: Significance of sublight microscopic mineral particles. *Am J Med* 50:395–402, 1971.
85. Craighead JE, Mossman BT: Pathogenesis of asbestos-associated diseases. *N Engl J Med* 306:1446–1455, 1982.
86. Roggli VL, Brody AR: Imaging techniques for application to lung toxicology. In: *Toxicology of the Lung* (Gardner DE, Crapo JD, Massaro EJ, eds.), New York: Raven Press, 1988, pp. 117–145.
87. Woitowitz H-J, Manke J, Brückel B, Rödelsperger K: Ferruginous bodies as evidence of occupational endangering by chrysotile asbestos? *Zbl Arbeitsmed Bd* 36:354–364, 1986.
88. Moulin E, Yourassowsky N, Dumortier P, De Vuyst P, Yernault JC: Electron microscopic analysis of asbestos body cores from the Belgian urban population. *Eur Respir J* 1:818–822, 1988.
89. Holden J, Churg A: Asbestos bodies and the diagnosis of asbestosis in chrysotile workers. *Environ Res* 39:232–236, 1986.
90. Crouch E, Churg A: Ferruginous bodies and the histologic evaluation of dust exposure. *Am J. Surg Pathol* 8:109–116, 1984.
91. Gross P, Tuma J, deTreville RTP: Unusual ferruginous bodies: Their formation from non-fibrous particulates and from carbonaceous fibrous particles. *Arch Environ Health* 22:534–537, 1971.
92. Roggli VL, Mastin JP, Shelburne JD, Roe MS, Brody AR: Inorganic particulates in human lung: Relationship to the inflammatory response. In: *Inflammatory Cells and Lung Disease* (Lynn WS, ed.), Boca Raton, FL: CRC Press, 1983, pp. 29–62.
93. Ramage JE, Roggli VL, Bell DY, Piantadosi CA: Interstitial pneumonitis and fibrosis associated with domestic wood burning. *Am Rev Respir Dis* 137:1229–1232, 1988.
94. Dodson RF, O'Sullivan MF, Corn CJ, Williams MG, Jr., Hurst GA: Ferruginous body formation on a nonasbestos mineral. *Arch Pathol Lab Med* 109:849–852, 1985.
95. Roggli VL: Analytical scanning electron microscopy in the investigation of unusual exposures. In: *Microbeam Analysis—1986* (Romig AD, Jr., Chambers WF, eds.), San Francisco: San Francisco Press, 1986, pp. 586–588.
96. Roggli VL, McGavran MH, Subach JA, Sybers HD, Greenberg SD: Pulmonary asbestos body counts and electron probe analysis of asbestos body cores in patients with mesothelioma: A study of 25 cases. *Cancer* 50:2423–2432, 1982.
97. Wright GW, Kuschner M: The influence of varying lengths of glass and asbestos fibres on tissue response in guinea pigs. In: *Inhaled Particles IV* (Walton WH, ed.), Oxford: Pergamon Press, 1977, pp. 455–474.
98. Morgan A, Holmes A, Davison W: Clearance of sized glass fibres from the rat lung and their solubility in vivo. *Ann Occup Hyg* 25:317–331, 1982.

99. Sebastien P, Gaudichet A, Bignon J, Baris YI: Zeolite bodies in human lungs from Turkey. *Lab Invest* 44:420–425, 1981.
100. Hayashi H, Kajita A: Silicon carbide in lung tissue of a worker in the abrasive industry. *Am J Ind Med* 14:145–155, 1988.
101. Funahashi A, Schlueter DP, Pintar K, Siegesmund KA, Mandel GS, Mandel NS: Pneumoconiosis in workers exposed to silicon carbide. *Am Rev Respir Dis* 129:635–640, 1984.

4. Asbestosis

VICTOR L. ROGGLI AND PHILIP C. PRATT

The term *pneumoconiosis* was originally coined by Zenker in 1866[1] to refer to disease processes related to the accumulation of dusts in the lung parenchyma. Since some dust (including asbestos fibers) can be found in the lungs of virtually all adults from the general population, *pneumoconiosis* has come to refer to the accumulation of excessive amounts of dust in the lung and the pathologic response to the presence of the accumulated dust.[2] *Asbestosis* is a form of pneumoconiosis that is related to the accumulation of abnormal amounts of asbestos fibers in the lung parenchyma. Indeed, asbestosis is the prototype of diseases caused by inhalation of mineral fibers. Although the mechanisms by which asbestos produces tissue injury are incompletely understood, much has been learned in the past several decades from experimental models. (This information is reviewed in detail in Chap. 10. Asbestos bodies, which are the hallmark of asbestos exposure and an important component of the histologic diagnosis of asbestosis, are discussed in Chap. 3. The results of quantitative tissue analysis for asbestos in cases with asbestosis are compared with those of other asbestos-related disorders and with normal and disease controls in Chap. 11.) The present chapter describes the morphologic features of asbestosis and relates these features to the clinical and radiographic manifestations of this disease.

HISTORICAL BACKGROUND

Health hazards related to exposure to asbestos dust have been recognized since ancient times. Pliny described sickness in slaves who worked with asbestos, but these descriptions received little attention.[3] With the widespread use of asbestos after the Industrial Revolution, the number of individuals exposed to asbestos dust increased dramatically. Dr. H. Montague Murray generally is credited with the first description of asbestos-related pulmonary disease, which occurred in a 33-year-old man who had been employed for 14 years in the carding section of an asbestos textile plant. The case was never published but was reported to a British parliamentary committee in 1906.[3,4] Eight years later, the German pathologist T. Fahr described diffuse interstitial fibrosis in the lungs of a 35-year-old asbestos worker, which he attributed to the patient's exposure to asbestos.[4,5] Fahr also called attention to crystals in the lung parenchyma. An additional case of pulmonary fibrosis in an asbestos worker was described in 1924 by Dr. W. E. Cooke,[6] who in a subsequent report coined the term *asbestosis*.[7] Subsequently, the medical literature has recorded numerous cases of asbestosis among workers exposed to asbestos through the mining and milling of asbestos-containing ores, the manufacture of asbestos-containing products, or the utilization of products composed entirely or partially of asbestos fibers.[4,8]

Asbestosis has been defined in pathologic terms by a number of investigators,[9–11] but these definitions have not been uniformly applied by pathologists. The most comprehensive description of the pathologic features of human asbestosis is that reported by the Pneumoconiosis Committee of the College of American Pathologists and the National Institute for Occupational Safety and Health.[12] This document set forth the *minimal histologic* criteria for the diagnosis of asbestosis. By *histologic criteria* is meant histologic observations that permit definitive diagnosis without requirement of clinical, radiographic, or exposure history. These were the "demonstration of discrete foci of fibrosis in the walls of respiratory bronchioles associated with accumulations of asbestos bodies." The wording of the definition is somewhat vague (perhaps intentionally) with respect to the numbers of asbestos bodies that must be found before a diagnosis of asbestosis can be made. The plural term *asbestos bodies* implies that at least two must be unequivocally identified, although other investigators have suggested that one is sufficient for the diagnosis in the presence of diffuse interstitial fibrosis,[13] whereas others have recommended that *clusters of three* bodies are necessary for a histologic diagnosis.[14] None of these studies specifies the number of slides to be examined, the magnification to be used, or the preferred staining procedure (hematoxylin and eosin vs. Prussian blue vs. Perls' iron stains).[8] Nonetheless, the crucial importance of the identification of asbestos bodies in histologic sections before a histologic diagnosis of asbestosis can be made is generally recognized, which in turn is a consequence of the nonspecificity of pulmonary interstitial fibrosis and the large number of disorders that can result in scarring of the lungs.[15–17]

CLINICAL FEATURES

Asbestosis generally occurs in individuals exposed to relatively large amounts of asbestos for extended periods of time,[18,19] and can occur after exposure to any of the three commercial forms of asbestos (chrysotile, amosite, or crocidolite) as well as the noncommercial amphibole, anthophyllite.[20] When levels of exposure are particularly heavy, as, for example, in spraying of asbestos insulation, disease may develop even if exposure is as brief as three years or less.[18] As is the case for other asbestos-related diseases, such as malignant mesothelioma or lung cancer, there is a long delay between initial exposure to asbestos and clinical manifestations of asbestosis. This interval is referred to as the latency period, and for asbestosis it is generally several decades.[21] Heavy exposures tend to have shorter latency periods, although rarely less than 15 years from initial exposure.[21] Epidemiological studies have shown a direct relationship between intensity and duration of asbestos exposure and the prevalence of asbestosis.[22] Furthermore, the attack rate appears to be greater for cigarette smokers than for nonsmokers among workers with similar levels of asbestos exposure.[23-27] Explanations offered for this observation include the inhibitory effect of cigarette smoking on pulmonary clearance mechanisms and direct enhancement by cigarette smoke of asbestos penetration of respiratory epithelium, resulting in retention of greater amounts of asbestos in the lungs of smokers.[28] In a recent case-control study of 487 autopsied asbestos miners in South Africa, no positive association between smoking and autopsy evidence of asbestosis was observed.[29] Asbestos fibers trapped within the pulmonary interstitium have a prolonged residence time in the lung; consequently, asbestosis may continue to progress many years after exposure has ceased.[25,30]

Many patients with asbestosis are asymptomatic.[31] In those with symptomatic disease, the most frequent complaints are dyspnea on exertion and dry, nonproductive cough.[18,31] In severe cases, the disease may progress to dyspnea even at rest, and the patient may note weight loss and chest pain. The most characteristic finding on physical examination is the presence of end-inspiratory basilar crepitations, or crackles.[18,19,31] Other signs that may be present, including digital clubbing, cyanosis, and tachypnea,[18,31] are generally indicative of advanced disease. Patients with long-standing hypoxia may develop cor pulmonale, with the accompanying signs of tall jugular "a" waves, right ventricular heave, and epigastric third and fourth heart sounds.[18]

RADIOGRAPHIC FINDINGS

Asbestosis is characterized radiographically by the presence of small irregular opacities, most prominent in the lung bases.[18,31] The number or profusion of these opacities increases with increasing severity or progression of the disease, resulting in obscuration of the vascular pattern and of the diaphragmatic and cardiac borders. The latter has been referred to as the "shaggy heart" sign of asbestosis. With increasing severity, there is a decrease in lung volumes and, in some cases, the appearance of honeycomb changes (Fig. 4-1). Large irregular opacities (greater than 1 cm in dimension) are an uncommon manifestation of asbestosis, and may in some cases be related to concomitant exposure to quartz.[31] The identification of pleural thickening or calcification aids in distinguishing asbestosis from the myriad other diseases that produce diffuse interstitial fibrosis.[15-17] The International Labor Office has developed a classification scheme for the radiographic assessment of pneumoconiosis that is based on the size and profusion of roentgenographically detected opacities.[32] The availability of standard films representing the various degrees of severity is necessary to enhance the reproducibility of the classification scheme.[18]

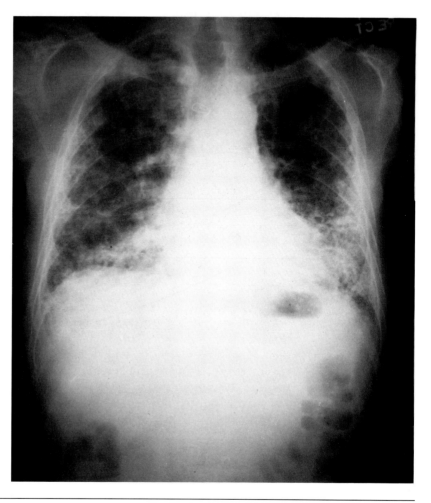

FIGURE 4-1. Posteroanterior chest radiograph from an insulator with asbestosis, showing small lung volumes and bilateral reticulonodular infiltrates most prominent in the lung bases. Courtesy of Dr. Colleen Bergin, Department of
Radiology, Duke University Medical Center. Reprinted from Ref. 8, with
permission.

Although chest roentgenography is a useful screening tool and an
important aid in epidemiologic surveys, the limitations of this diagnostic technique must be appreciated. Standard chest x-rays may
be negative in some individuals with histologically proven asbestosis,[33-35] so that a negative film does *not* exclude the presence of
disease. Also, some investigators have reported an excess of small,
irregular opacities in films from cigarette smokers who'd had no
exposure to asbestos,[29,36] although others have failed to confirm
this observation in population surveys.[24] Since standard chest
films can produce both false-positive and false-negative results, it is
of interest that computed tomography (CT) has been shown to

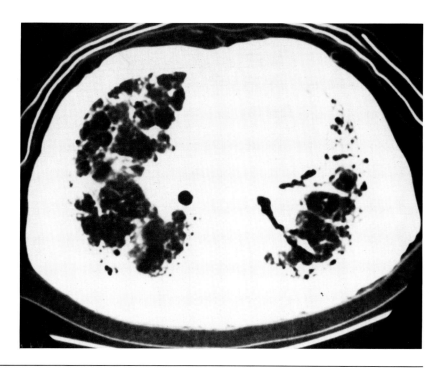

FIGURE 4-2. Computed tomography of the thorax from an insulator with asbestosis (same case as Fig. 4-1), showing prominent interstitial markings with honeycomb changes and peripheral accentuation. Courtesy of Dr. Colleen Bergin, Department of Radiology, Duke University Medical Center. Reprinted from Ref. 8, with permission.

have enhanced sensitivity and specificity for the recognition of asbestosis.[37] Furthermore, CT provides finer anatomic detail of the lesions of interstitial lung disease than can be achieved with routine chest roentgenograms[38,39] (Fig. 4-2). In addition, CT is a useful adjunct to conventional chest radiography in assessing the presence of emphysema,[40–42] which is often present in asbestos workers who smoke cigarettes (see later).

PULMONARY FUNCTION

Asbestosis classically produces a restrictive pattern on pulmonary function testing. The earliest changes include diminished vital capacity and diffusion capacity for carbon monoxide (D_LCO) with an increase in static lung recoil pressures.[18,31] As the disease progresses, there is an increase in resting and exercise minute ventilation, arterial desaturation with exercise (and later at rest), and diminishing total lung capacity (TLC).[18] TLC, however, should be interpreted cautiously as an indicator of the severity of asbestosis.[43] This is again related to the fact that many asbestos workers are cigarette smokers and thus prone to develop centrilobular emphysema, which tends to increase TLC whereas asbestosis has the opposite effect. Thus some individuals with severe asbestosis and severe emphysema may have a near normal TLC due to these opposing effects.[43]

There is also accumulating evidence that exposure to asbestos and a variety of other mineral dusts can contribute to chronic obstructive pulmonary disease.[44] Obstructive changes in pulmonary function tests occur in only a portion of exposed workers,[45] and are best demonstrated in nonsmoking asbestos workers.[46] The morphological correlate of this functional abnormality apparently is fibrosis and distortion of respiratory and membranous bronchioles with consequent interference with normal air flow.[47,48] Whether this lesion can produce clinically significant impairment is controversial. At any rate, the effect of cigarette smoking on obstruction is so overwhelming that, in asbestos workers who smoke, any contribution of dust exposure to their obstructive changes is negligible.[49,50] There is no evidence that asbestos exposure contributes to clinically significant emphysema.[8,51]

BRONCHOALVEOLAR LAVAGE
Bronchoalveolar lavage is a powerful investigative technique that provides a window for observing the events occurring in the most distal anatomic regions of the lung.[52] Aliquots of sterile saline are instilled into the airway through a fiber-optic bronchoscope and then retrieved by suction. This recovered bronchoalveolar lavage fluid (BALF) can then be analyzed for its asbestos and inflammatory cell content. Asbestos bodies can be found in BALF in more than 95% of patients with asbestosis, but are considered to be a marker of exposure rather than of disease (see Chap. 9). Nonetheless, pulmonary fibrosis due to asbestos exposure follows a dose-response relationship,[20] and the number of asbestos bodies per milliliter of BALF correlates with the degree of exposure as well as with the tissue asbestos burden. Thus the more asbestos bodies recovered from BALF, the greater the exposure and the greater the likelihood that the patient has asbestosis.[53] Examination of the cellular component can provide information regarding disease activity, and preliminary data in patients with asbestosis show an increased number of cells as well as an increased percentage of neutrophils, similar to the profile observed in idiopathic pulmonary fibrosis.[52] The greatest potential for bronchoalveolar lavage as a diagnostic tool with regard to asbestosis lies in combined examination of BALF for asbestos content and inflammatory cellular response.

PATHOLOGIC FINDINGS

GROSS MORPHOLOGY
In the earliest stages of asbestosis, the lungs may appear normal upon gross inspection. As the disease progresses in severity, fine

gray streaks of fibrous tissue become visible to the naked eye and are most prominent in the lower lobes and at the lung periphery.[12] This may progress to more coarse linear scarring often accompanied by loss of lung volume (Fig. 4-3). These linear areas of fibrosis are the pathologic correlate of the increased reticular markings and small irregular opacities observed in conventional radiographs of the chest. The interstitial fibrosis in addition is the morphologic counterpart of the restrictive functional abnormalities, which include stiff and noncompliant lungs with reduced volumes and diminished capacity for gaseous diffusion. The excessive collagen deposition results in an increase in lung weight as well as an increase in its consistency. In the most advanced stages of asbestosis, honeycomb changes are observed, and again are most prominent subpleurally and in the lower lobes.[12] These consist of cystlike spaces up to 1 cm in maximum dimension in areas of dense fibrosis (Fig. 4-4). In rare instances, progressive massive fibrosis has been described in individuals with asbestosis, probably attributable to mixed dust exposures (i.e., asbestos and silica). In exceptional cases, for reasons that are obscure, the fibrosis of asbestosis is more severe in the upper lobes.[54] There are no characteristic changes observed in the tracheobronchial tree in asbestosis,[12] although traction bronchiectasis may occur in densely scarred areas. Similarly, the regional lymph nodes are usually unremarkable on gross inspection.

The changes just described are not specific for asbestosis and may be observed in a wide variety of chronic interstitial lung diseases.[15–17] A useful feature that may aid in distinguishing asbestosis from other fibrotic lung diseases is the frequent association of pleural abnormalities (see Chap. 6). Diffuse thickening of the visceral pleura is often present (Figs. 4-3 and 4-5), whereas fibrous adhesions between the visceral and parietal pleura are variable. An even more characteristic finding related to asbestos exposure is the parietal pleural plaque, which appears as a circumscribed area of ivory-colored pleural thickening over the domes of the diaphragm or on the posterolateral chest wall running along the direction of the ribs.[55,56] Pleural plaques may be smooth or knobby on inspection (so-called "candle-wax dripping" appearance), have a cartilagenous consistency, and are often calcified. Not all patients with asbestosis have associated plaques, and certainly not all patients with pleural plaques manifest the morphologic changes of asbestosis.[55,56] Indeed, the term *asbestosis* should not be used to refer to the benign asbestos-related pleural abnormalities, since these lesions differ from the parenchymal disease in terms of clinical features, epidemiology, and prognosis.[51,57] Although some have argued that there is no need to distinguish between pleural and parenchymal fibrosis, since both derive from asbestos exposure,[58] the fallacy in this argument becomes clear when one considers that asbestos exposure can produce either asbestosis or malignant mesothelioma or both. Certainly there is no rationale for including malignant mesotheliomas within the purview of the term *asbestosis*.

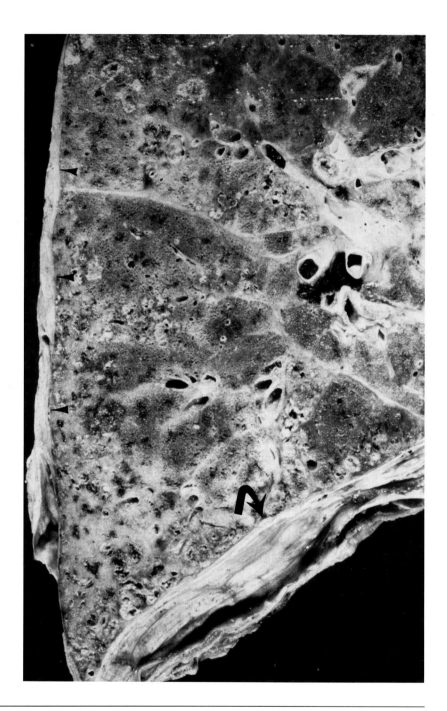

FIGURE 4-3. Coronal section of the lower portion of the lung of an insulator with asbestosis. There is pale gray, linear interstitial fibrosis especially prominent in the lower lobe. Note the visceral pleural thickening laterally (arrowheads) and adhesion of the diaphragm to the undersurface of the lung (curved arrow).

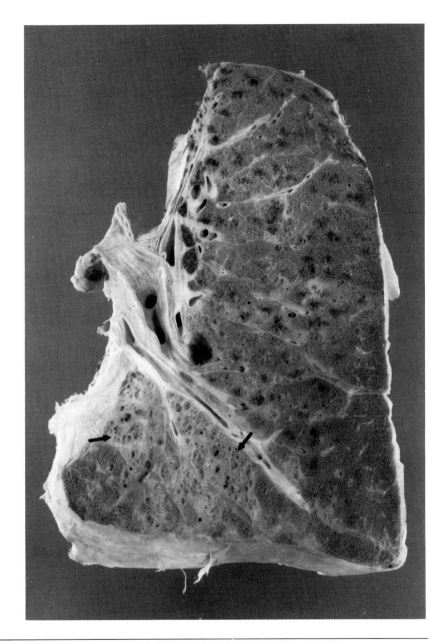

FIGURE 4-4. Coronal section of the left lung of an insulator with asbestosis and cavitary squamous cell carcinoma of the right lower lobe. Note the honeycomb changes in the medial portion of the lower lobe (arrows). Reprinted from Ref. 8, with permission.

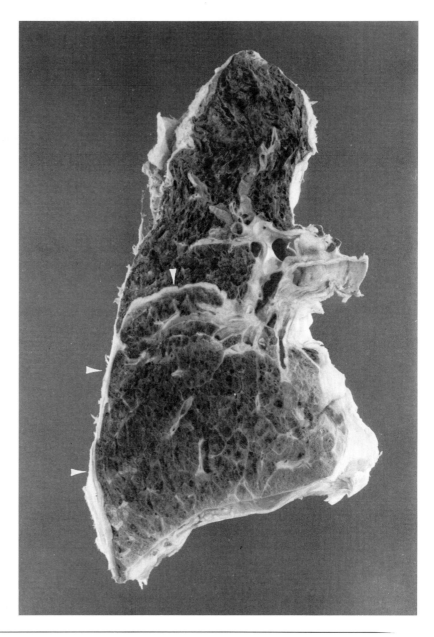

FIGURE 4-5. Coronal section of lung from an insulator and cigarette smoker showing
moderate asbestosis and severe centrilobular emphysema (compare with
honeycomb changes in Fig. 4-4). Note the visceral pleural thickening
enveloping the lung and extending into the interlobular fissure (arrowheads). Reprinted from Ref. 8, with permission.

Due to the high rate of cigarette smoking among asbestos workers, these patients often exhibit changes in the lung related to exposure to tobacco smoke. Therefore the pathologist must take care to distinguish abnormalities related to smoking from those caused by asbestos exposure. Centrilobular emphysema is frequently observed in the lungs of cigarette smokers,[59] and may be of such a severe degree as to overshadow the fibrosis of asbestosis (see Fig. 4-5). Emphysema must be distinguished from the honeycomb changes observed in advanced asbestosis. The distribution of the lesions is often helpful in this regard, with emphysema tending to be most severe in the upper lobes whereas honeycomb changes are more severe in the lower lobes. In addition, the cystic spaces of honeycombing are all roughly the same size (approximately 5 mm in diameter) and have thickened, fibrotic walls. On the other hand, emphysematous spaces are of variable size (from just grossly visible up to several centimeters in diameter) and have no "walls," since they represent areas of destruction of lung tissue and are not accompanied by grossly visible fibrosis.[59] Another helpful feature is the presence of thin, delicate tissue strands that traverse the emphysematous spaces. These represent remnants of blood vessels that persist following the destruction of lung parenchyma. The presence of significant amounts of emphysema (i.e., involvement of 25% or more of the lung parenchyma) is usually associated with obstructive changes on pulmonary function tests.[59] The lesions of asbestosis and emphysema are best assessed by careful inspection of slices prepared from lungs that have been inflated and fixed in distension by intrabronchial instillation of fixative solutions for at least two days.[12,59]

HISTOPATHOLOGY

The histologic hallmarks of asbestosis are the presence of excess amounts of collagen in the pulmonary interstitium, *and* the occurrence of asbestos bodies in paraffin sections.[12] Observations of lung tissue obtained at autopsy from asbestos workers, as well as experimental animal studies, have demonstrated that the earliest abnormality microscopically is the deposition of increased amounts of collagen in the walls of respiratory bronchioles.[12,60] With more extensive disease, fibrosis is observed to involve the walls of terminal bronchioles proximal to the respiratory bronchiole, as well as alveolar ducts distal to the respiratory bronchiole. Ultimately, the fibrotic process extends to involve the alveolar septa surrounding these structures (Fig. 4-6). The most extensive involvement is usually observed subpleurally and in those alveoli in closest proximity to the bronchioles. In the most advanced cases, large zones of lung parenchyma consist of alveoli with fibrotic walls, and honeycomb changes may be present. Characteristically, honeycomb changes consist of cystlike spaces with fibrotic walls. These cystic spaces range in diameter from 1–15 mm, are lined by cuboidal to low columnar epithelium, and frequently contain pools of mucus that accumulate within the spaces. Often

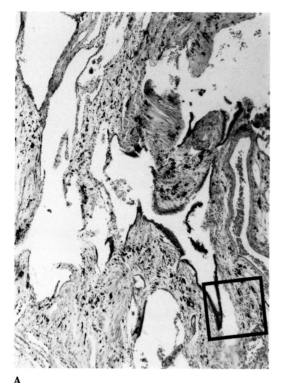

A

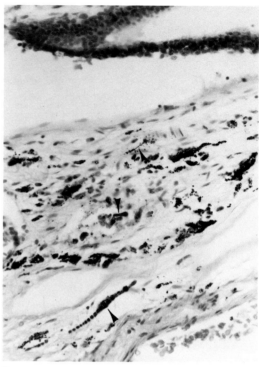

B

C

FIGURE 4-6. (A) Low-power photomicrograph of a bronchiole from an insulator with asbestosis. There is peribronchiolar fibrosis with distortion of the bronchiole. The fibrosis extends to involve adjacent alveoli. (B) Higher magnification of rectangular area marked in part (A) shows asbestos bodies embedded within fibrotic peribronchiolar connective tissue (arrowheads). (C) Elsewhere, clusters of asbestos bodies are embedded within fibrotic pulmonary interstitium. Hematoxylin and eosin, (A) ×52, (B) ×250, (C) ×325. Reprinted from Ref. 8, with permission.

TABLE 4-1. Histologic findings in 100 cases of asbestosis

Histologic feature	Percent
Always Present	
Asbestos bodies	100%
Peribronchiolar fibrosis	100
Often Present	
Alveolar septal fibrosis	82
Occasionally Present	
Honeycomb changes	15
Foreign-body giant cells	15
Pulmonary adenomatosis	10
Cytoplasmic hyalin	7
Desquamative interstitial pneumonitis-like areas	6
Rarely Present	
Osseous metaplasia (dendriform pulmonary ossification)	2
Pulmonary blue bodies	1

SOURCE: Reproduced from Ref. 8, with permission.

scattered within the fibrotic interstitium is a background of chronic inflammatory cells, mainly lymphocytes and plasma cells. The secondary lobular septa may also be markedly thickened by fibrous tissue, and there is often diffuse fibrotic thickening of the visceral pleura as well (see Chap. 6). The fibrotic process in asbestosis tends to be patchy, especially in early cases, so that many sections may have to be examined in order to find the diagnostic features.[12,61] Masson's trichrome stains can facilitate the assessment of the extent and distribution of the pulmonary interstitial fibrosis.

The second component required for the histologic diagnosis of asbestosis is the identification of asbestos bodies in paraffin sections. Asbestos bodies may be found lying free within alveolar spaces or embedded within the fibrotic pulmonary interstitium[8,12,61] (see Fig. 4-6). (The morphologic appearance of asbestos bodies and their distinction from other ferruginous bodies are described in detail in Chap. 3.) Occasionally, asbestos bodies are observed within foreign-body giant cells. The authors have also observed asbestos bodies within hilar or mediastinal lymph nodes, often associated with fibrosis of the lymph node parenchyma. This curious observation is largely confined to patients with a heavy asbestos lung burden, and is probably related to overloading of the clearance mechanisms.[62] Among 20 patients with asbestos bodies observed in thoracic lymph nodes, 17 had histologically confirmed asbestosis.[63] The detection of asbestos bodies in histologic sections can often be enhanced by iron stains such as Prussian blue, especially when the bodies are present in the sections in relatively low numbers.[8]

Other histologic changes have also been described in asbestosis, but are seen less commonly (Table 4-1). Foreign-body giant cells are observed within alveoli or, less commonly, within the fibrotic interstitium in about 15% of cases. Scarring and distortion of bronchioles

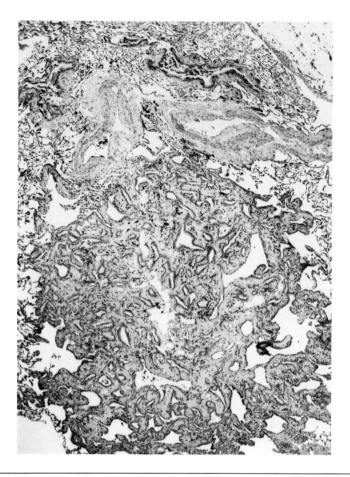

FIGURE 4-7. Area of so-called "pulmonary adenomatosis" shows scarring and distortion of bronchiole with lining of adjacent fibrotic alveolar septa by cuboidal bronchiolar epithelium. Hematoxylin and eosin, ×40.

with necrosis and disruption of the transitional zone from the respiratory bronchiole to the alveolar duct occasionally results in the lining of adjacent alveoli by cuboidal bronchiolar epithelium (Fig.4-7). This process, sometimes referred to as "pulmonary adenomatosis," occurs in about 10% of cases. Pulmonary adenomatosis is a misnomer, since this process is a hyperplastic response to tissue injury rather than a true neoplastic process. Hyperplastic alveolar Type II cells may also line the fibrotic alveolar septa in asbestosis, and in roughly 7% of cases these cells contain irregular, waxy-appearing, deeply eosinophilic material (Fig. 4-8). This so-called cytoplasmic hyalin has identical tinctorial and ultrastructural characteristics to those observed in hepatocytes in alcoholic hepatitis.[64] However, this abnormality is not specific for asbestos exposure and probably represents a nonspecific (albeit unusual) reaction to injury.[16,65] Alveolar macro-

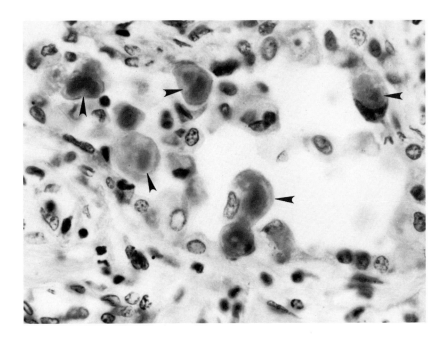

FIGURE 4-8. Photomicrograph of lung parenchyma in patient with asbestosis, showing hyperplastic alveolar Type II pneumocytes. Many of these cells contain cytoplasmic hyalin (arrowheads), which has the same tinctorial characteristics as the hyalin found within hepatocytes in patients with alcoholic hepatitis. Hematoxylin and eosin, ×680. Reprinted from Ref. 8, with permission.

phages are present in increased numbers in the alveoli of patients with asbestosis, and in about 6% of cases they are so numerous that the alveoli are packed with these cells in a pattern similar to desquamative interstitial pneumonitis[8,12,16] (Fig. 4-9). These uncommon histologic abnormalities are generally observed in the more advanced histologic stages of asbestosis.

Rarely observed in patients with asbestosis is dendriform pulmonary ossification,[66] which was observed in 2% of cases in the authors' series. This process is characterized by branching spicules of bone, often containing bone marrow, embedded within the fibrotic pulmonary interstitium (Fig. 4-10). It is thought that this unusual phenomenon results from metaplasia of interstitial fibroblasts to osteoblasts.[67] An additional unusual process that is observed in patients with asbestosis is the occurrence of the so-called pulmonary blue bodies. These basophilic, laminated concretions consist primarily of calcium carbonate[68] and are present within alveolar spaces in about 1% of cases[8] (see Table 4-1). They are not visualized with polarizing microscopy in hematoxylin- and eosin-stained sections, but are brightly birefringent in unstained paraffin sections[68] or in filter preparations of tissue digests[8] (Fig. 4-11). The mechanism of formation of

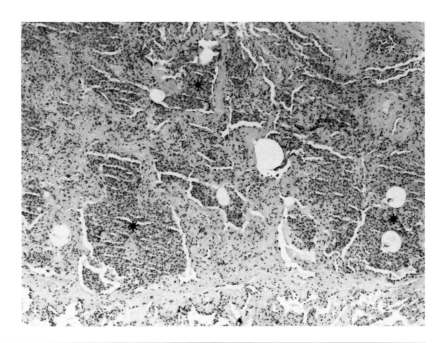

FIGURE 4-9. Low-power photomicrograph of lung in patient with asbestosis, showing alveoli packed with sheets of alveolar macrophages (asterisks). This pattern resembles that seen in desquamative interstitial pneumonitis. Hematoxylin and eosin, ×68. Reprinted from Ref. 8, with permission.

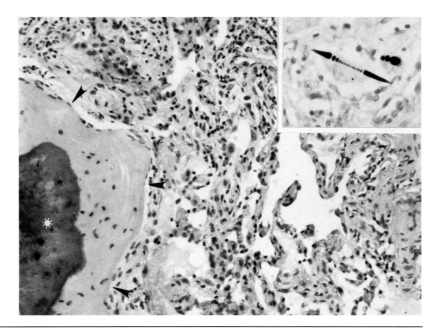

FIGURE 4-10. Pulmonary ossification in a patient with asbestosis, showing spicule of bone (arrowheads) with central calcification (asterisk) embedded within fibrotic interstitium. Inset shows asbestos bodies found elsewhere in the same section. Hematoxylin and eosin, ×175; inset, Prussian blue, ×325. Reprinted from Ref. 66, with permission.

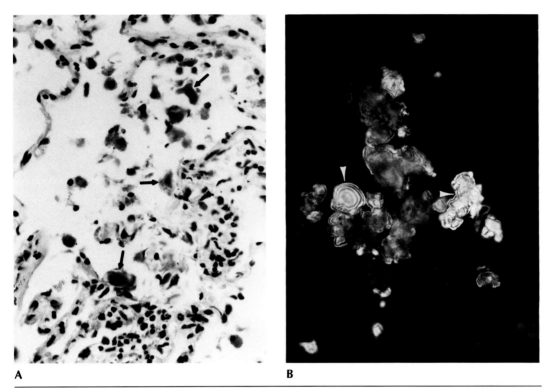

FIGURE 4-11. (A) Intraalveolar pulmonary blue bodies exhibit a somewhat laminated appearance (arrows) and consist primarily of calcium carbonate. Hematoxylin and eosin. (B) Nuclepore filter preparation of lung tissue digested in sodium hypochlorite [same case illustrated in part (A)] shows brightly birefringent "blue bodies" with clearly visible laminations (arrowheads). Unstained filter, polarizing microscopy. Part (A) ×400; part (B) ×325. Courtesy of Dr. Fred Askin, Department of Pathology, University of North Carolina, Chapel Hill, NC. Reprinted from Ref. 8, with permission.

blue bodies is unknown, but calcium salts have been observed to accumulate in the pulmonary interstitium in experimental animals exposed to aerosolized asbestos fibers[69] (see Chap. 10). Pulmonary blue bodies are not specific for asbestos exposure, and, like cytoplasmic hyalin, probably represent an unusual but nonspecific reaction to injury.[68]

Another peculiar association with asbestosis is pulmonary infections with aspergillus species. Hillerdal and Hecksher reported four cases of this unusual association,[70] and suggested that it was due to anatomical alterations of the bronchial tree or lung parenchyma resulting from the asbestos exposure. One of the authors (VLR) has personally observed five additional cases[71] (and unpublished observations) (Fig. 4-12), one of which was first diagnosed by fine-needle-aspiration cytology (see Chap. 9). No other opportunistic fungal

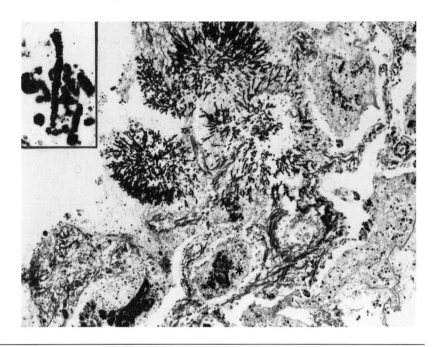

FIGURE 4-12. Numerous acutely branching, septate hyphae are present within the lung parenchyma. A clump of asbestos bodies can be seen in a nearby alveolus (asterisk). Grocott's methenamine silver technique, ×100. *Inset:* detailed view of clump of asbestos bodies. Hematoxylin and eosin, ×250. Reprinted from Ref. 71, with permission.

infections associated with asbestosis have been reported or observed by the authors.[8] The mechanism may involve suppression of the cell-mediated immune system by asbestos,[72] although the reason for the specificity for aspergillus is obscure.

ULTRASTRUCTURAL FEATURES

Few ultrastructural studies of the lung have been reported in patients with asbestosis. Shelburne et al.[73] observed that transmission electron microscopy (TEM) is an inefficient way to look for asbestos bodies, even in patients with a heavy tissue asbestos burden. This observation is related to the minute volume of tissue that is examined by TEM. Corrin et al.[74] studied eight cases of asbestosis via TEM, and observed a number of ultrastructural abnormalities, especially within the pulmonary interstitium. Within the alveolar spaces, excess numbers of alveolar macrophages were observed. There was patchy loss of Type I alveolar epithelium, and the thickened alveolar septa demonstrated interstitial edema and collagen deposition. Changes were also observed in the capillary compartment, consisting of endothelial swelling and endothelial basement-membrane thickening and reduplication. The changes observed were similar to those seen in the 17 cases of idiopathic pulmonary fibrosis (cryptogenic fibrosing alveolitis) except for a paucity of interstitial inflammatory cells and the presence of asbestos fibers in the patients with asbestosis.[74] There was no ultrastructural evidence of immune complex deposition.

DIFFERENTIAL DIAGNOSIS

Asbestosis must be distinguished from pulmonary injury related to inhalation of other toxic dusts and also from other forms of diffuse pulmonary fibrosis.[8] Silicosis can readily be distinguished from asbestosis, since it produces a circumscribed nodular pattern of fibrosis as opposed to the irregular linear interstitial fibrosis of asbestosis.[2] Furthermore, the changes of silicosis are most severe in the upper lobes, whereas asbestosis involves primarily the lower lobes. In addition, silicotic nodules are invariably present in the hilar lymph nodes, and pleural involvement, when it occurs, consists of circumscribed subpleural nodules beneath the visceral pleura, which are a few millimeters in diameter.[75] On the other hand, diffuse interstitial fibrosis similar to that seen in asbestosis can be observed with exposure to a variety of inorganic particulates.[2,75] This is also true for idiopathic pulmonary fibrosis of the usual or desquamative type, each of which displays many features overlapping with those of asbestosis. The distinction of asbestosis from these other conditions can be made by the identification of asbestos bodies in histologic sections and the tendency for asbestosis to preferentially involve the walls and adventitia of small airways. Also, in cases of fibrosis due to exposure to dusts other than asbestos, analysis of the mineral content of lung tissue can be quite helpful (see Chap. 11). Another useful feature is the frequent occurrence of visceral pleural fibrosis and parietal pleural plaques in patients with asbestosis.[8]

In the earlier stages of the disease, the diagnosis of asbestosis may be subtle and the distinction must be made from other causes of peribronchiolar fibrosis. Inhalation of other mineral dusts, such as silica, iron oxides, or aluminum oxides,[76] as well as exposure to cigarette smoke,[48] have been associated with peribronchiolar fibrosis. However, the degree of involvement of the small airways due to these exposures is in general less than that observed with asbestos exposure.[48,76] Again, the distinction is made by the identification of asbestos bodies in histologic sections. Furthermore, the small-airway lesions in cigarette smokers are most often characterized by goblet cell metaplasia, mucous plugging, and peribronchiolar inflammation.[59] Since many asbestos workers are also smokers, the small-airway lesions due to smoking and the peribronchiolar fibrosis of asbestosis often coexist in the same individual.

Asbestos workers are often exposed to other dusts as well, so that pathologic changes due to each dust may be manifested in the same individual. For example, shipyard workers in the course of their occupation may be exposed to substantial amounts of silica, talc, or welding fumes in addition to asbestos.[8] Crystalline silica is used in sandblasting and also constitutes one component of the lining of steam boilers in ships. Individuals engaged in sandblasting or boiler-scaling or even working in the vicinity of these operations often exhibit silicotic nodules within hilar lymph nodes and may also have similar nodules in the lung parenchyma, especially the upper lobes.[2] Similarly, shipyard welders are invariably exposed to some asbestos, so that the pathologist must take care to distinguish asbestosis from welder's pneumoconiosis. The latter is characterized by interstitial deposits of iron oxides, which appear as dark brown to black spherical particles, often with a golden brown rim.[2] Another frequent finding is the presence of pseudoasbestos bodies (see Chap. 3) with broad yellow or black cores. Very little collagen deposition is observed in response to the dust in welder's pneumoconiosis. Indeed, the presence of substantial amounts of interstitial fibrosis in a shipyard welder should raise one's suspicion of concomitant asbestosis. Among 28 cases of welder's pneumoconiosis in shipyard workers from the consultation files of one of the authors, only 11 cases satisfied criteria for the histologic diagnosis of asbestosis, i.e., peribronchiolar fibrosis and true asbestos bodies. In extreme example, isolated instances have been reported of asbestosis, silicosis, talcosis, and berylliosis in a single individual.[77]

Asbestosis must also be distinguished from organizing pneumonia, a well-known radiographic mimicker of carcinoma of the lung.[78] Because of the increased risk of lung cancer in asbestos workers (see Chap. 7), organizing pneumonia may lead to thoracotomy in these individuals and create a potentially confusing picture. The authors have observed several such instances, and it is not clear whether organizing pneumonia has an increased incidence in patients with asbestosis or whether these patients are merely followed more closely because of the increased risk of malignancy. Organizing pneumonia is characterized by plugs of young edematous connective tissue filling the alveolar spaces and alveolar ducts (Fig. 4-13). Varying numbers of chronic inflammatory cells are present within the plugs. A useful feature to remember is that organizing pneumonia is generally a localized process, whereas asbestosis is bilateral and diffuse. Organizing pneumonia is associated with some fibrotic thickening and edema of alveolar septa, often associated with Type II cell hyperplasia, so that the diagnostic features of asbestosis are frequently overshadowed or obscured in areas with superimposed organizing pneumonia.

Asbestosis must similarly be distinguished from iatrogenic pulmonary disease related to treatment for carcinoma of the lung. Because of the high rate of lung cancer among individuals with asbestosis (see Chap. 7), this is not an infrequent problem, particularly in examining lungs at autopsy. Radiation and chemotherapy both can result in pulmonary interstitial fibrosis. Radiation pneumonitis can be distinguished by its gross distribution, which is generally confined to the

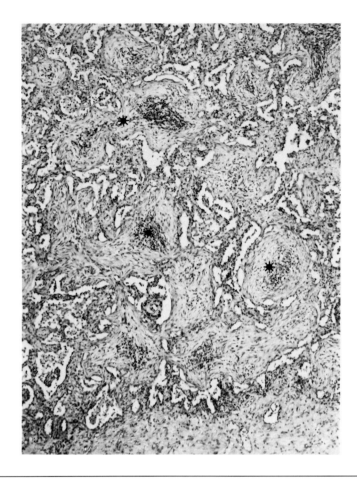

FIGURE 4-13. Photomicrograph of an area of organizing pneumonia in a patient with asbestosis. The patient had undergone resection of a lobe for a mass suspected to be carcinoma. Note the plugs of young, edematous connective tissue filling alveolar ducts and adjacent alveolar spaces (asterisks). Hematoxylin and eosin, ×52.

irradiated lung.[79] Furthermore, the vascular changes in radiation pneumonitis, including thickened and fibrotic vascular walls and endothelial vacuolization, are usually prominent. Drug-induced pulmonary cytotoxicity is more diffuse in its effects than asbestosis, and atypical hyperplastic Type II cells are frequently a prominent feature.[79] When pulmonary fibrosis due to administration of cytotoxic agents is superimposed on asbestosis, it may be necessary to refer to chest radiographs taken prior to administration of chemotherapy to confirm a diagnosis of asbestosis.

Some investigators have suggested that transbronchial biopsy may be useful for the diagnosis of asbestosis.[80,81] The authors have observed rare cases in which several asbestos bodies and clear-cut interstitial fibrosis (with Type II cell hyperplasia) were observed on a transbronchial biopsy specimen. When this observation is made in the setting of diffusely increased interstitial markings on chest x-ray, a diagnosis of asbestosis can be made with reasonable assurance. However, in most cases transbronchial biopsies are inadequate for the diagnosis of asbestosis,[12,51] and generous sampling from an open lung biopsy or autopsy tissue is normally required to make the subtle and intricate histologic distinctions just outlined.

SYSTEMIC MANIFESTATIONS

Asbestosis is uncommonly associated with systemic manifestations. In patients with advanced disease, digital clubbing or cyanosis may be observed,[18] as is the case for other types of diffuse pulmonary fibrosis. Kobayashi et al.[82] described a case of asbestosis in which interstitial fibrosis was also observed in the liver, kidney, myocardium, and thyroid gland. Asbestos fibers were also identified in each of these sites by electron microscopy. Such an occurrence is analogous to the phenomenon of extrapulmonary silicotic nodules, which may be found in the liver, spleen, bone marrow, and abdominal lymph nodes in patients with heavy exposures to silica and usually advanced silicosis.[83] Experimental studies showing that asbestos inhalation can result in the translocation of sufficient amounts of fibers to produce fibrosis in distant sites have not been reported, to our knowledge. A more plausible alternative explanation is that the case reported by Kobayashi et al.[82] represents coincident asbestosis and progressive systemic sclerosis (scleroderma). Scleroderma is an uncommon but well-recognized complication of exposure to crystalline silica,[84] and although the pathogenetic mechanism is poorly understood, a similar reaction may be possible in some individuals who are heavily exposed to asbestos. Asbestos exposure is known to produce immunologic alterations in the host that effect both humoral and cell-mediated immunity.[85,86] However, it is not known whether or how often these perturbations of the immune system result in clinical manifestations. Maguire et al.[87] reported a case of immunoblastic lymphadenopathy in a 71-year-old man with asbestosis. Cooke et al.[88] described another patient with lymphomatoid granulomatosis and proliferative glomerulonephritis in which asbestos fibers were observed in the renal mesangial matrix. However, the published gross and microscopic photographs of the lung more closely resembled pulmonary lymphoma.[89,90] The latter has been described in association with asbestos exposure[91] (see Chap. 8).

ASSESSMENT OF DIAGNOSTIC CRITERIA

The histologic diagnosis of asbestosis is important, because it provides independent confirmation of the presence or absence of a fibrotic pulmonary interstitial process that can be related to inhalation of asbestos-containing dust. As outlined earlier, asbestosis can be defined *histologically* as the presence of peribronchiolar fibrosis and asbestos bodies in tissue sections, with or without accompanying alveolar septal fibrosis.[8,12] Since exposure to toxic products other than asbestos can produce some peribronchiolar fibrosis,[48,76] it is recommended that, in the absence of alveolar septal fibrosis, a histologic diagnosis of asbestosis should be made only when a majority of the bronchioles show excessive amounts of connective tissue in their walls.[8] The assessment of fibrosis can be difficult when there is atelectasis, congestion, or consolidation of the lung with pneumonia, and care should be taken not to overinterpret such sections as showing interstitial fibrosis.[92] If assessment of the presence and extent of fibrosis is not straightforward on routinely prepared histologic sections, then Masson's trichrome-stained sections should be prepared and examined to assist in this evaluation. Furthermore, ferruginous bodies in histologic sections should be examined critically so that true asbestos bodies are not confused with pseudoasbestos bodies that have broad yellow or black cores (see Chap. 3). In cases for which there is a high index of suspicion for asbestosis but asbestos bodies are not readily identified on routinely stained sections, it is recommended that iron-stained sections be prepared and examined systematically at 200× magnification using a mechanical stage.[93,94] With this approach, five or more asbestos bodies per cm^2 of tissue section area examined was observed in 95% of our cases of asbestosis, and two or more asbestos bodies per cm^2 in all of our cases[8] (see Chap. 11). Since asbestos bodies are not necessarily evenly distributed in histologic sections,[12,93] more than one section should be examined when asbestos bodies are sparse.[8]

Fibrosis was confined to the walls of bronchioles in 18% of our cases (see Table 4-1), and some investigators have challenged the inclusion of such cases in the definition of asbestosis. The reasons given for excluding such cases include the observation that dusts other than asbestos can result in peribronchiolar fibrosis, and a lack of direct evidence that such lesions actually progress to alveolar septal fibrosis.[48,76] However, dusts other than asbestos can also produce alveolar septal fibrosis,[2] in which case the finding of asbestos bodies in histologic sections provides evidence that the fibrosis is secondary to asbestos exposure.[8,13] Restriction of the definition of asbestosis to cases in which the majority of bronchioles are involved greatly reduces the chances of overdiagnosing such lesions as being asbestos-related. Furthermore, experimental animal studies have demonstrated that the peribronchiolar region is an early site of asbestos-induced fibrosis.[60] The most compelling argument for including isolated peribronchiolar fibrosis (in the presence of asbestos bodies) within the scope of the definition of asbestosis is that asbestos exposure can produce increased fibrous tissue deposition in all portions of the pulmonary interstitium, which include the interstitium of the alveolar septa, subpleural connective tissue, secondary lobular septa, and the connective tissue sheath surrounding bronchovascular and bronchiolovascular bundles. Therefore, the authors believe that the preponderance of the evidence does not justify exclusion of pure peribronchiolar fibrosis from the definition of asbestosis.

The requirement for the identification of asbestos bodies in histologic sections before a diagnosis of asbestosis can be made has similarly not gone unchallenged. Arguments against this requirement include, first, the observation that chrysotile forms asbestos bodies poorly as compared to the amphiboles and many workers are exposed primarily to chrysotile asbestos,[95] and, second, that there is great variability from one individual to another in the efficiency with which fibers are coated to make asbestos bodies, some individuals apparently being poor asbestos-body formers.[96,97] However, Holden and Churg have shown that in at least one population of workers exposed exclusively to chrysotile ore, i.e., chrysotile miners, individuals with asbestosis do have asbestos bodies identified in histologic sections, and these bodies have chrysotile cores.[98]

The second argument is a more difficult problem, which will likely become more common as the number of cases with overt asbestosis decreases, due to diminished numbers of survivors of the heavy exposures of the past, and the relative proportion of patients with idiopathic pulmonary fibrosis will thus necessarily increase. There has been a handful of cases reported of patients with pulmonary fibrosis with low asbestos-body counts (less than 100 per gram of wet lung tissue) but an elevated tissue content of uncoated asbestos fibers as assessed by electron microscopy.[96,97] Such an occurrence is apparently rare, for no such case was encountered in our series of 76 patients with asbestosis. Furthermore, in a study of 16 patients with idiopathic pulmonary fibrosis[8] (see Chap. 11), both asbestos-body and uncoated-fiber content of the lung parenchyma were low. Whether or not the uncommon case with interstitial fibrosis, absence of asbestos bodies in histologic sections, and elevated tissue asbestos burden should be classified as asbestosis is controversial. However, a role of the asbestos fibers in the production of the fibrosis cannot at present be excluded.

Until a uniform method of analysis of tissue mineral fiber burden is established along with a proper quality control program, it is impractical and unrealistic to recommend a specific tissue asbestos-fiber content as a diagnostic criterion for asbestosis.[8] Nonetheless, the analysis presented in Chap. 11 indicates that *clinically significant* interstitial pulmonary fibrosis is unlikely to be the result of asbestos exposure when there are fewer than one million fibers 5 μ or greater in length per gram of dry lung tissue. The fibrogenicity of fibers in this size range is well established,[60,99–102] whereas that of fibers less than 5 μ in length remains unproven[103] (see Chap. 10). Therefore, no tissue level of fibers in the latter size range can at present be used as evidence for a diagnosis of asbestosis.[8]

GRADING SCHEME

A number of protocols have been published for the histologic grading of asbestosis.[11,12,104-107] One of the most recently reported grading schemes is that proposed by the College of American Pathologists and the National Institute for Occupational Safety and Health in 1982.[12] The interobserver and intraobserver variability for pathologists using this scheme was assessed, and application of the criteria to a set of cases was found to be reasonably reproducible. Universal application of such a scheme would be highly desirable for epidemiologic studies as well as for comparison with the already established radiologic scheme for classification of the pneumoconioses[32] (see earlier section on "Radiographic Findings"). It should be noted that the diagnosis of asbestosis must be established using the criteria outlined in the previous section prior to any attempt at grading.

Accurate histologic grading depends on adequate tissue sampling, preferably including sections from the central and peripheral regions from each lobe of both lungs.[12] Grading may be applied to samples obtained by open lung biopsy, although the limitations of sampling should be recognized. The grading scheme of the CAP-NIOSH includes a score for both severity and extent of disease.[12] A score for each of these parameters is determined for each slide, the two values multiplied to give a single value for each slide, and the individual values obtained for each slide averaged to give an average histologic grade for each case. Grading of severity is as follows:

Grade 0 = No peribronchiolar fibrosis
Grade 1 = Fibrosis confined to the walls of respiratory bronchioles and the first adjacent tier of alveoli
Grade 2 = Fibrosis extending to involve alveolar ducts or two or more tiers of alveoli adjacent to the bronchiole, with sparing of some alveoli between adjacent bronchioles
Grade 3 = Fibrotic thickening of the walls of all alveoli between at least two adjacent respiratory bronchioles
Grade 4 = Honeycomb changes (see earlier section on "Histopathology")

Grading of extent of disease is classified according to the percentage of bronchioles showing excessive peribronchiolar connective tissue:

Grade A = Only occasional bronchioles involved
Grade B = More than occasional involvement, but less than half
Grade C = More than half of all bronchioles involved by the fibrotic process[12]

This scheme allows 12 possible grades for each slide. However, practical application of the scheme by the authors indicates that certain combinations occur rarely or not at all. Virtually all cases with

TABLE 4-2. Histologic grading scheme for asbestosis*

Grade 0	No appreciable peribronchiolar fibrosis, or less than half of bronchioles involved
Grade 1	Fibrosis confined to the walls of respiratory bronchioles and the first tier of adjacent alveoli, with involvement of more than half of all bronchioles on a slide
Grade 2	Extension of fibrosis to involve alveolar ducts and/or two or more tiers of alveoli adjacent to the respiratory bronchiole, with sparing of at least some alveoli between adjacent bronchioles
Grade 3	Fibrotic thickening of the walls of all alveoli between at least two adjacent respiratory bronchioles
Grade 4	Honeycomb changes

SOURCE: Modified from the scheme presented in Ref. 12.
*An average score is obtained for an individual case by adding the scores for each slide (0 to 4), then dividing by the number of slides examined.

severity Grade 3 or 4 show Grade C profusion on the same slide, as do most of the cases with severity Grade 2. Furthermore, if one restricts the diagnosis of asbestosis in cases with severity Grade 1 to those in which most of the bronchioles are involved (see earlier section on "Assessment of Diagnostic Criteria"), then one is left with only four severity grades to consider. We recommend adoption of this simplified version of the CAP-NIOSH grading scheme,[12] the details of which are summarized in Table 4-2 and illustrated in Fig. 4-14. Others have proposed a similar scheme and applied it to experimental models of asbestosis.[108] Because of the reasonably good interobserver and intraobserver agreement obtained with the more extensive scheme,[12] similar or better agreement should be possible with this modified (and simplified) version.

FIGURE 4-14. Photomicrographs illustrating the grading scheme for asbestosis outlined in Table 4-2. Each of the cases satisfied the histologic criteria for the diagnosis of asbestosis outlined in the text. (A) *Grade 1:* Fibrosis is confined to the walls of respiratory bronchioles. *Inset:* Enlargement of area indicated by box shows several asbestos bodies embedded in fibrous tissue of bronchiolar wall. (B) *Grade 2:* Fibrosis extends to involve alveolar ducts and two or more tiers of adjacent alveoli. (C) *Grade 3:* All alveoli between adjacent bronchioles show fibrotic thickening. (D) *Grade 4:* Honeycomb changes, consisting of cystic spaces lined by bronchiolar type epithelium and with fibrotic walls. Hematoxylin and eosin; part (A) ×52, inset ×520; part (B) ×62; part (C) ×32; part (D) ×40.

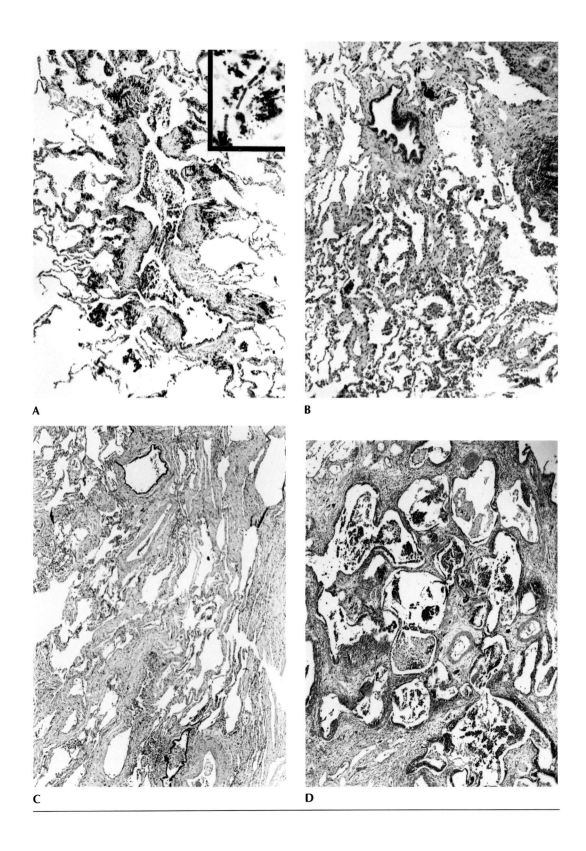

A

B

C

D

REFERENCES

1. Zenker FA: Staubinhalations Krankheiten der Lungen. 1866.
2. Roggli VL, Shelburne JD: Mineral Pneumoconioses. Ch. 21, In: *Pulmonary Pathology* (Dail DH, Hammar SP, eds.), New York: Springer-Verlag, 1988, pp. 589–617.
3. Lee DHK, Selikoff IJ: Historical background to the asbestos problem. *Environ Res* 18:300–314, 1979.
4. Castleman BI: *Asbestos: Medical and Legal Aspects.* New York: Harcourt Brace Jovanovich, 1984.
5. Craighead JE: Eyes for the epidemiologist: The pathologist's role in shaping our understanding of the asbestos-associated diseases. *Am J Clin Pathol* 89:281–287, 1988.
6. Cooke WE: Fibrosis of the lungs due to the inhalation of asbestos dust. *Br Med J* II:147, 1924.
7. Cooke WE: Pulmonary asbestosis. *Br Med J* II:1024–1025, 1927.
8. Roggli VL: Pathology of human asbestosis: A critical review. In: *Advances in Pathology*, vol. 2 (Fenoglio-Preiser, CM, ed.), Chicago: Year Book Med. Pub., 1989, pp. 31–60.
9. McCullough, SF, Aresini G, Browne K, et al.: Criteria for the diagnosis of asbestosis and considerations in the attribution of lung cancer and mesothelioma to asbestos exposure. *Int Arch Occup Environ Health* 49:357–361, 1982.
10. Kannerstein M, Churg J: *Pathology of Asbestos-Related Diseases.* Washington, DC: Armed Forces Institute of Pathology, 1979.
11. Hinson KFW, Otto H, Webster I, et al.: Criteria for the diagnosis and grading of asbestosis. In: *Biological Effects of Asbestos* (Bogovski P, ed.), Lyon, France: World Health Organization, 1973.
12. Craighead JE, Abraham JL, Churg A, et al.: The pathology of asbestos-associated diseases of the lungs and pleural cavities: Diagnostic criteria and proposed grading schema (Report of the Pneumoconiosis Committee of the College of American Pathologists and the National Institute for Occupational Safety and Health). *Arch Pathol Lab Med* 106:544–596, 1982.
13. Churg A: Analysis of asbestos fibers from lung tissue: Research and diagnostic uses. *Sem Respir Med* 7:281–288, 1986.
14. Warnock ML, Prescott BT, Kuwahara TJ: Correlation of asbestos bodies and fibers in lungs of subjects with and without asbestosis. *Scanning Electron Microsc.*/II:845–857, 1982.
15. Spencer H, ed.: *Pathology of the Lung*, 4th ed. Oxford: Pergamon Press, 1985.
16. Katzenstein A-L A, Askin FB: *Surgical Pathology of Non-Neoplastic Lung Disease.* Philadelphia: Saunders, 1982.
17. Dail DH, Hammar SP, eds.: *Pulmonary Pathology.* New York: Springer-Verlag, 1988.
18. Seaton A: Asbestos-related diseases. Ch. 13, In: *Occupational Lung Diseases*, 2nd ed. (Morgan WKC, Seaton A, eds.), Philadelphia: Saunders, 1984, pp. 323–376.
19. Beljan JR, Cooper T, Dolan WD, et al.: A Physician's Guide to Asbestos-Related Diseases: Council on Scientific Affairs. *JAMA* 252:2593–2597, 1984.
20. Selikoff IJ, Lee DHK: *Asbestos and Disease.* New York: Academic Press, 1978.
21. Selikoff IJ, Hammond EC, Seidman H: Latency of asbestos disease among insulation workers in the United States and Canada. *Cancer* 46:2736–2740, 1980.
22. Segarra F, Monte MB, Ibanez LP, Nicolas JP: Asbestosis in a Barcelona fibrocement factory. *Environ Res* 23:292–300, 1980.

23. McMillan GHG, Pethybridge RJ, Sheers G: Effect of smoking on attack rates of pulmonary and pleural lesions related to exposure to asbestos dust. *Br J Ind Med* 37:268–272, 1980.

24. Kilburn KH, Lilis R, Anderson HA, Miller A, Warshaw RH: Interaction of asbestos, age, and cigarette smoking in producing radiographic evidence of diffuse pulmonary fibrosis. *Am J Med* 80:377–381, 1986.

25. Finkelstein MM, Virgilis JJ: Radiographic abnormalities among asbestos-cement workers: An exposure-response study. *Am Rev Respir Dis* 129:17–22, 1984.

26. Ducatman AM, Withers BF, Yang WN: Smoking and roentgenographic opacities in US Navy asbestos workers. *Chest* 97:810–813, 1990.

27. Barnhart S, Thornquist M, Omenn GS, Goodman G, Feigl P, Rosenstock L: The degree of roentgenographic parenchymal opacities attributable to smoking among asbestos-exposed subjects. *Am Rev Respir Dis* 141:1102–1106, 1990.

28. Hobson J, Gilks B, Wright J, Churg A: Direct enhancement by cigarette smoke of asbestos fiber penetration and asbestos-induced epithelial proliferation in rat tracheal explants. *J Natl Cancer Inst* 80:518–521, 1988.

29. Hnizdo E, Sluis-Cremer GK: Effect of tobacco smoking on the presence of asbestosis at postmortem and on the reading of irregular opacities on roentgenograms in asbestos-exposed workers. *Am Rev Respir Dis* 138:1207–1212, 1988.

30. Cookson W, DeKlerk N, Musk AW, Glancy JJ, Armstrong B, Hobbs M: The natural history of asbestosis in former crocidolite workers of Wittenoom Gorge. *Am Rev Respir Dis* 133:994–998, 1986.

31. Fraser RG, Paré JAP: The Pneumoconioses and Chemically Induced Lung Diseases. Ch. 12 In: *Diagnosis of Diseases of the Chest*, 2nd ed., Vol. 3, Philadelphia: Saunders, 1979.

32. International Labour Organisation: International Classification of Radiographs of the Pneumoconioses. Occupational Safety and Health Series. No. 22 (Rev). Geneva: ILO, 1980.

33. Rockoff SD, Schwartz A: Roentgenographic underestimation of early asbestosis by International Labor Organization Classification: Analysis of data and probabilities. *Chest* 93:1088–1091, 1988.

34. Epler GR, McLoud TC, Gaensler EA, Mikus JP, Carrington CB: Normal chest roentgenograms in chronic diffuse infiltrative lung disease. *N Engl J Med* 298:934–939, 1978.

35. Kipen HM, Lilis R, Suzuki Y, Valciukas JA, Selikoff IJ: Pulmonary fibrosis in asbestos insulation workers with lung cancer: A radiological and histopathological evaluation. *Br J Ind Med* 44:96–100, 1987.

36. Weiss W: Cigarette smoke, asbestos, and small irregular opacities. *Am Rev Respir Dis* 130:293–301, 1984.

37. Friedman AC, Fiel SB, Fisher MS, Radekci PD, Lev-Toaff A-S, Caroline DF: Asbestos-related pleural disease and asbestosis: A comparison of CT and chest radiography. *Am J Roentgenol* 150:269–275, 1988.

38. Bergin CJ, Müller NL: CT in the diagnosis of interstitial lung disease. *Am J Roentgenol* 145:505–510, 1985.

39. Aberle DR, Gamsu G, Ray CS: High-resolution CT of benign asbestos-related diseases: Clinical and radiographic correlation. *Am J Roentgenol* 151:883–891, 1988.

40. Pratt PC: Role of conventional chest radiography in diagnosis and exclusion of emphysema. *Am J Med* 82:998–1006, 1987.

41. Foster WL, Pratt PC, Roggli VL, Godwin JD, Halvorsen RA, Putman CE: Centrilobular emphysema: CT-Pathologic correlation. *Radiology* 159:27–32, 1986.

42. Bergin C, Müller N, Nichols DM, Lillington G, Hogg JC, Mullen B, Grymaloski MR, Osborne S, Paré PD: The diagnosis of emphysema:

A computed tomographic-pathologic correlation. *Am Rev Respir Dis* 133:541–546, 1986.

43. Barnhart S, Hudson LD, Mason SE, Pierson DJ, Rosenstock L: Total lung capacity: An insensitive measure of impairment in patients with asbestosis and chronic obstructive pulmonary disease? *Chest* 93:299–302, 1988.

44. Becklake MR: Chronic airflow limitation: Its relationship to work in dusty occupations. *Chest* 88:608–617, 1985.

45. Churg A, Wright JL, Wiggs B, Paré PD, Lazar N: Small airways disease and mineral dust exposure: Prevalence, structure, and function. *Am Rev Respir Dis* 131:139–143, 1985.

46. Kilburn KH, Warshaw RH, Einstein K, Bernstein J: Airway disease in non-smoking asbestos workers. *Arch Environ Health* 40:293–295, 1985.

47. Churg A, Wright JL: Small airways disease and mineral dust exposure. *Pathol Annu*, Part 2, Vol. 18, pp. 233–251, 1983.

48. Wright JL, Churg A: Morphology of small-airway lesions in patients with asbestos exposure. *Hum Pathol* 15:68–74, 1984.

49. Kilburn KH, Warshaw R, Thornton JC: Asbestosis, pulmonary symptoms, and functional impairment in shipyard workers. *Chest* 88:254–259, 1985.

50. Sue DY, Oren A, Hansen JE, Wasserman K: Lung function and exercise performance in smoking and non-smoking asbestos-exposed workers. *Am Rev Respir Dis* 132:612–618, 1985.

51. Churg A: Nonneoplastic diseases caused by asbestos. In: *Pathology of Occupational Lung Disease* (Churg A, Green FHY, eds.), New York: Igaku-Shoin, 1988, pp. 213–277.

52. Hunninghake GW, Gadek JE, Kawanami O, Ferrans VJ, Crystal RG: Inflammatory and immune processes in the human lung in health and disease: Evaluation by bronchoalveolar lavage. *Am J Pathol* 97:149–205, 1979.

53. DeVuyst P, Dumortier P, Moulin E, Yourassowsky N, Yernault JC: Diagnostic value of asbestos bodies in bronchoalveolar lavage fluid. *Am Rev Respir Dis* 136:1219–1244, 1987.

54. Hillerdal G: Asbestos exposure and upper lobe involvement. *Am J Roentgenol* 139:1163–1166, 1982.

55. Hillerdal G: Pleural plaques: Occurrence, exposure to asbestos, and clinical importance. *Acta Univ Upsaliensis* 363:1–227, 1980.

56. Wain SL, Roggli VL, Foster WL: Parietal pleural plaques, asbestos bodies, and neoplasia: A clinical, pathologic, and roentgenographic correlation of 25 consecutive cases. *Chest* 86:707–713, 1984.

57. Murphy RL, Becklake MR, Brooks SM, et al.: The diagnosis of non-malignant diseases related to asbestos. *Am Rev Respir Dis* 134:363–368, 1986.

58. Franzblau A, Lilis R: The diagnosis of non-malignant diseases related to asbestos. *Am Rev Respir Dis* 136:790–791, 1987.

59. Pratt PC: Emphysema and chronic airways disease. Ch. 24 In: *Pulmonary Pathology* (Dail DH, Hammar SP, eds.), New York: Springer-Verlag, 1988, pp. 651–669.

60. Vorwald AJ, Durkan TM, Pratt PC: Experimental studies of asbestosis. *Arch Ind Hyg Occup Med* 3:1–43, 1951.

61. Greenberg SD: Asbestos. Ch. 22 In: *Pulmonary Pathology* (Dail DH, Hammar SP, eds.), New York: Springer-Verlag, 1988, pp. 619–635.

62. Vincent JH, Jones AD, Johnston AM, McMillan C, Bolton RE, Cowie H: Accumulation of inhaled mineral dust in the lung and associated lymph nodes: Implications for exposure and dose in occupational lung disease. *Ann Occup Hyg* 31:375–393, 1987.

63. Roggli VL, Benning TL: Asbestos bodies in pulmonary hilar lymph nodes. *Mod Pathol* 3:513–517, 1990.

64. Kuhn C, Kuo T-T: Cytoplasmic hyalin in asbestosis: A reaction of injured alveolar epithelium. *Arch Pathol* 95:190–194, 1973.

65. Warnock ML, Press M, Churg A: Further observations on cytoplasmic hyaline in the lung. *Hum Pathol* 11:59–66, 1980.
66. Joines RA, Roggli VL: Dendriform pulmonary ossification: Report of two cases with unique findings. *Am J Clin Pathol* 91:398–402, 1989.
67. Ndimbie OK, Williams CR, Lee MW: Dendriform pulmonary ossification. *Arch Pathol Lab Med* 111:1062–1064, 1987.
68. Koss MN, Johnson FB, Hochholzer L: Pulmonary blue bodies. *Hum Pathol* 12:258–266, 1981.
69. Brody AR, Hill LH: Interstitial accumulation of inhaled chrysotile asbestos fibers and consequent formation of microcalcifications. *Am J Pathol* 109:107–114, 1982.
70. Hillderdal G, Hecksher T: Asbestos exposure and aspergillus infection. *Eur J Respir Dis* 63:420–424, 1982.
71. Roggli VL, Johnston WW, Kaminsky DB: Asbestos bodies in fine needle aspirates of the lung. *Acta Cytol* 28:493–498, 1984.
72. Kagan E: Current perspectives in asbestosis. *Ann Allergy* 54:464–474, 1985.
73. Shelburne JD, Wisseman CL, Broda KR, Roggli VL, Ingram P: Lung—Nonneoplastic conditions. In: *Diagnostic Electron Microscopy*, Vol. IV (Trump BF, Jones RJ, eds.), New York: Wiley, 1983, pp. 475–538.
74. Corrin B, Dewar A, Rodriguez-Roisin R, Turner-Warwick M: Fine structural changes in cryptogenic fibrosing alveolitis and asbestosis. *J Pathol* 147:107–119, 1985.
75. Craighead JE, Kleinerman J, Abraham JL, et al.: Diseases associated with exposure to silica and nonfibrous silicate minerals. *Arch Pathol Lab Med* 112:673–720, 1988.
76. Churg A, Wright JL: Small-airway lesions in patients exposed to nonasbestos mineral dusts. *Hum Pathol* 14:688–693, 1983.
77. Mark GJ, Monroe CB, Kazemi H: Mixed pneumoconiosis: Silicosis, asbestosis, talcosis, and berylliosis. *Chest* 75:726–728, 1979.
78. Ackerman LV, Elliott GV, Alanis M: Localized organizing pneumonia: Its resemblance to carcinoma: A review of its clinical, roentgenographic and pathologic features. *Am J Roentgenol Radium Ther Nucl Med* 71:988–996, 1954.
79. Bedrossian CWM: Iatrogenic and Toxic Injury. Ch. 19 In: *Pulmonary Pathology* (Dail DH, Hammar SP, eds.), New York: Springer-Verlag, 1988, pp. 511–534.
80. Kane PB, Goldman SL, Pillai BH, Bergofsky EH: Diagnosis of asbestosis by transbronchial biopsy: A method to facilitate demonstration of ferruginous bodies. *Am Rev Respir Dis* 115:689–694, 1977.
81. Dodson RF, Hurst GA, Williams MG, Corn C, Greenberg SD: Comparison of light and electron microscopy for defining occupational asbestos exposure in transbronchial lung biopsies. *Chest* 94:366–370, 1988.
82. Kobayashi H, Okamura A, Ohnishi Y, Kondo A, Yamamoto T, Ozawa H, Morita T: Generalized fibrosis associated with pulmonary asbestosis. *Acta Pathol Jpn* 33:1223–1231, 1983.
83. Slavin RE, Swedo JL, Brandes D, Gonzalez-Vitale JC, Osornio-Vargas A: Extrapulmonary silicosis: A clinical, morphologic, and ultrastructural study. *Hum Pathol* 16:393–412, 1985.
84. Cowie RL: Silica-dust-exposed mine workers with scleroderma (systemic sclerosis). *Chest* 92:260–262, 1987.
85. Kagan E, Solomon A, Cochrane JC, Beissner EI, Gluckman J, Rocks PH, Webster I: Immunological studies of patients with asbestosis. I. Studies of cell-mediated immunity. *Clin Exp Immunol* 28:261–267, 1977.
86. Kagan E, Solomon A, Cochrane JC, Kuba P, Rocks PH, Webster I: Immunological studies of patients with asbestosis. II. Studies of circulating lymphoid cell numbers and humoral immunity. *Clin Exp Immunol* 28:268–275, 1977.

87. Maguire FW, Mills RC, Parker FP: Immunoblastic lymphadenopathy and asbestosis. *Cancer* 47:791–797, 1981.
88. Cooke CT, Matz LR, Armstrong JA, Pinerua RF: Asbestos-related interstitial pneumonitis associated with glomerulonephritis and lymphomatoid granulomatosis. *Pathology* 18:352–356, 1986.
89. Colby TV, Carrington CB: Pulmonary lymphomas simulating lymphomatoid granulomatosis. *Am J Surg Pathol* 6:19–32, 1982.
90. Churg A: Pulmonary angiitis and granulomatosis revisited. *Hum Pathol* 14:868–883, 1983.
91. Kagan E, Jacobson RJ: Lymphoid and plasma cell malignancies: Asbestos-related disorders of long latency. *Am J Clin Pathol* 80:14–20, 1983.
92. Churg A: An inflation procedure for open lung biopsies. *Am J Surg Pathol* 7:69–71, 1983.
93. Roggli VL, Pratt PC: Numbers of asbestos bodies on iron-stained tissue sections in relation to asbestos body counts in lung tissue digests. *Hum Pathol* 14:355–361, 1983.
94. Vollmer RT, Roggli VL: Asbestos body concentrations in human lung: Predictions from asbestos body counts in tissue sections with a mathematical model. *Hum Pathol* 16:713–718, 1985.
95. Becklake MR: Asbestosis criteria. *Arch Pathol Lab Med* 108:93, 1984.
96. Dodson RF, Williams MG, O'Sullivan MF, Corn CJ, Greenberg SD, Hurst GA: A comparison of the ferruginous body and uncoated fiber content in the lungs of former asbestos workers. *Am Rev Respir Dis* 132:143–147, 1985.
97. Warnock ML, Wolery G: Asbestos bodies or fibers and the diagnosis of asbestosis. *Environ Res* 44:29–44, 1987.
98. Holden J, Churg A: Asbestos bodies and the diagnosis of asbestosis in chrysotile workers. *Environ Res* 39:232–236, 1986.
99. Wright GW, Kuschner M: The influence of varying lengths of glass and asbestos fibers on tissue response in guinea pigs. In: *Inhaled Particles IV* (Walton WH, ed.), Oxford: Pergamon Press, 1977, pp. 455–474.
100. Davis JMG, Beckett ST, Bolton RE, Collins P, Middleton AP: Mass and number of fibres in the pathogenesis of asbestos-related lung disease in rats. *Br J Cancer* 37:673–688, 1978.
101. Crapo JD, Barry BE, Brody AR, O'Neil JJ: Morphological, morphometric, and X-ray microanalytical studies on lung tissue of rats exposed to chrysotile asbestos in inhalation chambers. In: *Biological Effects of Mineral Fibers*, Vol. 1 (Wagner JC, ed.), IARC Scientific Publications No. 30:Lyon, 1980, pp. 273–283.
102. Lee KP, Barras CE, Griffith FD, Waritz RS, Lapin CA: Comparative pulmonary responses to inhaled inorganic fibers with asbestos and fiberglass. *Environ Res* 24:167–191, 1981.
103. Gross P: Is short-fibered asbestos dust a biological hazard? *Arch Environ Health* 29:115–117, 1974.
104. Report and recommendations of the working group on asbestos and cancer. *Br J Ind Med* 22:165–171, 1965.
105. Warnock ML, Kuwahara TJ, Wolery G: The relation of asbestos burden to asbestosis and lung cancer. *Pathol Annu*, Part 2, Vol. 18, 1983, pp. 109–145.
106. Wagner JC, Moncrief CB, Coles R, Griffiths DM, Munday DE: Correlation between fibre content of the lungs and disease in naval dockyard workers. *Br J Ind Med* 43:391–395, 1986.
107. Davis JMG: The pathology of asbestos related disease. *Thorax* 39:801–808, 1984.
108. Smith CM, Batcher S, Catanzaro A, Abraham JL, Phalen R: Sequence of bronchoalveolar lavage and histopathologic findings in rat lungs early in inhalation asbestos exposure. *J Toxicol Environ Health* 20:147–161, 1987.

5. Mesothelioma

Victor L. Roggli, Fred Sanfilippo, and John D. Shelburne

Mesothelioma means, literally, "tumor of the mesothelium." The term is often used synonymously with *malignant* (diffuse) *mesothelioma*, a malignancy arising from the serosal lining of one of the three major body cavities—the pleural, peritoneal, or pericardial cavities. These cavities are lined by a single layer of flattened-to-cuboidal cells of mesodermal origin that constitutes the mesothelium proper.[1] The membrane forming the lining of the serous body cavities includes not only the mesothelial cells but the underlying basement membrane, elastic and connective tissue, and scattered mesenchymal cells as well. Mesothelial cells possess a complex cytoskeletal network of intermediate filaments, produce hyaluronic acid, and express long surface microvilli that project into the serous cavities (Fig. 5-1).[2] Numerous pinocytotic vesicles may be observed in association with the plasma membrane.[3] There is still some uncertainty as to whether mesotheliomas result from neoplastic transformation of differentiated mesothelial cells or from a more primitive progenitor such as the submesothelial mesenchymal cell (or from both).[4]

Malignant (diffuse) mesothelioma is a rare neoplasm. Its rarity combined with its strong association with asbestos exposure makes it a signal malignancy, i.e., an epidemiologic marker for exposure to asbestos.[5] The mechanism by which asbestos induces mesothelioma is not completely understood. (This mechanism is considered in detail in Chap. 10. The results of quantitative tissue analysis for asbestos content in cases with malignant mesothelioma are compared with those of other asbestos-related disorders and with normal controls in Chap. 11.) The present chapter reviews the pathologic features of malignant mesothelioma of the serous cavities, the means of distinguishing mesothelioma from other conditions with which it may be confused, and the various agents that have been implicated in the etiology of mesothelioma. Benign tumors arising from the serosal membranes have sometimes been referred to as mesotheliomas, and these exceedingly rare tumors have been reviewed elsewhere.[2] Such tumors are not related to asbestos exposure, and they will not be considered further other than to note the features that permit their distinction from malignant (diffuse) mesotheliomas.

HISTORICAL BACKGROUND

Mesotheliomas are uncommon tumors, and until this century there were few descriptions of this disease in the literature. In 1767, Joseph Lieutand described, from a series of 3000 autopsies, two pleural tumors that might have been mesotheliomas.[6] The detailed description by E. Wagner published in 1870[7] leaves little doubt that he was describing what we now recognize as malignant pleural mesothelioma.[8,9]

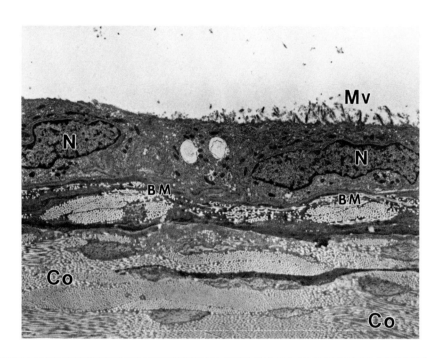

FIGURE 5-1. Transmission electron micrograph of normal mesothelium. Note flattened mesothelial cells, one of which has long surface microvilli (Mv). BM = basement membrane, N = nucleus, Co = collagen. Magnified ×3430. Reprinted from Ref. 2, with permission.

In 1924, Robertson reviewed earlier reports in the literature and concluded that only sarcomatous tumors could be regarded as primary pleural malignancies.[10] He believed that pleural tumors with an epithelial pattern represented metastases from other sites. In 1931, Klemperer and Rabin[11] described five pleural tumors, four of which were localized and one of which was diffuse. These authors separated the localized tumors of the pleura from diffuse pleural malignancies, and used the term *mesothelioma* to refer to the entire histologic spectrum of epithelial and spindle-cell primary malignancies that diffusely involve the pleura.[8,9] By the 1950s, growing numbers of diffuse primary peritoneal tumors were recognized, and malignant mesothelioma became generally accepted as a distinct clinicopathologic entity.[12]

The British pathologist S. R. Gloyne is credited with the first description of pleural malignancy in an individual occupationally exposed to asbestos.[13] This report, appearing in 1933, referred to a case of "squamous carcinoma of the pleura," which Professor Gloyne did not believe was related to the patient's asbestosis.[14] This was followed by reports from Germany in 1943 by Wedler[15] and from the United States in 1947 by Mallory[16] of further cases of pleural malignancy associated with exposure to asbestos. Additional reports appeared in the 1940s and '50s,[13,17] and by 1960 Keal had described the association between peritoneal mesothelioma and asbestos exposure.[18] Any remaining doubt concerning the association between asbestos exposure and malignant mesothelioma was dispelled by the classic study of J. C. Wagner's in 1960,[19] which described 33 cases of diffuse pleural mesothelioma occurring in the Northwestern Cape Province of South Africa, in 32 of which there was a documented exposure to asbestos. In some instances the patient's only exposure was living in proximity to an asbestos mine. Since 1960, numerous studies have appeared in the literature confirming the association between asbestos exposure and malignant mesothelioma of the pleura, the peritoneum, and even the pericardium.[2]

ETIOLOGIC CONSIDERATIONS

ASBESTOS

Since the publication of the study by Wagner et al. in 1960,[19] epidemiologic studies from many industrialized countries have documented rising rates of malignant mesothelioma following the heavy commercial use of asbestos.[20-27] A large proportion of cases in these studies have derived from shipyard workers[20,26,28] and insulators,[29,30] where large numbers of workers had heavy exposures. Other occupational exposures to asbestos, including miners and millers,[19,27,31] railroad machinists and steam locomotive repair workers,[32,33] and workers in asbestos factories,[34] have also resulted in appreciable numbers of cases. In addition to occupational exposures, some cases have resulted from indirect exposures, such as living near an asbestos factory or mine,[19] or from household exposures in which family members come into contact with asbestos-contaminated clothing of an asbestos worker.[35,36] Some unusual exposures to asbestos associated with mesothelioma also have been documented, such as manufacturers of asbestos-containing cigarette filters,[37] or members of a Native American pueblo where asbestos was used in the preparation of silver jewelry and in whitening of ceremonial leggings and moccasins,[38] or children exposed to diapers made from cotton cloth sacks in which asbestos insulation had been transported.[39]

A prolonged period between initial exposure to asbestos and manifestation of disease, known as the *latent interval*, is typically observed for most asbestos-associated diseases, and malignant mesothelioma is no exception. The latent interval for mesothelioma is usually 20 or more years after the initial exposure, and virtually never less than 15 years.[40] The latent interval peaks at 30–40 years postexposure, and may extend to 70 or more years in some cases.[29,41] Furthermore, the risk appears to increase dramatically with time from initial exposure. Peto et al.[42] have examined this relationship mathematically and found that the available data are best explained by a model in which mesothelioma risk increases with the third or fourth power of time from first exposure. These investigators also concluded that there is a linear dose–response relationship between the amount of asbestos to which an individual is exposed and the risk of developing mesothelioma.[42] In addition, a threshold level of exposure below which mesothelioma will not occur has not yet been identified.[43] Peritoneal mesotheliomas appear to be associated with heavier and more prolonged exposure to asbestos than is the case for pleural mesotheliomas,[2,35,44] although the latent interval is similar for both sites.[42] This observation is consistent with the finding that asbestosis can be diagnosed clinically in 50% of patients with peritoneal mesothelioma but in only 20% of patients with pleural mesothelioma.[2,35]

The various types of asbestos fibers do not appear to have the same potential for the production of malignant mesothelioma in humans. Of the commercially valuable forms of asbestos, crocidolite appears to pose the greatest risk, amosite a somewhat lesser risk, and chrysotile the least risk.[45–50] Furthermore, individuals with mesothelioma who are exposed to chrysotile through the mining and milling of asbestos have more tremolite than chrysotile in their lung tissues, even though tremolite (a noncommercial amphibole) accounts for only a small percentage of the chrysotile ore.[51,52] This observation has led some investigators to suggest that it is the amphibole component of chrysotile ore that is responsible for the increased risk of malignant mesothelioma in chrysotile miners and millers.[52,53] Several studies have shown that environmental exposures to tremolite asbestos can result in an increased risk of developing mesothelioma, particularly where the tremolite fibers have a high aspect ratio (i.e., length:diameter).[54–56] In this regard, it is of interest that anthophyllite, which consists of relatively broad fibers with a low aspect ratio, has not been implicated as a cause of malignant mesothelioma in humans.[36] (The relationship between fiber dimensions and other characteristics and their carcinogenic potential is discussed in greater detail in Chap. 10.)

Although the association between asbestos and malignant mesothelioma is indisputable, only a small proportion (10% or less) of asbestos workers develop mesothelioma,[29,35] and about half of the reported cases of mesothelioma have no documented exposure to asbestos.[21,35,57] In areas where no substantial asbestos-using industry exists, as few as 10% of patients with malignant mesothelioma have a history of exposure to asbestos; whereas in areas where shipyards or asbestos mines are located, 70% or more of mesothelioma patients have a positive exposure history.[35] In some instances, the apparent absence of exposure is due to inadequate historical information. Nonetheless, the observation that a substantial proportion of patients with malignant mesothelioma have no identifiable exposure to asbestos has led investigators to look for other potential etiologic or predisposing factors. These are reviewed in the following sections.

ZEOLITES

The discovery of an epidemic of malignant pleural mesothelioma in two small Anatolian villages in Turkey[58] has largely been responsible for the current interest in the pathologic effects of zeolites.[2] These two villages, Karain and Tuskoy, are situated on volcanic tuffs rich in fibrous erionite, a hydrated aluminum silicate belonging to the family of zeolite minerals. Erionite is ubiquitous in the local environment of these villages,[59] and the fiber has been recovered from lung tissues of villagers,[60] although some asbestos fibers can be identified as well.[61] These villagers have the highest rates of mesothelioma of any population yet encountered, while similar villages only a short distance away have had no reported cases. Erionite has physical properties and dimensions that closely resemble those of commercial amphiboles, and injection of erionite fibers into the pleural and peritoneal cavities of experimental animals has resulted in the development of pleural and peritoneal mesotheliomas.[62,63] No cases of human mesothelioma due to erionite exposure have as yet been reported from the United States.

RADIATION

There have been a number of case reports in which radiation administered to the thorax or abdomen preceded by many years the development of malignant mesothelioma of the pleura or peritoneum.[64] Radiation in these cases has been administered as internal or external radiotherapy, and some cases have followed the intravascular administration of thorium dioxide (Thorotrast). The latent interval is generally prolonged, ranging from 7–36 years from the initial exposure to radiation until the diagnosis of malignant mesothelioma.[64] One of the strongest arguments favoring a role of radiation in mesothelioma induction derives from several recent reports of malignant pleural mesothelioma developing in young adults who had received intensive radiotherapy and chemotherapy in childhood for Wilms' tumor.[65–67] In these cases, a portion of the lung parenchyma (and hence pleura) was included in the radiation fields of the abdomen and renal bed. Lung tissue analysis for asbestos was performed in one of these cases and gave values within the range expected for a reference population.[67] Experimental animal studies have also implicated radiation as a causative factor in the development of malignant mesothelioma.[68]

OTHER FACTORS

Additional factors implicated as possible contributing causes to the development of malignant mesothelioma in humans include chronic inflammation and scarring of the pleura, chemical carcinogens, viruses, and hereditary predisposition.[64] A number of cases have been reported in which chronic empyema or therapeutic pneumothorax preceded by several decades the development of malignant pleural mesothelioma.[69] In one instance, malignant mesothelioma developed

20 years after the instillation of leucite spheres in the ipsilateral pleural cavity as a treatment for tuberculosis.[57] The identification of malignant mesothelioma in oil refinery and petrochemical plant workers suggests the possibility that asbestos might interact with certain chemical carcinogens in the production of mesothelioma.[57] However, cigarette smoking has not been implicated as a risk factor for mesothelioma.[35] One epidemiologic study showed a slightly increased risk of malignant mesothelioma in fiberglass workers,[21] although this finding has not been confirmed. Several reports of familial aggregations of malignant mesothelioma indicate that host genetic factors may contribute to the development of mesothelioma, perhaps by rendering the host more susceptible to asbestos exposure.[70-72] Finally, reports of mesothelioma developing in childhood[73] or even in utero[74] for which none of these risk factors could be identified indicate that there are probably as-yet-unknown factors involved in the pathogenesis of this rare malignancy.

PATHOLOGIC FEATURES

PLEURAL MESOTHELIOMA

Gross Morphology

The most common site of origin of malignant (diffuse) mesothelioma is the pleura. In large series, the ratio of pleural to peritoneal locations is approximately 10:1.[75] Pleural mesotheliomas characteristically involve both visceral and parietal pleura, with a tendency to spread over the surface of the lung, eventually encasing it in a rind of tumor.[75-77] The tumor may occur in sheets of varying thickness or as nodular masses. In exceptional cases, malignant mesothelioma may present as a pleural-based localized mass.[78,79] Pleural mesotheliomas often invade the chest wall or mediastinum; in advanced cases, the tumor may invade the opposite pleural cavity or the peritoneum. Superficial invasion of the underlying lung parenchyma is often present (Fig. 5-2). Occasionally, the tumor may also invade along needle tracks subsequent to biopsy procedures.[12]

The gross pathologic features of malignant pleural mesothelioma correlate well with the clinical symptoms at initial presentation. Invasion of parietal pleura and chest wall is associated with chest pain. Encasement of the lung can restrict ventilation, resulting in dyspnea. Extensive thoracic involvement by tumor is often accompanied by weight loss. A large, often bloody, pleural effusion is usually present at the time of initial diagnosis,[80] but late in the course of the disease the pleural space may be obliterated.[2] Large effusions can also contribute to the patient's dyspnea. Although it is distinctly unusual for distant metastases to be clinically evident at the time of initial presentation, metastases are found in over half of the cases at

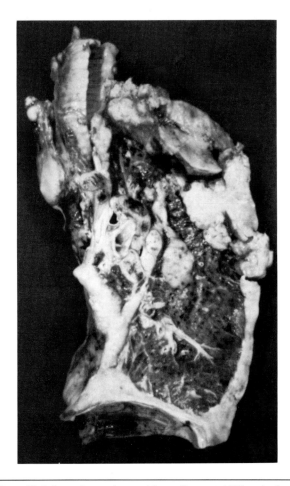

FIGURE 5-2. Coronal slice of left lung in patient with malignant (diffuse) pleural mesothelioma shows encasement of lung by rind of tumor. Note superficial invasion of underlying parenchyma (arrow). Reprinted from Ref. 2, with permission.

autopsy.[57] Mesotheliomas may metastasize by either lymphatic or hematogenous pathways, and lymph nodes are the most common site of metastatic disease.[57,75] In rare instances, extensive lymphangitic pulmonary spread is present at the time of diagnosis.[81]

The gross morphologic features are very important in the diagnosis of malignant (diffuse) pleural mesothelioma. When this information is not available directly, it may be obtained through observations by the surgeon or from radiographic studies. Massive pleural effusion may obscure details of tumor distribution on plain films, but computed tomography or magnetic resonance imaging of the thorax can provide detailed information regarding these important gross pathologic features (Fig. 5-3).[82–84] Although the gross distribution of malignant mesothelioma is characteristic, it is not pathognomonic:

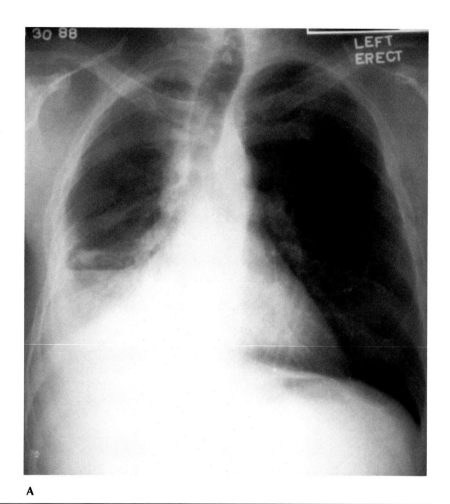

A

FIGURE 5-3. (A) Posteroanterior chest x-ray shows a unilateral pleural effusion. (B) Computed tomography of the thorax from the same patient shows irregular pleural thickening with encasement of the lung. These radiographic features are typical for malignant (diffuse) pleural mesothelioma. Courtesy Dr. Caroline Chiles, Duke University Medical Center, Durham, NC.

Other malignancies may directly invade or metastasize to the pleural cavity. At autopsy, therefore, it is important to inspect carefully the viscera in order to exclude a primary malignancy with secondary involvement of the pleura. For example, small peripheral lung carcinomas can initially invade the pleura and closely mimic the gross appearance of malignant pleural mesothelioma (Fig. 5-4).[85]

The diagnosis of malignant pleural mesothelioma depends not only on the typical gross features but also on the identification of a histologic pattern compatible with mesothelioma and the exclusion of metastatic tumor. In some cases, this may require additional histochemical, immunohistochemical, or ultrastructural studies (see upcoming sections). Studies describing the cytologic features of

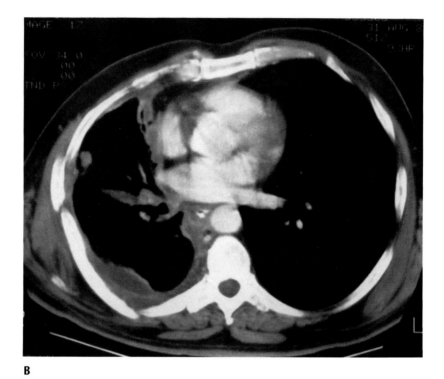

B

mesothelioma in pleural effusions and needle biopsies have been published, [86-88] but the distinction from reactive mesothelial hyperplasia or metastatic adenocarcinoma may be difficult or impossible based on such limited samples (see Chap. 9).[2] Therefore, most investigators believe that generous sampling of tumor at thoracotomy is usually required for an unequivocal premortem pathologic diagnosis of malignant pleural mesothelioma.[2,8,76-78]

Histopathology
Malignant mesothelioma is characterized histologically by a broad range of microscopic appearances, both from one tumor to another and frequently within a single tumor.[8] Mesotheliomas are conventionally classified into three histologic patterns: (1) epithelial, (2) sarcomatous, and (3) mixed or biphasic. These patterns occur in approximately 50, 20, and 30% of cases, respectively.[2,57,75] The histologic classification of 200 pleural mesotheliomas in the authors' series is summarized in Table 5-1. The most common variant is the epithelial pattern, which is composed of cuboidal or polyhedral tumor cells with central nuclei and often prominent nucleoli. Eosinophilic cytoplasm is moderately abundant, and cytoplasmic vacuoles may be identified in some cases. Multinucleated forms and occasional mitoses may be observed, but anaplasia, extreme pleomorphism, and atypical mitotic

TABLE 5-1. Histopathologic classification of 200 cases
of malignant pleural mesothelioma

Histologic pattern		Percent
Epithelial		40%
Biphasic (mixed epithelial and sarcomatous)		37
Sarcomatous		23
Desmoplastic	8 %	
Lymphohistiocytoid	0.5%	_____
TOTAL		100%

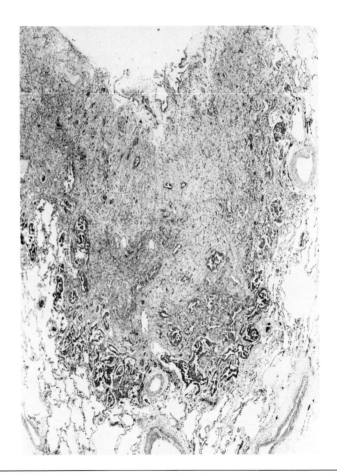

FIGURE 5-4. Low-power photomicrograph of a small peripheral scar carcinoma found at
autopsy that measured 5 mm in maximum dimension. Multiple pleural
deposits of tumor histologically identical to the adenocarcinoma at the periphery of the central scar resulted in a pattern mimicking mesothelioma.
H&E ×24.

figures are distinctly uncommon.[2,89] One cytologic feature that has been reported to be characteristic of epithelial tumor cells of malignant mesothelioma is a constant nuclear-to-cytoplasmic ratio.[90] The neoplastic cells in the epithelial variant may be arranged in papillary, tubular, or solid nest configurations[2] [Fig. 5-5 (A) through (C)]. They may also line cleftlike spaces or grow as solid sheets of tumor cells. Often several of these patterns may be observed in different areas of a single tumor. The epithelial variant is most readily confused with metastatic adenocarcinoma, and this difficulty increases as the epithelial tumor cells become more anaplastic.[2]

The sarcomatous, or spindle-cell, pattern of malignant mesothelioma is the least common of the three major histologic variants. The tumor cells are elongated or spindle-shaped and may show considerable pleomorphism and mitotic activity.[2] Most commonly the pattern resembles that of fibrosarcomas of soft tissues, although additional patterns have been described, including neurogenic sarcoma, leiomyosarcoma, chondrosarcoma, and osteosarcoma[75,91,92] [Fig. 5-6 (A) through (C)]. We have also observed cases in which the spindle cells have a storiform arrangement and are intermixed with bizarre tumor giant cells in a pattern reminiscent of malignant fibrous histiocytoma [see Fig. 5-6 (D)]. Mesenchymal malignancies frequently exhibit considerable histologic plasticity; and in addition, osteosarcomatous and chondrosarcomatous foci have been described in otherwise-typical mesotheliomas.[78] The authors therefore accept the various sarcomatous patterns just listed as mesothelioma provided that the gross appearance is characteristic and there is no evidence of a primary soft-tissue sarcoma elsewhere in the patient.[2] However, this view is not shared by all investigators.[75]

The most distinctive pattern of malignant mesothelioma is the biphasic or mixed pattern.[76] These tumors have areas that exhibit one or more of the epithelial patterns described earlier, and in addition have areas that exhibit a spindle-cell or sarcomatous appearance [see Fig. 5-5 (D)]. Transition from the epithelial to the spindle-cell component may be gradual or abrupt. Metastases may contain either component alone, or both may be present together.[2] The frequency of the biphasic pattern ranges from 25–50% in various series of malignant pleural mesothelioma and depends somewhat on how extensively the tumor is sampled.[57,76] The identification of a biphasic pattern on a needle biopsy of the pleura may be sufficient to make a diagnosis of malignant mesothelioma in a patient whose tumor has the typical gross distribution. However, the pathologist must be careful to differentiate a true sarcomatous component (see Fig. 5-6) from a cellular fibroblastic response to metastatic carcinoma.[2]

A particularly deceptive pattern is the desmoplastic variant of malignant mesothelioma.[93,94] The individual neoplastic cells in this variant are widely separated by thick bands of hyalinized collagen, often arranged in interweaving bundles or whorls, or in a storiform pattern (Fig. 5-7). This pattern can be found as a component of a large percentage of malignant mesotheliomas,[90] so the term is restricted to cases in which this pattern predominates.[93,94] In the authors' series of 200 malignant pleural mesotheliomas, a desmoplastic pattern predominated in 16 cases (8%). The majority of desmoplastic malignant mesotheliomas are associated with the sarcomatous cell type; indeed, with thorough sampling, frankly sarcomatous areas are invariably found.[94] However, biphasic and, rarely, epithelial mesotheliomas in which a desmoplastic pattern predominated have been described.[93,94] In small biopsy specimens or even open biopsies, one must use caution not to confuse the desmoplastic variant with nonspecific pleural fibrosis or parietal pleural plaques. The latter contain very few cells and the collagen bundles are parallel with a "basket-weave" pattern (see Chap. 6), never in a storiform pattern. Features that favor a diagnosis of desmoplastic mesothelioma over a reactive fibrotic process include increased cellularity, usually with some plump and hyperchromatic nuclei, haphazardly arranged collagen bundles, and areas of bland necrosis.[12] Patients with malignant pleural mesothelioma often have parietal pleural plaques, and these may be sampled by the surgeon at the time of open biopsy. In the authors' series, the characteristic morphologic features of parietal pleural plaques were identified in biopsy material from 21 of 200 patients with malignant pleural mesothelioma.

Another uncommon histologic variant of malignant mesothelioma, recently described by Henderson et al.,[95] is the so-called lymphohistiocytoid mesothelioma. These authors describe three cases in a series of 394 malignant mesotheliomas that were characterized by an intense lymphoplasmacytic infiltration superimposed on scattered neoplastic cells with a histiocytoid appearance. As a result, these tumors bore a striking resemblance to malignant lymphomas of the non-Hodgkins type (Fig. 5-8). The true nature of the underlying neoplastic cells in such cases becomes apparent with immunohistochemical and ultrastructural studies[95] [see Fig. 5-8 (B)] (vide infra).

Metastases from malignant mesothelioma generally resemble the histologic appearance of the primary tumor. Although it has been suggested that distant metastases occur more frequently with the sarcomatous variant,[96] a recent review of 42 cases of pleural mesothelioma showed no difference in the frequency of blood-borne or lymphatic metastases among the three major histologic types.[97] It is interesting to note that, whereas lymph node metastases are

---

FIGURE 5-5. Histologic patterns of malignant (diffuse) pleural mesothelioma with predominately epithelial components: (A) papillary pattern; (B) tubular pattern; and (C) solid sheets. The tumor cells have fairly uniform central nuclei with prominent nucleoli. (D) Biphasic pattern showing epithelial area (*top*) with acinar formation adjacent to an area of sarcomatous differentiation (*bottom right*). Hematoxylin and eosin: Parts (A) through (C) ×170; part (D) ×100. Parts (C) and (D) reprinted from Ref. 2, with permission.

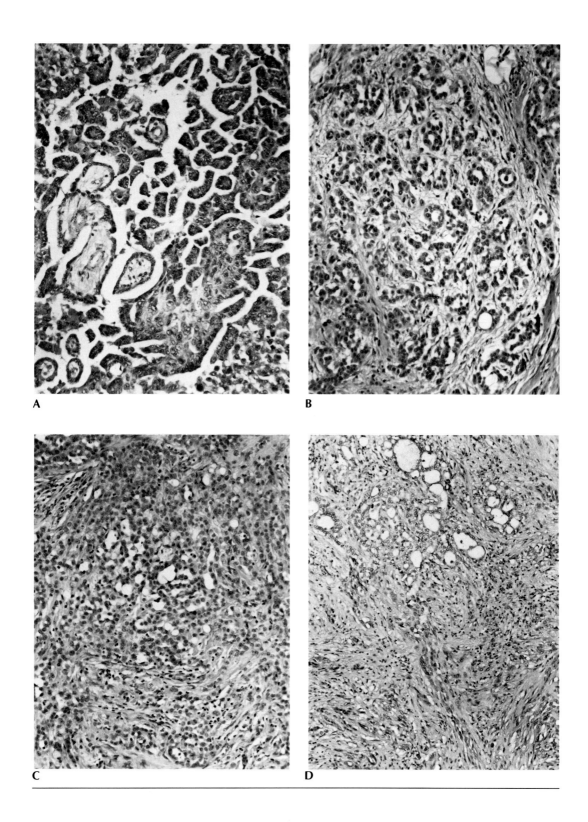

commonly identified,[57,75] metastases to extrathoracic lymph nodes are rather uncommon, occurring in eight of 77 cases of malignant pleural mesothelioma in one series.[98] In exceptional cases, osseous metastases have been described as the initial clinical evidence of tumor dissemination in desmoplastic pleural mesothelioma.[99] Hematogenous metastases of desmoplastic mesothelioma sometimes exhibit the curious phenomenon of central hyalinization with a peripheral cellular storiform pattern.[2] Finally, rare cases have been reported in which liver metastases from a malignant pleural mesothelioma underwent dystrophic calcification and presented with hepatic calcification initially detected roentgenographically.[100]

Histochemistry

The histochemical basis for distinguishing malignant pleural mesothelioma from metastatic adenocarcinoma rests on the identification of hyaluronic acid production in the former instance and neutral mucin in the latter.[2] Neutral mucin may be identified histochemically by means of the periodic acid Schiff (PAS) stain. The specificity of the PAS reaction for neutral mucin is increased by prior digestion of the section with diastase in order to remove glycogen, which may be abundant in some epithelial mesotheliomas as well as in some adenocarcinomas. The demonstration of PAS-positive, diastase-resistant intraluminal secretions or cytoplasmic vacuoles within a tumor is indicative of adenocarcinoma and essentially excludes a diagnosis of mesothelioma.[2,12,57,75,76,89,101] The granular cytoplasmic staining of glycogen in some epithelial mesotheliomas should be eliminated by digesting the section with diastase prior to PAS staining (Fig. 5-9). A false positive reaction with the PAS stain in mesotheliomas may occur if removal of glycogen by diastase is incomplete; therefore, simultaneous controls should always be performed. In addition, basement membrane material, which may be prominent in epithelial mesotheliomas, will stain with the PAS reaction. Careful attention to the pattern of staining will usually prevent the confusion of residual glycogen or basement membrane material with positive staining for neutral mucins. The PAS stain is generally negative and of no use in the diagnosis of sarcomatous mesotheliomas.[2] The mucicarmine stain, sometimes used for the identification of neutral mucin, will occasionally react with hyaluronic acid and thus give a false positive

---

FIGURE 5-6. Histologic patterns of malignant (diffuse) pleural mesothelioma with predominately sarcomatoid components: (A) fibrosarcomatous pattern; (B) osteosarcomatous pattern with osteoid formation (*center*) and well-formed ossification (*bottom*); (C) neurogenic sarcomatous pattern; and (D) malignant fibrous histiocytoma-like pattern, with numerous tumor giant cells. H&E: Part (A) ×250; part (B) ×32; part (C) ×52; part (D) ×130. Parts (A) and (B) reprinted from Ref. 2, with permission.

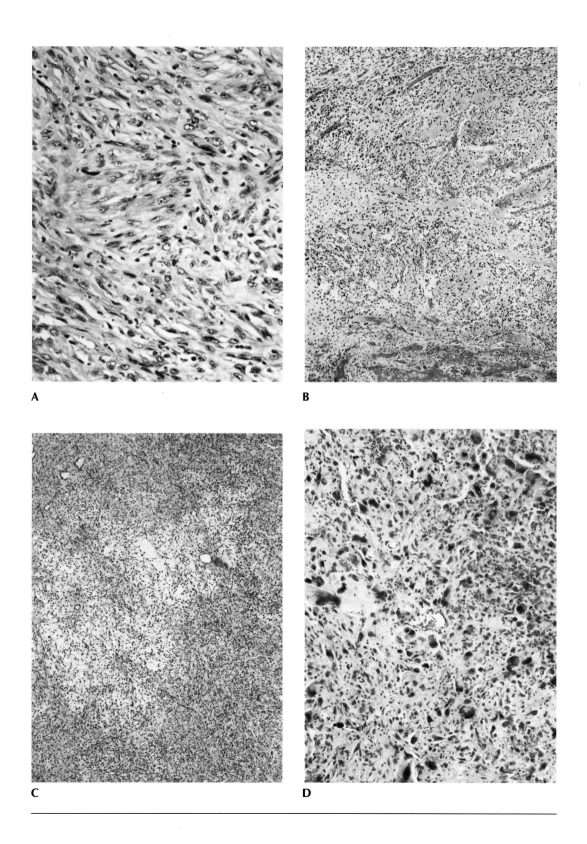

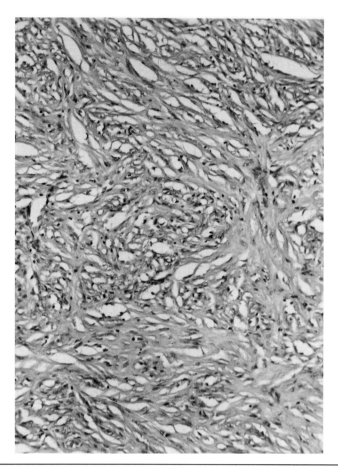

FIGURE 5-7. Desmoplastic malignant pleural mesothelioma consisting of thick bundles of collagen arranged in a storiform pattern with scattered, rather inconspicuous tumor cells in spaces between the fiber bundles. Such a pattern would be difficult to recognize as malignant on a small biopsy specimen. H&E ×130. Reprinted from Ref. 2, with permission.

result.[102] The specificity of the mucicarmine stain may be improved by prior digestion of the section with hyaluronidase.[103]

Identification of hyaluronic acid as the sole or major acid mucopolysaccharide in an epithelial tumor has also been proposed as a useful histochemical feature for the diagnosis of malignant mesothelioma.[2,12,75,76,89,101] Acid mucopolysaccharides, including hyaluronic acid, are identified histochemically with the alcian blue or colloidal iron stains. The specificity of the reaction for hyaluronic acid is then determined by digestion of a serial section with hyaluronidase prior to staining. The result depends to some degree on the hyaluronidase used, since Streptomyces hyaluronidase is specific for hyaluronic acid, whereas testicular hyaluronidase digests chondroitin

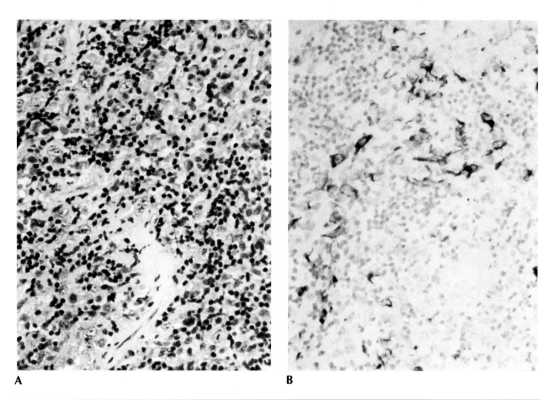

A   B

FIGURE 5-8. (A) Lymphohistiocytoid malignant pleural mesothelioma, showing large pale neoplastic nuclei (arrowheads) in a background of small lymphocytes. The pattern resembles that of mixed small- and large-cell lymphomas. (B) Adjacent serial section stained for cytokeratins shows positive staining of the large neoplastic cells. Part (A) H&E, ×325; part (B) immunoperoxidase (cytokeratins), ×325.

sulfate as well as hyaluronic acid.[104] In using the alcian blue or colloidal iron stains as a diagnostic tool, only intracytoplasmic or intraluminal material associated with epithelial cells should be considered (Fig. 5-10), since abundant hyaluronic acid may be present in the sarcomatous component of a mesothelioma as well as in the reactive stroma surrounding nests of metastatic adenocarcinoma.[2,89,101] Alcian-blue–positive intracytoplasmic or intraluminal material that is entirely removed by hyaluronidase treatment strongly supports a diagnosis of malignant mesothelioma, whereas staining unaffected by hyaluronidase treatment favors a diagnosis of adenocarcinoma. Simultaneous controls should always be performed to ensure that the stains and enzyme are working properly.

Pleural effusions in patients with malignant mesothelioma may be rich in hyaluronic acid,[80,105] and electrophoresis of glycosaminoglycans in pleural effusions has been proposed as a diagnostic aid.[106] In patients with mesothelioma, hyaluronic acid is usually the sole or

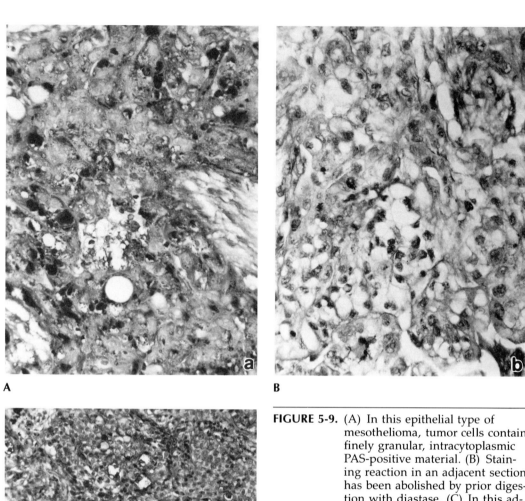

A

B

C

FIGURE 5-9. (A) In this epithelial type of mesothelioma, tumor cells contain finely granular, intracytoplasmic PAS-positive material. (B) Staining reaction in an adjacent section has been abolished by prior digestion with diastase. (C) In this adenocarcinoma metastatic to the pleura, PAS-positive material within glandular lumens remains following digestion by diastase, indicating the presence of neutral mucin. Reprinted from Ref. 2, with permission.

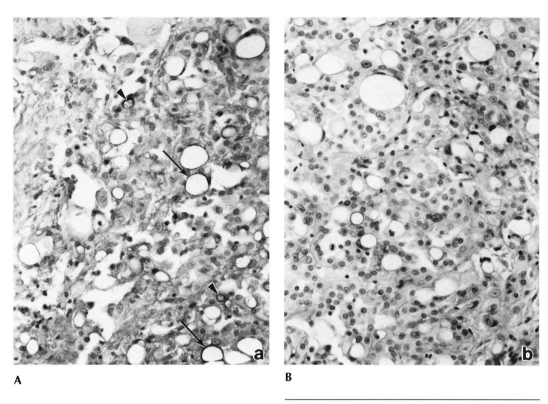

A

B

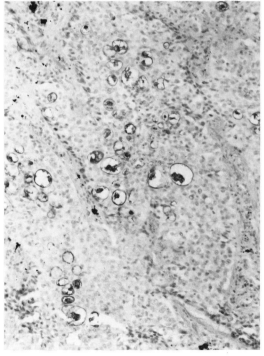

C

FIGURE 5-10. (A) In this epithelial pleural mesothelioma, tumor cells are forming nests with lumens that are filled with (arrowheads) or rimmed by (arrows) alcian-blue–positive material. (B) This material is completely removed from a serial section by prior digestion with hyaluronidase. (C) In this adenocarcinoma metastatic to the pleura, alcian-blue–positive material persists in the lumens following digestion with hyaluronidase. Reprinted from Ref. 2, with permission.

predominant acid mucopolysaccharide (glycosaminoglycan) identified electrophoretically in the effusion, whereas a mixture of glycosaminoglycans is generally found in malignant effusions associated
with adenocarcinoma. However, rare instances of metastatic pancreatic carcinoma have been reported in which the resultant pleural
effusion contained predominantly hyaluronic acid.[76] In addition,
rare cases of pleural mesothelioma have been reported in which
chondroitin sulfate was the predominant acid mucopolysaccharide
in the effusion.[107] Some studies have suggested that electrophoresis of glycosaminoglycans extracted from a tumor is diagnostically
useful.[106,108] Other investigators have observed that hyaluronic acid is
neither the sole nor the predominant glycosaminoglycan in most
mesotheliomas.[104,109] Obviously, studies on whole-tumor extracts include both epithelial tumor cells as well as extracellular stroma, the
relative proportions of which will influence the distribution and frequency of the various glycosaminoglycans obtained.[2]

A recent study examined the content of six enzymes from various
metabolic pathways in 16 surgically resected mesotheliomas and
compared the results to those in 56 adenocarcinomas.[110] Interestingly, the level of gamma-glutamyl transpeptidase was significantly
lower in mesothelial tumors than in carcinomas, and there was very
little overlap between the two groups. The level of another enzyme,
thymidine kinase, which correlates well with tumor-volume-doubling
times, was inversely related to postdiagnosis survival time.[110] This is
a fertile area for investigation, and other useful enzyme markers may
be forthcoming.

In summary, histochemistry may be useful in discriminating between adenocarcinoma and mesothelioma: Positive staining with PAS
that persists following diastase is indicative of adenocarcinoma, and
positive staining with alcian blue in an epithelial tumor that is abolished by hyaluronidase treatment strongly supports a diagnosis of
malignant mesothelioma (Table 5-2). However, a substantial proportion of adenocarcinomas fail to produce detectable amounts of neutral mucin, and only about half of epithelial mesotheliomas produce
histochemically detectable quantities of hyaluronic acid.[2] Therefore,
negative histochemical studies provide no diagnostically useful information; and in a substantial proportion of cases, histochemical stains
will not discriminate between malignant mesothelioma and metastatic adenocarcinoma.

Immunohistochemistry
Mesothelial cells contain a complex cytoskeleton composed of intermediate filaments that have been shown by means of the indirect
immunofluorescence technique and by two-dimensional gel electrophoresis to include cytokeratin and vimentin.[111] Cytokeratins are a
complex group of proteins consisting of at least 19 structurally distinct polypeptides. These proteins are produced to varying degrees
within epithelial cells.[112] Vimentin is an intermediate filament that

TABLE 5-2. Histochemical features of malignant mesothelioma and adenocarcinoma

	Adenocarcinoma	Epithelial and biphasic mesothelioma	Sarcomatous mesothelioma
DPAS*	Positive-staining cytoplasmic vacuoles or luminal spaces in 40–70% of cases	Basement membrane staining in some cases; no cytoplasmic or intraluminal mucin positivity	Negative; incomplete basement membrane material may stain in some cases
Alcian blue with and without hyaluronidase	Positive-staining cytoplasmic vacuoles or luminal spaces resistant to hyaluronidase treatment (about 60% of cases)	Positive-staining cytoplasmic vacuoles or luminal spaces sensitive to hyaluronidase treatment (about 50–60% of cases)	Extracellular (stromal) positivity only (not of diagnostic value)

*DPAS = Periodic acid Schiff stain with diastase predigestion

is generally found in cells of mesenchymal origin. Recent studies have shown a range of expression of these intermediate filament proteins, from the quiescent submesothelial mesenchymal cells to the fully differentiated mesothelial cell lining the pleural cavity.[113] The quiescent mesenchymal cell expresses only vimentin, whereas in reactive mesothelium, the submesothelial mesenchymal cells express both vimentin and low-molecular-weight cytokeratins. Moreover, fully differentiated mesothelial cells express both high- and low-molecular-weight cytokeratins, but have lost the ability to express vimentin.[113] These observations suggest that submesothelial mesenchymal cells are pluripotent and capable of surface differentiation.

Neoplasms often express the same pattern of intermediate filaments as their normal tissue of origin,[114] so a number of studies have investigated the utility of immunohistochemistry to recognize these filaments in malignant mesotheliomas to aid in the distinction of mesothelioma from other malignancies with which it may be confused. Early studies using polyclonal antikeratin antibodies showed intense staining of mesotheliomas for keratin proteins as compared to weak or absent staining for adenocarcinomas.[115,116] Immunoelectron microscopy techniques demonstrated that the keratin antiserum was in fact labeling intermediate filaments.[117] Subsequent studies reported that some epithelial mesotheliomas stained weakly for cytokeratins,[118] and the current consensus of most investigators appears to be that cytokeratin immunoperoxidase techniques have no discriminating value in differentiating epithelial malignant mesotheliomas from metastatic adenocarcinoma.[90,119–123] When monoclonal antibodies to both high- and low-molecular-weight keratins (e.g., AE_1/AE_3, Hybritech) are applied to properly fixed tissues, both epithelial mesotheliomas and adenocarcinomas generally show moderate to strong staining (Fig. 5-11).

A number of cytokeratin proteins have been identified in epithelial or biphasic mesotheliomas, including cytokeratins 4–8, 14, 17, 18,

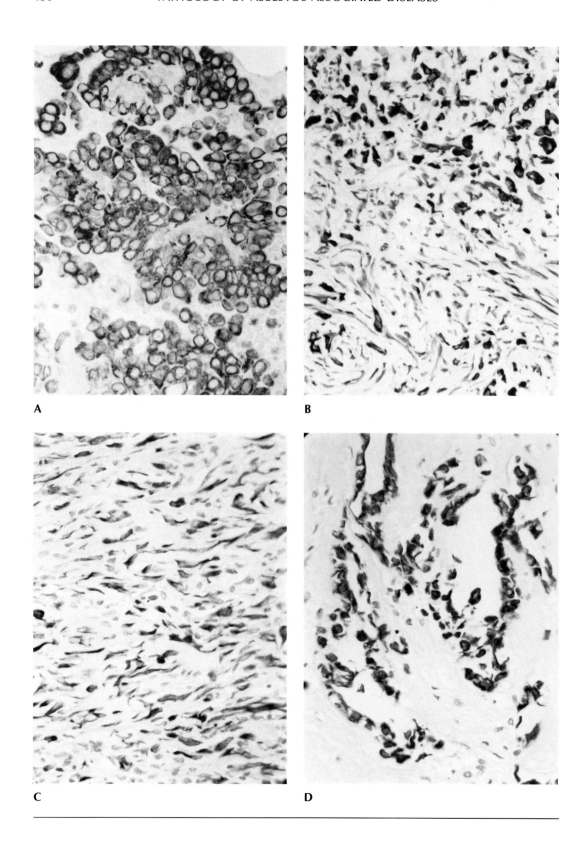

and 19. Four of these (7, 8, 18, and 19) are also found in adeno-carcinomas.[124] Panels of monoclonal antibodies directed against subsets of the 19 known keratins are available, and these may prove useful in discriminating between patterns of cytokeratin production in mesotheliomas as compared to adenocarcinomas of various origins.[112] For example, a monoclonal antibody (AE-14) directed against cytokeratin 5 has shown promising results in discriminating between epithelial and biphasic mesotheliomas (12 of 13 cases staining positively) as compared to pulmonary adenocarcinomas (negative staining in 15 cases and staining of only a few cells in an additional six cases). However, this antibody does not work on formalin-fixed, paraffin-embedded tissues.[125]

Some authors have claimed that the pattern of keratin immuno-reactivity is of diagnostic utility. Kahn et al.[126] studied the distribution of cytoplasmic keratin staining in 10 adenocarcinomas and four mesotheliomas using a number of polyclonal and monoclonal anti-keratin antibodies. A perinuclear pattern of staining was observed in mesotheliomas, whereas a weblike pattern occurred in adenocarcinomas. These different staining patterns were visualized when the di-aminobenzidine color reaction was allowed to proceed for less than two minutes. Further studies are necessary to confirm the diagnostic utility of these observations.

Recently, investigators have turned their attention toward examining the utility of antikeratin antibodies in the diagnosis of sarcomatous mesotheliomas. We have previously reported that none of seven sarcomatous mesotheliomas was positive for cytokeratins.[2] However, this study employed a polyclonal antibody prepared against human callus keratins, and only 39% of adenocarcinomas examined (7 of 18) showed positive staining with this antibody.[2] In contrast, Bolen et al.[113] used a number of different monoclonal antikeratin antibodies on acid ethanol-fixed, paraffin-embedded sections and found positive staining for cytokeratins in all seven cases of sarcomatous mesothelioma they examined. Subsequent studies have confirmed the positive staining of the spindle-cell component of mesotheliomas for cytokeratins when sensitive monoclonal antibodies are used, and documented the usefulness of this technique for distinguishing sarcomatoid mesothelioma from other spindle-cell malignancies.[127,128] We have similarly observed positive staining of the spindle-cell component of the vast majority of mesotheliomas, using monoclonal antibodies AE_1/AE_3 (see Fig. 5-11). Reactive fibrous pleural lesions,

FIGURE 5-11. Immunohistochemical staining for cytokeratins using a cocktail of monoclonal antibodies to high- and low-molecular-weight keratins. (A) Diffuse cytoplasmic staining in a predominately epithelial mesothelioma. (B) Staining of epithelial components (*top*) and spindle-cell components (*bottom*) of a biphasic mesothelioma. (C) Cytoplasmic staining of spindle cells in a predominately sarcomatous mesothelioma. (D) Diffuse cytoplasmic staining in an adenocarcinoma metastatic to pleura.

including parietal pleural plaques and fibrosis induced by metastases, also show positive staining of spindle cells for cytokeratins; therefore, this technique is of no use in distinguishing between reactive and neoplastic mesothelial proliferations.[113,128] Furthermore, other sarcomas, including synovial sarcoma and epithelioid sarcoma, demonstrate positive staining for cytokeratins,[8] and recent reports indicate that some leiomyosarcomas and malignant fibrous histiocytomas may show positive staining as well.[129,130] In addition, cytokeratin antibodies will not discriminate between the spindle-cell component of malignant mesothelioma and that of spindle-cell squamous carcinomas of the lung.[131]

Vimentin is the other intermediate filament that forms part of the cytoskeletal network of mesothelial cells. A number of studies have examined the possibility of using antibodies to vimentin as an aid in the diagnosis of malignant mesothelioma. Churg[132] reported that coexpression of vimentin and cytokeratin in tumor cells is a useful feature for distinguishing malignant mesothelioma from adenocarcinoma, although fixation in acid-alcohol solution is necessary for optimal detection of vimentin. Mullink et al.[133] used a double immunoenzyme staining technique to detect coexpression of vimentin and keratin within individual tumor cells, and also concluded that this finding was useful in making the distinction between mesothelioma and adenocarcinoma. On the other hand, Hammar[8] reported that most epithelial mesotheliomas are negative for vimentin, whereas some large-cell carcinomas of the lung coexpress vimentin and cytokeratins. Other neoplasms also have been reported to coexpress these two types of intermediate filaments, including carcinomas of the kidney and thyroid gland, pleomorphic adenomas of the salivary gland, and metastatic carcinoma cells within effusions.[2,124] It is also a widespread phenomenon in cell cultures. Expression of vimentin does not aid in the differentiation of reactive from neoplastic mesothelium.[113]

Carcinoembryonic antigen (CEA) has proven to be a most useful marker for distinguishing malignant epithelial mesotheliomas from adenocarcinomas. CEA is an oncofetal protein that is often abundant in neoplasms of endodermal origin, including carcinomas of the lung and the gastrointestinal tract. Wang et al.[134] were the first to report that mesotheliomas fail to express CEA as determined by the immunoperoxidase method. Corson and Pinkus,[118] using a polyclonal anti-CEA antibody, observed that some epithelial mesotheliomas stain weakly for CEA, but that the intensity was less than that observed in adenocarcinomas. This observation has since been confirmed by others for both epithelial and sarcomatous mesotheliomas.[2,135,136] Immunoperoxidase staining for CEA (along with pattern of cytokeratin immunoreactivity and mucin histochemistry) has also been reported useful for distinguishing adenocarcinoma from malignant mesothelioma in cell blocks of malignant effusions.[137] Monoclonal antibodies to CEA have been reported to give cleaner backgrounds, less nonspecific cross-reactivity, and higher specificity for mesotheliomas, with no false positives in 28 pleural mesotheliomas.[138] However, the sensitivity of this antibody is also reduced, with only 72% of 50 adenocarcinomas showing positive staining. When polyclonal commercial CEA antibodies are employed, the results should be interpreted with caution, since inflammatory cells, areas of necrosis, and lung tissue will stain positive with polyclonal anti-CEA[2] (Fig. 5-12).

None of these immunohistochemical techniques has proven totally satisfactory in all cases, so other approaches have been investigated. Singh et al.[139] prepared a polyclonal antibody by injecting cells cultured from human serous effusions into rabbits and rats, and showed that the antibody reacted with tumor cells of malignant mesotheliomas in an indirect immunofluorescence assay. Donna et al.[140,141] prepared a polyclonal antibody against a protein isolated from the cytoplasm of mesothelioma cells. This antibody was used in an immunoperoxidase procedure on formalin-fixed, paraffin-embedded tissue sections, and was shown to react with all tumors derived from coelomic surfaces but not with a wide variety of other tumors. Anderson et al.[142] isolated a monoclonal antibody derived from mice immunized with a human mesothelioma cell line, and showed that this antibody bound to biphasic mesotheliomas but not to normal lung and pleura using an immunoperoxidase technique. The antibody reacted with only four of seven mesothelioma cell lines and showed some reactivity against a few carcinoma, sarcoma, and melanoma cell lines. Stahel et al.[143,144] prepared monoclonal antibodies against a mesothelioma cell line that distinguished malignant mesothelioma from pulmonary adenocarcinoma on cryostat sections. However, some lung squamous cell carcinomas, breast carcinomas, and ovarian carcinomas also showed focal staining. Hsu et al.[145] prepared a monoclonal antibody against a mesothelial cell line that reacted with all five mesotheliomas tested but with none of 26 carcinomas from various sites (including seven pulmonary adenocarcinomas). This antibody worked well on frozen cryostat sections but failed to stain formalin-fixed or paraffin-embedded tissue sections.

Other investigators have studied monoclonal antibodies that react with adenocarcinomas but not with mesotheliomas and therefore demonstrate differential diagnostic potential. Szpak et al.[146] reported that monoclonal antibody B72.3, generated against a membrane-enriched fraction of human metastatic breast carcinoma, gave positive results with the immunoperoxidase technique in 19 of 22 pulmonary adenocarcinomas but in none of 20 cases of malignant mesothelioma. This specificity of monoclonal antibody B72.3 was confirmed by Otis et al.,[147] although only half of their cases of adenocarcinoma were positive. Sheibani et al.[138] found that a monoclonal antibody directed against the Leu-M1 antigen reacted with 47 of 50 primary adenocarcinomas of the lung but with none of 28 pleural mesotheliomas. Wick et al.[148] reported similar findings in a study of 41 epithelial malignant mesotheliomas and 43 adenocarcinomas involving serosal surfaces. The specificity of the Leu-M1 monoclonal antibody was also confirmed by Otis et al.;[147] but again, only half of the

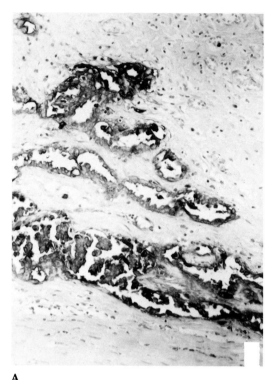

A

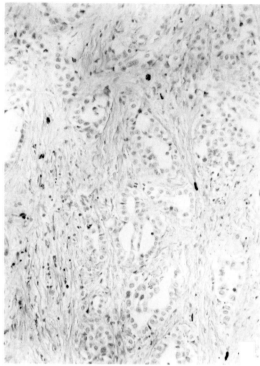

B

C

FIGURE 5-12. Immunohistochemical staining for carcinoembryonic antigen (CEA) using a polyclonal commercial antibody. (A) In this adenocarcinoma metastatic to the pleura, the tumor cells are strongly positive for CEA. (B) In this epithelial mesothelioma, the tumor cells are negative for CEA. (C) Nests of mesothelial tumor cells have invaded alveolar spaces (arrowheads). Note strong positivity of alveolar septa and type II cells for CEA, but negative staining of tumor cells. Reprinted from Ref. 2, with permission.

adenocarcinomas tested were positive. A subsequent study by War-nock et al.[149] confirmed the differential diagnostic utility of both B72.3 and Leu M1 monoclonal antibodies, with none of 38 mesotheliomas staining with either antibody. However, B72.3 reacted with 86%, whereas Leu M1 reacted with 57% of 44 lung carcinomas tested in this study. Similar results were reported by Ordóñez.[150]

Lee et al.[151] studied two monoclonal antibodies raised against human pulmonary carcinoma cell lines and compared them with broad-spectrum antikeratin antibody and polyclonal anti-CEA for their ability to discriminate between malignant mesothelioma and metastatic pulmonary adenocarcinoma involving the pleura. These investigators found that one monoclonal antibody (624 A12) reacted with 9 of 10 metastatic adenocarcinomas but none of 43 mesotheliomas, whereas the other antibody (44–3A6) strongly stained all 10 adenocarcinomas but showed focal weak immunoreactivity for only 10 of 43 mesotheliomas. The combined use of these monoclonal antibodies was deemed superior to anti-CEA and antikeratin for this differential diagnosis.

Another novel approach is the use of lectin immunohistochemistry to distinguish the surface glycoconjugate profiles of malignant mesothelioma and pulmonary adenocarcinoma. Kawai et al.[152] report that stains for Ricinus communis (RCA–1) and succinylated wheat germ agglutinin are potentially useful in this regard. In addition, Noguchi et al.[153] report that the majority of peripheral pulmonary adenocarcinomas of the non-mucus-producing type react with antibodies directed against surfactant apoprotein or certain blood group antigens (Lewis[a] and Tn antigen), whereas mesotheliomas, with rare exceptions, did not stain with these antibodies.

Antibodies that appear of no use in distinguishing mesothelioma from adenocarcinoma include antibodies to epithelial membrane antigen and human milk-fat globule. Battifora and Kopinski[119] reported that a monoclonal antibody directed against human milk-fat globule (MFG-2) reacted with all 64 adenocarcinomas originating in the breast, lung, or ovary, but with none of 12 malignant mesotheliomas. On the other hand, Bolen et al.[113] found no discriminating utility of two different monoclonal antibodies directed against human milk-fat globule, a finding since confirmed by others.[137,150,154] Pinkus and Kurtin,[155] using a monoclonal antibody against epithelial membrane antigen (EMA), found equal reactivity against mesotheliomas (six of six) and a wide variety of carcinomas. These observations have also been confirmed.[8,137,150] In addition, antibodies directed against laminin, laminin receptors, or Type IV collagen do not distinguish malignant mesotheliomas from adenocarcinomas of the lung or breast.[156]

The immunohistochemical staining reactions of mesotheliomas, reactive mesothelium, adenocarcinomas, and most sarcomas for cytokeratins, vimentin, and CEA are summarized in Table 5-3. Antibodies to CEA appear useful for distinguishing epithelial mesotheliomas from adenocarcinomas, whereas antikeratin antibodies assist

TABLE 5-3. Immunohistochemical staining for some common antigens in malignant mesothelioma, reactive mesothelium, and other neoplasms[a]

	Cytokeratins[b]	Vimentin	CEA
Malignant mesothelioma			
Epithelial	+	±	−[c]
Biphasic	+	+	−
Sarcomatous	+	+	−
Reactive mesothelium	+	±	−
Adenocarcinomas	+	±	+[c]
Soft-tissue sarcomas	−[d]	+	−

[a]+ = Positive; − = Negative; ± = Variable staining
[b]Monoclonal antibody "cocktail" for high and low molecular weight keratins
[c]A few epithelial mesotheliomas show focal staining with polyclonal anti-CEA, and some adenocarcinomas are negative, esp. with monoclonal anti-CEA
[d]See text for exceptions

in the distinction between sarcomatous mesotheliomas and most soft-tissue sarcomas. Monoclonal antibodies to vimentin, Leu M1, and tumor-associated glycoprotein (B72.3) also appear to have some discriminating value. None is 100% accurate, and results should be interpreted in conjunction with other histopathologic findings. Some investigators prefer to use panels composed of specific monoclonal antibodies directed against a variety of antigens,[8,147,154,157] and this approach may hold the greatest promise for accurate diagnosis.

Ultrastructural Features
There is no single ultrastructural hallmark that is unique to mesothelioma. Rather, there is a constellation of ultrastructural findings characteristic of malignant mesotheliomas.[2,8] These findings include: abundant intermediate filaments often organized into tonofibrillar bundles; long, sinuous, slender surface microvilli with a tendency to branch; and often prominent accumulations of intracytoplasmic glycogen[158–163] [Fig. 5-13 (A)]. In contrast, adenocarcinomas have relatively few intermediate filaments and short, blunt microvilli [see Fig. 5-13 (B)]. The subjective differences in microvillus structure between mesotheliomas and adenocarcinomas have resulted in attempts by several investigators to establish more objective criteria by measuring the length-to-diameter ratio of the five to 10 longest microvilli in a field.[161–163] For epithelial mesotheliomas, this ratio is greater than 10 in most cases that have been studied. Conversely, for adenocarcinomas the ratio is less than 10 in almost all reported cases.[2,157,161–163] Intracellular lumina of epithelial mesotheliomas often are lined by these long microvilli, which are sometimes embedded in electron-dense deposits of hyaluronic acid that has been secreted by the tumor cell.[8] On the other hand, surface microvilli of adenocarcinoma cells often have prominent rootlets and glycocalyx, sometimes associated with glycocalyceal bodies.[8] Another interesting observation is the presence of microvilli making direct contact with

collagen fibers through basement membrane defects on the abluminal side of tumor cells, a finding that was noted in 10 of 12 mesotheliomas but in none of 20 adenocarcinomas.[164]

Intercellular junctions of the macula adherens type (true desmosomes) are found with equal frequency in epithelial mesotheliomas and adenocarcinomas.[2] However, there are some qualitative differences that have been reported in the junctions found in these two types of malignancies. Burns et al.[165] used transmission electron microscopic morphometry to measure desmosomes in epithelial malignant mesotheliomas and adenocarcinomas, and found that "giant" desmosomes (i.e., desmosomes greater than $1\,\mu$ in length) were more frequent in the former than in the latter. Nevertheless, the mean desmosomal length was not significantly different between the two groups.[165] Mukherjee et al.[166] reported a freeze-fracture study of intercellular junctions in two cases of pleural mesothelioma obtained by biopsy, and noted that both tight and gap junctions were less well developed and less numerous than in exfoliated mesothelioma cells in effusions or benign mesothelial cells. It would be of interest to perform similar studies comparing the freeze-fracture characteristics of intercellular junctions in epithelial mesotheliomas versus adenocarcinomas obtained by biopsies as well as effusions.

In a recent review, Dardick et al.[167] emphasized that all of the fine structural diagnostic criteria of malignant epithelial mesothelioma are expressed to varying degrees in individual cases, and the absence of any one feature (such as long surface microvilli) does not preclude a diagnosis of mesothelioma. Tonofibrillar bundles are present in significantly greater numbers in epithelial mesotheliomas as compared to adenocarcinomas,[2,161] and are often found in a perinuclear distribution [see Fig. 5-13 (A)]. However, they may be absent in some epithelial mesotheliomas,[8,161] and they may be prominent in squamous cell carcinomas or adenosquamous carcinomas of the lung [see Fig. 5-13 (C)]. Certain ultrastructural features when present will confirm a diagnosis of adenocarcinoma and exclude mesothelioma. These include the identification of mucous granules, Clara cell granules, and lamellar bodies.[8] In addition, dense-core neuroendocrine-type granules occur in some pulmonary carcinomas but have not been reported in mesotheliomas.

Sarcomatous mesotheliomas generally have ultrastructural features that resemble those of soft-tissue fibrosarcoma[2] [see Fig. 5-13 (D)]. The tumor cells are elongated or spindle-shaped with elongated nuclei, prominent nucleoli, short cytoplasmic fragments of distended rough endoplasmic reticulum, occasionally prominent intermediate cytoplasmic filaments, and variable amounts of extracellular collagen. In some cases, the tumor cells resemble myofibroblasts, with peripherally located actin filaments[8] occasionally associated with dense bodies.[168] Cells with transitional features intermediate between epithelial and mesenchymal cells have also been described.[168] These features include the presence of intercellular junctions, occasional

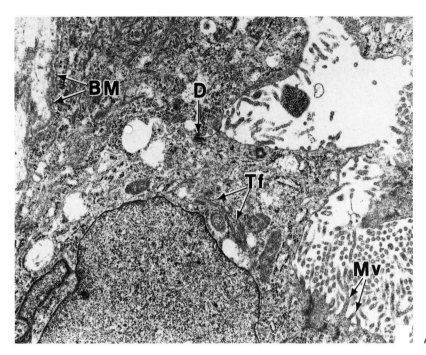

A

FIGURE 5-13. (A) This epithelial mesothelioma illustrates long, slender microvilli (Mv), tonofibrillar bundles (Tf), desmosomes (D), and basement membrane (BM).(B) Blunt surface microvilli (Mv) and a junctional complex (JC) are observed in this adenocarcinoma metastatic to the pleura. Intermediate filaments and tonofibrillar bundles are not identified. (C) Numerous tonofibrillar bundles (Tf) and prominent desmosomes (D) are present in this squamous cell carcinoma of the lung. (D) This sarcomatous mesothelioma demonstrates spindle cells with cytoplasmic filaments (F) and abundant extracellular collagen (Co), N = nucleus. Transmission electron micrographs, part (A) ×10,000, part (B) ×6000, part (C) ×6000, part (D) ×4000. Parts (A), (B), and (D) reprinted from Ref. 2, with permission.

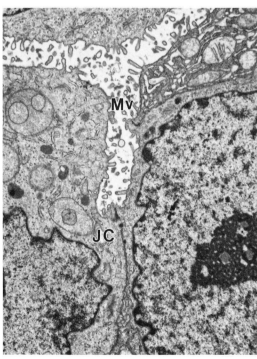

B

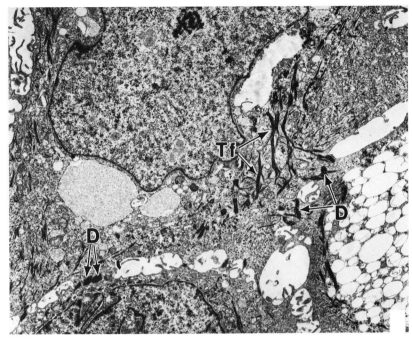

C

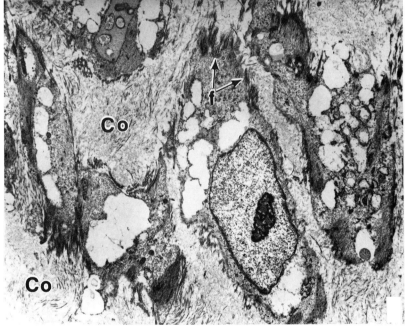

D

surface microvilli, incomplete basement membrane, and even a few tonofibrillar bundles.

In summary, ultrastructural features of a tumor may be quite useful in the diagnosis of malignant mesothelioma[2,8] (Table 5-4). However, since there are no ultrastructural hallmarks for mesothelioma that are invariably present in all cases, the ultrastructural features of a tumor need to be considered in the context of the surgical, radiographic, and histologic findings.[167]

Differential Diagnosis

Malignant mesothelioma must be distinguished on the one hand from benign reactive pleural abnormalities, and on the other from various metastatic and primary neoplasms involving the pleura.

The distinction between reactive mesothelial hyperplasia and an early or well-differentiated epithelial mesothelioma can be quite difficult to make, especially when dealing with small samples (e.g., needle biopsy). The formation of tumor masses or the presence of true pleural invasion (being careful to avoid the pitfall of tangential sections!) establishes the diagnosis of malignancy. The findings of necrosis and cytologic atypia are also useful features, although reactive mesothelial cells have a wide range of nuclear variability, and there is some overlap histologically between reactive and neoplastic mesothelial cells.[12] In some cases, sampling may show obvious malignant mesothelioma at one site and atypical reactive changes at another. With generous sampling and careful attention to cytologic details, the distinction between malignant epithelial mesothelioma and reactive mesothelial hyperplasia is readily apparent in most instances.[2]

Similar difficulty may arise when attempting to distinguish between reactive fibroblastic pleural lesions and the desmoplastic variant of malignant pleural mesothelioma. Storiform arrangement of the collagen bundles, focal areas of bland necrosis within the thickened pleura, and frankly sarcomatous areas are features indicative of mesothelioma. Invasion into skeletal muscle fibers in the chest wall or into subpleural fat also establishes a diagnosis of malignancy [Fig. 5-14 (A)].[169] On the other hand, reactive processes usually have a fibrinous surface exudate and show a tendency for maturation [see Fig. 5-14 (B)]; that is, the most cellular areas are adjacent to the fibrin-covered inner surface (nearest the pleural space), and the least cellular areas adjacent to the chest wall (furthest from the pleural space).[170] Cytokeratin immunohistochemistry is of limited utility, since the spindle cells in reactive fibrous pleural lesions are invariably positive for keratins[128,169,171] [see Fig. 5-14 (C)]. However, immunostaining for cytokeratins may be helpful in difficult cases by demonstrating subtle invasion of adipose tissue by keratin-positive spindle cells.[103] A feature that favors a benign, reactive process is the presence of capillaries almost completely traversing the thickened pleura in a direction perpendicular to the pleural surface [see Fig. 5-14 (D)].

TABLE 5-4. Ultrastructural features of malignant mesothelioma and adenocarcinoma*

	Adenocarcinoma	Malignant mesothelioma, epithelial component	Malignant mesothelioma, sarcomatous component
Microvilli	Short, blunt microvilli; LDR < 10; may have prominent rootlets, glycocalyx, and glycocalyceal bodies	Long, sinuous, often branching microvilli; LDR usually > 10; may have microvilli contacting collagen fibers thru BM discontinuities on abluminal side	Generally absent; occasional cell may show a few short surface microvilli
Intermediate filaments	Generally sparse; occasional to rare tonofibrillar bundles	Generally abundant; tonofibrillar bundles numerous in about 70% of cases	May be abundant in some cells; tonofibrillar bundles sparse to absent
Intercellular junctions	Desmosomes and junctional complexes regularly present; rare "giant" desmosomes	Desmosomes and junctional complexes regularly present; occasional "giant" desmosome	Desmosomes generally absent; occasional intermediate-type junctions in some cases
Other features	Mucous granules, Clara cell granules, or lamellar bodies frequently present; intracellular lumina common	Occasional lysosomes; intracellular lumina common, sometimes with electron-dense secretion	Peripheral actin filaments may be present; short cytoplasmic fragments of distended RER

SOURCE: Modified from Refs. 2 and 8.
*LDR = Average length-to-diameter ratio of microvilli (see text); RER = Rough endoplasmic reticulum; BM = Basement membrane

Distinguishing between metastatic adenocarcinoma and malignant epithelial mesothelioma is the most common diagnostic problem facing the surgical pathologist confronted with a biopsy of a pleural malignancy. The difficulty of the problem increases as the tumor cells become more anaplastic.[2] The techniques available to the pathologist to assist in making this distinction include histochemistry, immunohistochemistry, and electron microscopy, and the discriminating features are discussed in detail in their respective sections (see earlier) and are summarized in Tables 5-2 through 5-4. In brief, epithelial mesotheliomas tend to contain hyaluronic acid, abundant tonofilaments, and long microvilli, whereas adenocarcinomas often exhibit neutral mucins, acid mucopolysaccharides other than hyaluronic acid, CEA, short microvilli, and scanty intermediate filaments by electron microscopy.[2] Metastatic renal cell carcinoma involving the pleura may be particularly difficult to distinguish from a biphasic mesothelioma.[172] These tumors may also be biphasic and often exhibit histochemical and immunohistochemical features similar to those of biphasic mesothelioma (e.g., tumor cells may be positive for both vimentin and cytokeratin). However, the presence of a substantial clear-cell component to the tumor is an important clue, since a clear-cell pattern is not a prominent feature of malignant mesothelioma.

Other neoplasms that can involve the pleura include localized fibrous tumors of the pleura, angiosarcoma of the pleura, lymphomas and leukemias, and soft-tissue sarcomas (either from the chest wall or metastatic from a distant site).[8,12] Localized fibrous tumors of the pleura have histological features that overlap to some degree with those of sarcomatous pleural mesotheliomas. They are distinguished by their gross appearance, which is that of a circumscribed spherical mass or cushion, often with a pedunculated attachment to the pleura.[2] The spindle-shaped tumor cells of localized fibrous tumors of the pleura have been negative for cytokeratins in most cases that have been examined immunohistochemically.[8,173–176] Angiosarcomas of the pleura are exceedingly rare[12] and consist of pleomorphic malignant endothelial cells lining irregular vascular spaces. The tumor cells of angiosarcoma are often positive for Factor VIII antigen immunohistochemically and contain diagnostic Weibel-Palade bodies ultrastructurally. Lymphomas and leukemias involving the pleura must

FIGURE 5-14. (A) Invasion of skeletal muscle fibers of chest wall (arrowheads) by sarcomatous pleural mesothelioma. (B) Chronic organizing pleuritis shows a fibrinous surface exudate and markedly thickened parietal pleura. (C) Immunoperoxidase staining for cytokeratins shows positive-staining spindle cells in chronic organizing pleuritis. (D) Immunoperoxidase staining for Factor VIII antigen delineates capillaries oriented perpendicular to the pleural surface almost completely traversing the fibrotic, thickened pleura. [Parts (B), (C), and (D) from same case.] Part (A) ×130, part (B) ×40, part (C) ×325, and part (D) ×40.

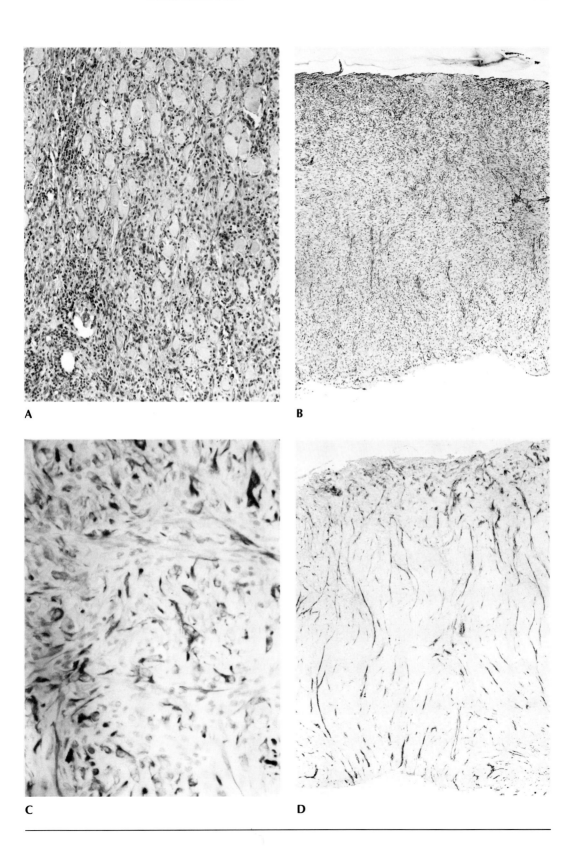

A

B

C

D

be distinguished from the lymphohistiocytoid variant of malignant mesothelioma.[95] In such cases, the underlying neoplastic mesothelial cells can be recognized by their cytokeratin positivity by immunohistochemistry and their ultrastructural features.[95] Soft-tissue sarcomas involving the chest wall and secondarily invading the pleura may rarely pose a diagnostic problem; keratin-positivity of the spindle cells may be useful in confirming a diagnosis of sarcomatous pleural mesothelioma and excluding a chest wall sarcoma.[176] Metastases from soft-tissue sarcomas to the thorax are usually due to hematogenous spread, and appear as spherical intrapulmonary masses that are bilateral and most prominent in the lower lobes. The pleura may on occasion be involved, but such metastatic deposits have not been observed to produce the diffuse pleural thickening seen in advanced mesothelioma.[12]

A proposed scheme for differentiating between malignant pleural mesothelioma and other malignancies involving the pleura is presented in Fig. 5-15. The suggested sequence of diagnostic procedures is based in part on the time and expense involved in performing ultrastructural studies. The diagnosis should be apparent in most instances without the requirement for electron microscopy.[2] Tumors displaying the typical gross features of mesothelioma with a biphasic or sarcomatous histologic pattern are, in the authors' opinion, diagnostic of mesothelioma. In doubtful cases, immunohistochemistry for cytokeratins may be beneficial by identifying keratin-positive spindle cells in the tumor. In attempting to distinguish malignant mesothelioma from other malignant tumors, it is important to consider that a patient may have both. We have observed four cases of dual primary malignancies in a series of 129 consecutive pleural mesotheliomas (3.1%). These included two cases of biphasic pleural mesothelioma and adenocarcinoma of the prostate, one case of granular cell variant of renal adenocarcinoma and desmoplastic mesothelioma, and one case of epithelial mesothelioma and metastatic melanoma. Careful attention to histologic patterns and additional studies such as immunohistochemistry may be necessary to ascertain whether two separate primary malignancies are in fact present. The frequency of a second primary malignancy in patients with pleural mesothelioma (3.1%) is not different from the rate of second primary malignancies in general (2–3%).[177]

PERITONEAL MESOTHELIOMA

The peritoneum is the second most common site of involvement by malignant (diffuse) mesothelioma, accounting for about 10% of cases.[75] Peritoneal mesotheliomas tend to spread over the surface of the abdominal viscera in a way similar to that in which pleural mesotheliomas spread over the surface of the lung. As a result, the tumor eventually encases the abdominal organs (Fig. 5-16). The tumor is generally firm and white, studding the peritoneal surface with numerous individual nodules in a pattern indistinguishable from

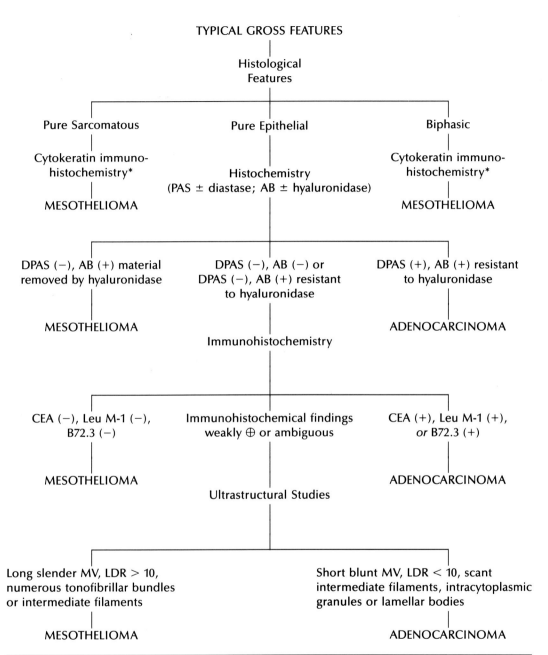

FIGURE 5-15. Diagnostic approach for distinguishing malignant mesothelioma and metastatic adenocarcinoma to the pleura (or peritoneum). Typical gross features include tendency to spread along visceral surfaces, as determined by radiographic or computed tomographic studies, direct observation at thoracotomy or laparotomy, or autopsy. Histologic recognition of a tumor as pure sarcomatous or pure epithelial presupposes adequate sampling.
*Optional studies reserved primarily for ambiguous cases.
DPAS = Periodic acid Schiff with prior diastase digestion; AB = Alcian blue; CEA = Carcinoembryonic antigen; MV = Microvilli; LDR = length-to-diameter ratio of MV. Modified from Ref. 2, with permission.

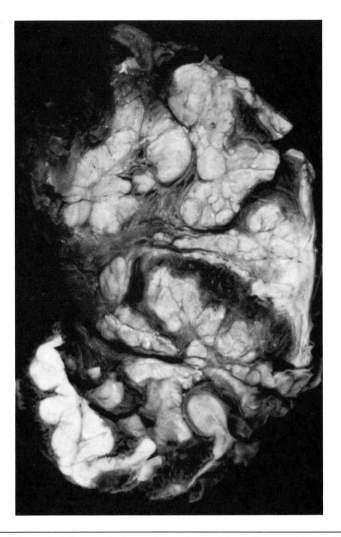

FIGURE 5-16. Coronal slice of abdominal viscera in patient with malignant (diffuse) peritoneal mesothelioma shows encasement and compression of bowel (dark areas) by confluent nodules of tumor. Reprinted from Ref. 2, with permission.

peritoneal carcinomatosis. Plaques of tumor or matted masses may also be seen. The omentum is often markedly thickened by infiltrating tumor, and adhesions may be prominent. These gross pathologic features correlate well with the clinical symptoms at presentation, which include cramping abdominal pain, weight loss, and increasing abdominal girth. The latter is related to the large amount of ascitic fluid that accumulates. In some cases, bowel obstruction may occur. As with pleural mesothelioma, clinically evident distant metastases are seldom noted at initial presentation, although they are commonly found at autopsy.[57,178] Extension to involve one or both pleural cavities may occur,[179] sometimes making it difficult to discern the exact site of origin.[12] At autopsy, careful inspection of the viscera is necessary in order to exclude a primary malignancy with secondary peritoneal involvement. This is most likely to occur with carcinomas of the stomach, pancreas, or ovaries.[2]

The diagnosis of malignant peritoneal mesothelioma depends on the finding of the typical gross features as described earlier, identification of a histologic pattern compatible with mesothelioma, and exclusion of metastatic tumor (peritoneal carcinomatosis). In surgical cases, information regarding the gross distribution of tumor can be obtained from computed tomography of the abdomen and/or direct observations by the surgeon at laparotomy. Surgical exploration is generally required in order to obtain sufficient quantities of tissue to permit an accurate pathologic assessment and to inspect carefully the abdominal viscera for the presence of an occult primary malignancy.[2] For example, in a report of 18 cases of peritoneal mesothelioma diagnosed by laparoscopy and peritoneal biopsy, eight were rejected on subsequent pathologic review.[180] Peritoneal mesotheliomas exhibit the same histologic spectrum as pleural mesotheliomas. In the authors' series of 27 peritoneal mesotheliomas, 18 were epithelial, eight were biphasic, and only one was purely sarcomatous (Fig. 5-17). Cases of diffuse peritoneal mesothelioma have also been reported in which the tumor presented with innumerable cysts involving the visceral and parietal peritoneum.[181–183] However, it has been argued that such cases do not represent mesotheliomas at all, but rather are examples of a nonneoplastic reactive mesothelial proliferation.[184] The histochemical, immunohistochemical, and ultrastructural features of peritoneal mesothelioma are similar to those of pleural mesothelioma, although fewer cases have been studied.[2,12,57,101,119,158,163,185,186]

Malignant peritoneal mesothelioma must be distinguished from reactive mesothelial hyperplasia, metastatic carcinoma with secondary involvement of the peritoneum, and other papillary peritoneal tumors in women.[2] The peritoneal mesothelium has a remarkable capacity for undergoing marked hyperplastic changes, with formation of papillary structures, pseudoacini, or squamous nests. Especially exuberant hyperplastic responses may occur in patients with cirrhosis and ascites.[187] The demonstration of invasion and the presence of focal necrosis and nuclear anaplasia permit the distinction between malignant mesothelioma and reactive hyperplasia. Metastatic carcinomas involving the peritoneum are frequently mucin positive [Fig. 5-18 (A)], and this finding can be confirmed by means of a positive PAS stain following diastase treatment, which essentially excludes the diagnosis of mesothelioma. A broad histologic spectrum of papillary tumors of the peritoneum occur in women, some of which behave aggressively and resemble serous papillary adenocarcinomas of the ovary, presumably deriving from extraovarian epithelium with Müllerian potential.[188,189] These serous papillary adenocarcinomas of

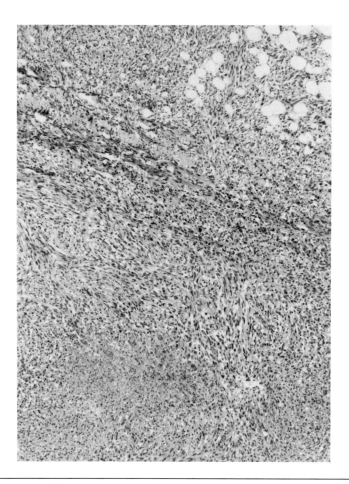

FIGURE 5-17. Sarcomatous diffuse peritoneal mesothelioma shows invasion of peritoneal fat (*upper right*) and a focus of necrosis (*lower left*). Extensive sampling at autopsy showed that the tumor had a sarcomatous appearance throughout. H&E ×68.

the peritoneum often show considerable nuclear anaplasia and mitotic activity, usually demonstrate scattered intracytoplasmic mucin vacuoles with the PAS stain, and may contain numerous psammoma bodies [see Fig. 5-18 (B)]. Peritoneal mesotheliomas of the papillary type may have scattered psammoma bodies, but they are usually not prominent.[12] Some well-differentiated epithelial mesotheliomas occurring predominately in women have been described that consist of a single layer of flattened-to-cuboidal mesothelial cells lining vascular papillary fibrous cores [see Fig. 5-18 (C)]. These tumors often follow an indolent course with prolonged survival.[2,12,188,190]

In some cases, immunohistochemical studies or electron microscopy may be required to distinguish between peritoneal mesothelioma and other malignant tumors involving the peritoneum. Epithelial mesotheliomas are generally negative for CEA[185,191] and

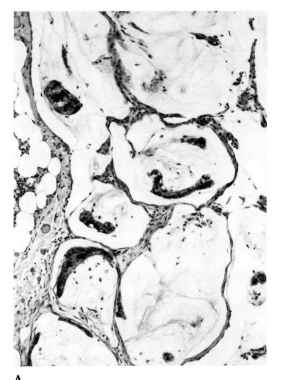

A

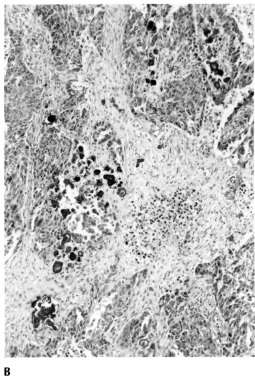

B

C

FIGURE 5-18. (A) Metastatic mucin-producing adenocarcinoma in the peritoneum consists of pools of mucin within spaces lined by delicate connective tissue stroma. Some of the spaces are partially lined by a layer of tall columnar tumor cells. (B) Serous papillary adenocarcinoma of the peritoneum contains numerous psammoma bodies (arrowheads) in this field. These tumors often have PAS-positive cytoplasmic mucin vacuoles as well. (C) Papillary peritoneal tumor, or well-differentiated epithelial mesothelioma, shows vascular papillary fibrous cores lined by a single layer of flattened-to-cuboidal epithelium. The tumor recurred 11 years later, and the patient was still alive 13 years after the initial diagnosis. H&E: Part (A) ×100, part (B) ×100, and part (C) ×170. Parts (A) and (C) reprinted from Ref. 2, with permission.

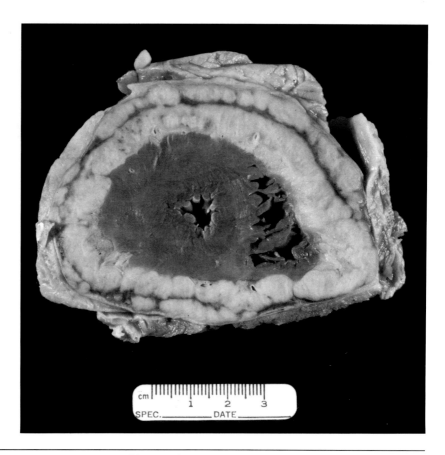

FIGURE 5-19. Transverse section of heart, showing complete encasement by malignant pericardial mesothelioma.

possess long, branching microvilli,[158,163,191] whereas metastatic adenocarcinomas are often positive for CEA[118] and possess short, stubby microvilli.[162]

PERICARDIAL MESOTHELIOMA

Pericardial mesotheliomas are the least common of the malignant (diffuse) mesotheliomas.[2,75] These tumors invade the parietal and visceral pericardium, eventually encasing the heart in a mass of tumor (Fig. 5-19). A pericardial effusion is often present and may be bloody. Clinically, these patients present with arrhythmias, cardiac failure, or pericardial constriction.[192–194] Weight loss and anorexia may also occur. Chest roentgenograms show cardiac enlargement or a mass, and low voltage in the anterior leads is demonstrable by electrocardiogram. One case report noted abnormal pericardial uptake by means of gallium-67 scintigraphy.[194] Magnetic resonance imaging may facilitate the delineation of the location and extent of tumor.[195] Microscopic examination has shown a biphasic pattern in most cases, but epithelial and sarcomatous variants have also been described.[75] Immunohistochemical and ultrastructural studies have only rarely been reported,[192,193,196] but these tumors appear to be morphologically identical to their pleural and peritoneal counterparts.[2] Pericardial mesotheliomas must be distinguished from the much more common metastatic carcinoma involving the pericardium or epicardium.[197,198] In addition, pleural mesotheliomas often extend to and invade the contiguous pericardium,[12] further complicating the diagnosis of primary pericardial mesothelioma. The so-called mesothelioma of the atrioventricular node is a benign tumor that is not derived from mesothelium at all but rather from endoderm.[2,199–201] Several cases of pericardial mesothelioma have been reported in individuals exposed to asbestos.[202–205]

MESOTHELIOMA OF THE TUNICA VAGINALIS TESTIS

The tunica vaginalis testis is an extension of the peritoneum, and as such is lined by a layer of mesothelial cells. Rare examples of malignant mesothelioma arising from the tunica vaginalis testis have been reported.[206] Clinically, these tumors present as a hydrocele or scrotal mass. The histologic spectrum is similar to that of other malignant mesotheliomas, ranging from sarcomatous to papillary epithelial variants.[206] Epithelial variants that have been examined ultrastructurally have features similar to those of mesothelioma occurring elsewhere. In a few cases, malignant mesothelioma of the tunica vaginalis testis has been associated with a history of exposure to asbestos.[206] These rare lesions may represent malignant counterparts of the benign adenomatoid tumor, for which there is also histochemical and ultrastructural evidence for a mesothelial derivation.[207]

TREATMENT AND PROGNOSIS

The prognosis for malignant (diffuse) mesothelioma is poor.[2] The median survival from the time of initial diagnosis in several large series has ranged from 7 to 15 months.[208–214] There seems general agreement that a good performance status[209,213] and early stage at time of diagnosis[209,212–214] are favorable prognostic factors. Several schemes for staging malignant pleural mesotheliomas have been proposed (Table 5-5),[215–217] and patients with early-stage disease are the most likely to benefit from aggressive therapy. Some studies have suggested that survival for peritoneal mesotheliomas is worse than that for pleural mesotheliomas,[209,210] although this observation was not confirmed in the large study of 1475 cases conducted by the Surveillance, Epidemiology and End Results (SEER) Program.[212] Similarly, it has been reported that the prognosis is better for epithelial versus sarcomatous mesotheliomas,[208,209,214] though this observation was not confirmed in a study of 262 patients from South Africa.[213] The

TABLE 5-5. Staging schemes for malignant pleural mesothelioma

	Butchart et al.[215]	Intergroup Mesothelioma Committee	Chahinian[217]
Stage I	Tumor confined to ipsilateral pleura, lung, and pericardium	Tumor limited to ipsilateral hemithorax (pleura, lung, pericardium, chest wall, mediastinum)	Tumor confined to ipsilateral parietal or visceral pleura
Stage II	Tumor invading chest wall or mediastinal structures (esophagus, heart, contralateral pleura); or metastases to thoracic lymph nodes	Involvement of contralateral pleura, mediastinal or contralateral hilar nodes	Superficial local invasion involving diaphragm, endothoracic fascia, or ipsilateral lung; or metastases to ipsilateral hilar nodes
Stage III	Tumor penetrating diaphragm to involve peritoneum; or involvement of contralateral pleura; or metastases to extrathoracic lymph nodes	Extrathoracic extension to lymph nodes or peritoneum	Deep local invasion involving chest wall, pericardium, or mediastinum; or metastases to mediastinal or contralateral hilar nodes
Stage IV	Distant blood-borne metastases	Distant blood-borne metastases	Distant blood-borne metastases; extension to contralateral pleura, peritoneum, or neck

two largest and most recent studies[212,213] have shown a better survival for women than for men. Also, age at time of diagnosis has been found to be a significant prognostic factor in some studies[209,212] (younger patients have a superior survival) but not in others.[213] In addition, duration of symptoms greater than six months at the time of diagnosis was found to be a favorable prognostic factor by Alberts et al.[213] but not by Chahinian et al.[209]

In evaluating the effects of treatment on survival in mesothelioma, it is important to take into account patient age and sex, and stage of disease.[212] Furthermore, a few five-year survivors have been recorded in most large series.[208,209,212,213,218] Death is usually secondary to complications of local disease, so surgical therapy has been advocated as a mainstay of treatment. Radical surgery in the form of extrapleural pneumonectomy has resulted in a few five-year disease-free survivals, but the role of curative surgery remains controversial.[35] This form of surgery is available only for patients with limited disease at the time of diagnosis, and it is associated with a significant morbidity and mortality.[214,219] Furthermore, the efficacy of this approach has not been evaluated in a randomized clinical trial. Radiotherapy and combination chemotherapy have produced clinical responses in isolated instances, but most large series indicate that malignant mesotheliomas are in general nonresponsive to therapy and that new treatment modalities will be required.[169,210,211,213,214] One report actually noted worse survival for patients treated with chemotherapy (with or without radiotherapy) as compared to untreated cases.[220]

Because of this bleak outlook for patients diagnosed with malignant mesothelioma, some investigators have emphasized the importance of early diagnosis combined with a multimodality therapeutic approach as the only means of improving patient survival.[221–223] A recent study of 37 patients with peritoneal mesothelioma reported a disease-free survival of 9 to 36 months in six patients with early disease who were treated intensively with combined therapy,[224] indicating that such an approach may eventually offer some hope for patients with this highly fatal disease. However, this optimism should be tempered with caution in light of occasional long-term survivors of untreated peritoneal mesothelioma.[225]

REFERENCES

1. *Stedman's Medical Dictionary*, 22nd ed. Baltimore: Williams & Wilkins, 1972.
2. Roggli VL, Kolbeck J, Sanfilippo F, Shelburne JD: Pathology of human mesothelioma: Etiologic and diagnostic considerations. *Pathol Annu*, Part 2, Vol. 22:91–131, 1987.
3. Kuhn C: The cells of the lung and their organelles. In: *The Biochemical Basis of Pulmonary Function* (Crystal RG, ed.), New York: Marcel Dekker, 1976, pp. 3–48.

4. Davis JMG: The histopathology and ultrastructure of pleural mesotheliomas produced in the rat by injections of crocidolite asbestos. *Br J Exp Pathol* 60:642–652, 1979.

5. McDonald JC: Health implications of environmental exposure to asbestos. *Environ Health Persp* 62:319–328, 1985.

6. Chahinian AP: Malignant mesothelioma. In: *Cancer Medicine* (Holland JF, Frei E III, eds.), Philadelphia: Lea & Febiger, 1982, pp. 1744–1751.

7. Wagner E: Das tuberkelahnliche lymphadenom. *Arch d Heilkunde* 11:497–526, 1870.

8. Hammar SP, Bolen JW: Pleural neoplasms. Ch. 30 In: *Pulmonary Pathology* (Dail DH, Hammar SP, eds.), New York: Springer-Verlag, 1988, pp. 973–1028.

9. Craighead JE: Eyes for the epidemiologist: The pathologist's role in shaping our understanding of the asbestos-associated diseases. *Am J Clin Pathol* 89:281–287, 1988.

10. Robertson HE: "Endothelioma" of the pleura. *J Cancer Res* 8:317–375, 1924.

11. Klemperer P, Rabin CB: Primary neoplasms of pleura: Report of five cases. *Arch Pathol* 11:385–412, 1931.

12. McCaughey WTE, Kannerstein M, Churg J: Tumors and pseudotumors of the serous membranes. *Atlas of Tumor Pathology,* 2nd Series, Fascicle 20. Washington, DC: Armed Forces Institute of Pathology, 1985.

13. Castleman BI: *Asbestos: Medical and Legal Aspects.* New York: Harcourt Brace Jovanovich, 1984.

14. Gloyne SR: The morbid anatomy and histology of asbestosis. *Tubercle* 14:550–558, 1933.

15. Wedler HW: Über den Lugenkrebs bei Asbestose. *Dtsch Arch Klin Med* 191:189–209, 1943.

16. Mallory TB, Castleman B, Parris EE: Case records of the Massachusetts General Hospital #33111. *N Engl J Med* 236:407–412, 1947.

17. Lee DHK, Selikoff IJ: Historical background to the asbestos problem. *Environ Res* 18:300–314, 1979.

18. Keal EE: Asbestosis and abdominal neoplasms. *Lancet* 2:1211–1216, 1960.

19. Wagner JC, Sleggs CA, Marchand P: Diffuse pleural mesothelioma and asbestos exposure in the Northwestern Cape Province. *Br J Ind Med* 17:260–271, 1960.

20. Edge JR, Choudhury SL: Malignant mesothelioma of the pleura in Barrow-in-Furness. *Thorax* 33:26–30, 1978.

21. McDonald AD, McDonald JC: Malignant mesothelioma in North America. *Cancer* 46:1650–1656, 1980.

22. Otto H: Das berufsbedingte mesotheliom in der BRD. *Pathologe* 2:8–18, 1980.

23. Churg A: Malignant mesothelioma in British Columbia in 1982. *Cancer* 55:672–674, 1985.

24. Andersson M, Olsen JH: Trend and distribution of mesothelioma in Denmark. *Br J Cancer* 51:699–705, 1985.

25. Malker HSR, McLaughlin JK, Malker BK, Stone BJ, Weiner JA, Erickson JLE, Blot WJ: Occupational risks for pleural mesothelioma in Sweden, 1961–79. *J Natl Cancer Inst* 74:61–66, 1985.

26. Connelly RR, Spirtas R, Myers MH, Percy CL, Fraumeni JF: Demographic patterns for mesothelioma in the United States. *J Natl Cancer Inst* 78:1053–1060, 1987.

27. Ferguson DA, Berry G, Jelihovsky T, Andreas SB, Rogers AJ, Fung SC, Grimwood A, Thompson R: The Australian Mesothelioma Surveillance Program 1979–1985. *Med J Australia* 147:166–172, 1987.

28. Sheers G, Coles RM: Mesothelioma risks in a naval dockyard. *Arch Environ Health* 35:276–282, 1980.

29. Selikoff IJ, Hammond EC, Seidman H: Mortality experience of insulation workers in the United States and Canada, 1943–1976. In: Health hazards of asbestos exposure (Selikoff IJ, Hammond EC, eds.), *Ann NY Acad Sci* 330:91–116, 1979.

30. Ribak J, Lilis R, Suzuki Y, Penner L, Selikoff IJ: Malignant mesothelioma in a cohort of asbestos insulation workers: Clinical presentation, diagnosis, and causes of death. *Br J Ind Med* 45:182–187, 1988.

31. Churg A: Analysis of asbestos fibers from lung tissue: Research and diagnostic uses. *Sem Respir Med* 7:281–288, 1986.

32. Schenker MB, Garshick E, Munoz A, Woskie SR, Speizer FE: A population-based case-control study of mesothelioma deaths among U.S. railroad workers. *Am Rev Respir Dis* 134:461–465, 1986.

33. Mancuso TF: Relative risk of mesothelioma among railroad machinists exposed to chrysotile. *Am J Ind Med* 13:639–657, 1988.

34. Wolf KM, Piotrowski ZH, Engel JD, Bekeris LG, Palacios E, Fisher KA: Malignant mesothelioma with occupational and environmental asbestos exposure in an Illinois community hospital. *Arch Intern Med* 147:2145–2149, 1987.

35. Antman KH: Malignant mesothelioma. *N Engl J Med* 303:200–202, 1980.

36. Craighead JE, Mossman BT: Pathogenesis of asbestos-associated diseases. *N Engl J Med* 306:1446–1455, 1982.

37. Talcott J, Thurber W, Gaensler E, Antman K, Li FP: Mesothelioma in manufacturers of asbestos-containing cigarette filters. *Lancet* I:392, 1987.

38. Driscoll RJ, Mulligan WJ, Schultz D, Candelaria A: Malignant mesothelioma: A cluster in a Native American pueblo. *N Engl J Med* 318:1437–1438, 1988.

39. Li FP, Dreyfus MG, Antman KH: Asbestos-contaminated nappies and familial mesothelioma. *Lancet* I:909–910, 1989.

40. McDonald AD, McDonald JC: Epidemiology of malignant mesothelioma. Ch. 2 In: *Asbestos-Related Malignancy* (Antman K, Aisner J, eds.), Orlando, FL: Harcourt Brace Jovanovich, 1987, pp. 31–55.

41. Selikoff IJ, Hammond EC, Seidman H: Latency of asbestos disease among insulation workers in the United States and Canada. *Cancer* 46:2736–2740, 1980.

42. Peto J, Seidman H, Selikoff IJ: Mesothelioma mortality in asbestos workers: Implications for models of carcinogenesis and risk assessment. *Br J Cancer* 45:124–135, 1982.

43. Chronic Hazard Advisory Panel on Asbestos: Report to the U.S. Consumer Product Safety Commission, Directorate for Health Sciences, Washington, D.C., 1983.

44. Browne K, Smither WJ: Asbestos-related mesothelioma: Factors discriminating between pleural and peritoneal sites. *Br J Ind Med* 40:145–152, 1983.

45. Dunnigan J: Linking chrysotile asbestos with mesothelioma. *Am J Ind Med* 14:205–209, 1988.

46. Churg A: On Dr. Dunnigan's commentary linking chrysotile asbestos with mesothelioma. *Am J Ind Med* 14:235–238, 1988.

47. Becklake MR: On Dr. Dunnigan's commentary linking chrysotile asbestos with mesothelioma. *Am J Ind Med* 14:239–240, 1988.

48. Craighead JE: Response to Dr. Dunnigan's commentary. *Am J Ind Med* 14:241–243, 1988.

49. Roggli VL, Pratt PC: Amphiboles and chrysotile asbestos exposure. *Am J Ind Med* 14:245–246, 1988.

50. McDonald JC: Tremolite, other amphiboles, and mesothelioma. *Am J Ind Med* 14:247–249, 1988.

51. Churg A, Wiggs B, Depaoli L, Kampe B, Stevens B: Lung asbestos content in chrysotile workers with mesothelioma. *Am Rev Respir Dis* 130:1042–1045, 1984.

52. McDonald AD, McDonald JC, Pooley FD: Mineral fiber content of lung in mesothelial tumours in North America. *Ann Occup Hyg* 26:417–422, 1982.
53. Churg A: Chrysotile, tremolite, and malignant mesothelioma in man. *Chest* 93:621–628, 1988.
54. Langer AM, Nolan RP, Constantopoulos SH, Moutsopoulos HM: Association of Metsovo lung and pleural mesothelioma with exposure to tremolite-containing whitewash. *Lancet* I:965–967, 1987.
55. McConnochie K, Simonato L, Mavrides P, Christofides P, Pooley FD, Wagner JC: Mesothelioma in Cyprus: The role of tremolite. *Thorax* 42:342–347, 1987.
56. Yazicioglu S, Ilcayto R, Balci K, Sayli BS, Yorulmaz B: Pleural calcification, pleural mesotheliomas, and bronchial cancers caused by tremolite dust. *Thorax* 35:564–569, 1980.
57. Roggli VL, McGavran MH, Subach J, Sybers HD, Greenberg SD: Pulmonary asbestos body counts and electron probe analysis of asbestos body cores in patients with mesothelioma: A study of 25 cases. *Cancer* 50:2423–2432, 1982.
58. Baris YI, Artvinli M, Sahin AA: Environmental mesothelioma in Turkey. *Ann NY Acad Sci* 330:423–432, 1979.
59. Pooley FD: Evaluation of fiber samples taken from the vicinity of two villages in Turkey. In: *Dusts and Disease: Occupational and Environmental Exposures to Selected Fibrous and Particulate Dusts* (Lemen R, Dement JM, eds.), Park Forest South, IL: Pathotox Publishing: 1979, pp. 41–44.
60. Sebastien P, Gaudichet A, Bignon J, Baris YI: Zeolite bodies in human lungs from Turkey. *Lab Invest* 44:420–425, 1981.
61. Rohl AN, Langer AM, Moncure G, Selikoff IJ, Fischbein A: Endemic pleural disease associated with exposure to mixed fibrous dust in Turkey. *Science* 216:518–520, 1982.
62. Maltoni C, Minardi F, Morisi L: Pleural mesotheliomas in Sprague-Dawley rats by erionite: First experimental evidence. *Environ Res* 29:238–244, 1982.
63. Suzuki Y, Kohyama N: Malignant mesothelioma induced by asbestos and zeolite in the mouse peritoneal cavity. *Environ Res* 35:277–292, 1984.
64. Peterson JT, Greenberg SD, Buffler PA: Non-asbestos-related malignant mesothelioma: A review. *Cancer* 54:951–960, 1984.
65. Antman KH, Ruxer RL, Aisner J, Vawter G: Mesothelioma following Wilms' tumor in childhood. *Cancer* 54:367–369, 1984.
66. Anderson KA, Hurley WC, Hurley BT, Ohrt DW: Malignant pleural mesothelioma following radiotherapy in a 16-year-old boy. *Cancer* 56:273–276, 1985.
67. Austin MB, Fechner RE, Roggli VL: Pleural malignant mesothelioma following Wilms' tumor. *Am J Clin Pathol* 86:227–230, 1986.
68. Warren S, Brown CE, Chute RN, Federman M: Mesothelioma relative to asbestos, radiation, and methylcholanthrene. *Arch Pathol Lab Med* 105:305–312, 1981.
69. Hillerdal G, Berg J: Malignant mesothelioma secondary to chronic inflammation and old scars: Two new cases and review of the literature. *Cancer* 55:1968–1972, 1985.
70. Risberg B, Nickels J, Wågermark J: Familial clustering of malignant mesothelioma. *Cancer* 45:2422–2427, 1980.
71. Lynch HT, Katz D, Markvicka SE: Familial mesothelioma: Review and family study. *Cancer Genet Cytogenet* 15:25–35, 1985.
72. Hammar SP, Bockus D, Remington F, Freidman S, LaZerte G: Familial mesothelioma: A report of two families. *Hum Pathol* 20:107–112, 1989.
73. Fraire AE, Cooper S, Greenberg SD, Buffler P, Langston C: Mesothelioma of childhood. *Cancer* 62:838–847, 1988.
74. Nishioka H, Furusho K, Yasunaga T, Tanaka K, Yamanouchi A, Yokota T, Ishihara T, Nakashima Y: Congenital malignant mesothelioma: A case report and electron-microscopic study. *Eur J Pediatr* 147:428–430, 1988.

75. Hillerdal G: Malignant mesothelioma 1982: Review of 4710 published cases. *Br J Dis Chest* 77:321–343, 1983.
76. McCaughey WTE: Criteria for diagnosis of diffuse mesothelial tumors. *Ann NY Acad Sci* 132:603–613, 1965.
77. Craighead JE, Abraham JL, Churg A, et al.: Pathology of asbestos-associated diseases of the lungs and pleural cavities: Diagnostic criteria and proposed grading schema (Report of the Pneumoconiosis Committee of the College of American Pathologists and the National Institute for Occupational Safety and Health). *Arch Pathol Lab Med* 106:544–596, 1982.
78. Adams VI, Unni KK, Muhm JR, Jett JR, Ilstrup DM, Bernatz PE: Diffuse malignant mesothelioma of pleura: Diagnosis and survival in 92 cases. *Cancer* 58:1540–1551, 1986.
79. Obers VJ, Leiman G, Girdwood RW, Spiro FI: Primary malignant pleural tumors (mesotheliomas) presenting as localized masses: Fine needle aspiration cytologic findings, clinical and radiologic features and review of the literature. *Acta Cytolog* 32:567–575, 1988.
80. Sahn SA: State of the Art: The pleura. *Am Rev Respir Dis* 138:184–234, 1988.
81. Solomons K, Polakow R, Marchand P: Diffuse malignant mesothelioma presenting as bilateral malignant lymphangitis. *Thorax* 40:682–683, 1985.
82. Alexander E, Clark RA, Colley DP, Mitchell SE: CT of malignant pleural mesothelioma. *AJR* 137:287–291, 1981.
83. Mirvis S, Dutcher JP, Haney PJ, Whitley NO, Aisner J: CT of malignant pleural mesothelioma. *AJR* 140:665–670, 1983.
84. Lorigan JG, Libshitz HI: MR imaging of malignant pleural mesothelioma. *J Comput Asst Tomogr* 13:617–620, 1989.
85. Harwood TR, Gracey DR, Yokoo H: Pseudomesotheliomatous carcinoma of the lung: A variant of peripheral lung cancer. *Am J Clin Pathol* 65:159–167, 1976.
86. Whitaker D, Shilkin KB: Diagnosis of pleural malignant mesothelioma in life: A practical approach. *J Pathol* 143:147–175, 1984.
87. Roberts GH, Campbell GM: Exfoliative cytology of diffuse mesothelioma. *J Clin Pathol* 25:577–582, 1972.
88. Sterrett GF, Whitaker D, Shilkin KB, Walters MNI: Fine needle aspiration cytology of malignant mesothelioma. *Acta Cytologica* 31:185–193, 1987.
89. Churg J, Rosen SH, Moolten S: Histological characteristics of mesothelioma associated with asbestos. *Ann NY Acad Sci* 132:614–622, 1965.
90. Adams VI, Unni KK: Diffuse malignant mesothelioma of pleura: Diagnostic criteria based on an autopsy study. *Am J Clin Pathol* 82:15–23, 1984.
91. Yousem SA, Hochholzer L: Malignant mesotheliomas with osseous and cartilaginous differentiation. *Arch Pathol Lab Med* 111:62–66, 1987.
92. Andrion A, Mazzucco G, Bernardi P, Mollo F: Sarcomatous tumor of the chest wall with osteochondroid differentiation: Evidence of mesothelial origin. *Am J Surg Pathol* 13:707–712, 1989.
93. Kannerstein M, Churg J: Desmoplastic diffuse malignant mesothelioma. In: *Progress in Surgical Pathology*, Vol. II (Fenoglio CM, Wolff M, eds.), New York: Masson Pub., 1980, pp. 19–29.
94. Cantin R, Al-Jabi M, McCaughey WTE: Desmoplastic diffuse mesothelioma. *Am J Surg Pathol* 6:215–222, 1982.
95. Henderson DW, Attwood HD, Constance TJ, Shilkin KB, Steele RH: Lymphohistiocytoid mesothelioma: A rare lymphomatoid variant of predominantly sarcomatoid mesothelioma. *Ultrastruct Pathol* 12:367–384, 1988.
96. Harrison RN: Sarcomatous pleural mesothelioma and cerebral metastases: Case report and review of eight cases. *Eur J Respir Dis* 65:185–188, 1984.
97. Huncharek M, Muscat J: Metastases in diffuse pleural mesothelioma: Influence of histologic type. *Thorax* 42:897–898, 1987.

98. Huncharek M, Smith K: Extrathoracic lymph node metastases in malignant pleural mesothelioma. *Chest* 93:443–444, 1988.

99. Machin T, Mashiyama ET, Henderson JAM, McCaughey WTE: Bony metastases in desmoplastic pleural mesothelioma. *Thorax* 43:155–156, 1988.

100. Campbell GD, Greenberg SD: Pleural mesothelioma with calcified liver metastases. *Chest* 79:229–230, 1981.

101. Kannerstein M, Churg J, Magner D: Histochemistry in the diagnosis of malignant mesothelioma. *Ann Clin Lab Sci* 3:207–211, 1973.

102. Churg A: Malignant mesothelioma. *Chest* 89:367S–368S, 1986.

103. Battifora H: The Pleura. Ch. 24 In: *Diagnostic Surgical Pathology* (Sternberg SS, ed.), New York: Raven Press, 1989, pp. 829–855.

104. Kawai T, Suzuki M, Shinmei M, Maenaka Y, Kageyama K: Glycosaminoglycans in malignant diffuse mesothelioma. *Cancer* 56:567–574, 1985.

105. Pettersson T, Fröseth B, Riska H, Klockars M: Concentration of hyaluronic acid in pleural fluid as a diagnostic aid for malignant mesothelioma. *Chest* 94:1037–1039, 1988.

106. Waxler B, Eisenstein R, Battifora H: Electrophoresis of tissue glycosaminoglycans as an aid in the diagnosis of mesotheliomas. *Cancer* 44:221–227, 1979.

107. Iozzo RV, Goldes JA, Chen W-J, Wight TN: Glycosaminoglycans of pleural mesothelioma: A possible biochemical variant containing chondroitin sulfate. *Cancer* 48:89–97, 1981.

108. Nakano T, Fujii J, Tamura S, Amuro Y, Nabeshima K, Horai T, Hada T, Higashino K: Glycosaminoglycan in malignant pleural mesothelioma. *Cancer* 57:106–110, 1986.

109. Chiu B, Churg A, Tengbled A, Rearce R, McCaughey WTE: Analysis of hyaluronic acid in the diagnosis of malignant mesothelioma. *Cancer* 54:2195–2199, 1984.

110. Greengard O, Head JF, Chahinian AP, Goldberg SL: Enzyme pathology of human mesotheliomas. *J Natl Cancer Inst* 78:617–622, 1987.

111. LaRocca PJ, Rheinwald JG: Coexpression of simple epithelial keratins and vimentin by human mesothelium and mesothelioma in vivo and in culture. *Cancer Res* 44:2991–2999, 1984.

112. Cooper D, Schermer A, Sun T-T: Classification of human epithelia and their neoplasms using monoclonal antibodies to keratins: Strategies, applications, and limitations. *Lab Invest* 52:243–256, 1985.

113. Bolen JW, Hammar SP, McNutt MA: Reactive and neoplastic serosal tissue: A light-microscopic, ultrastructural, and immunocytochemical study. *Am J Surg Pathol* 10:34–47, 1986.

114. Gown AM, Vogel AM: Monoclonal antibodies to human intermediate filament proteins: II. Distribution of filament proteins in normal human tissues. *Am J Pathol* 114:309–321, 1984.

115. Schlegel R, Banks-Schlegel S, McLeod JA, Pinkus GS: Immunoperoxidase localization of keratin in human neoplasms. *Am J Pathol* 101:41–50, 1980.

116. Said JW, Nash G, Banks-Schlegel S, Sasson AF, Murakami S, Shintaku IP: Keratin in human lung tumors: Patterns of localization of different-molecular-weight keratin proteins. *Am J Pathol* 113:27–32, 1983.

117. Warhol MJ: The ultrastructural localization of keratin proteins and carcinoembryonic antigen in malignant mesotheliomas. *Am J Pathol* 116:385–390, 1984.

118. Corson JM, Pinkus GS: Mesothelioma: Profile of keratin proteins and carcinoembryonic antigen: An immunoperoxidase study of 20 cases and comparison with pulmonary adenocarcinomas. *Am J Pathol* 108:80–87, 1982.

119. Battifora H, Kopinski MI: Distinction of mesothelioma from adenocarcinoma: An immunohistochemical approach. *Cancer* 55:1679–1685, 1985.

120. Gibbs AR, Harach R, Wagner JC, Jasani B: Comparison of tumour markers in malignant mesothelioma and pulmonary adenocarcinoma. *Thorax* 40:91–95, 1985.

121. Holden J, Churg A: Immunohistochemical staining for keratin and carcinoembryonic antigen in the diagnosis of malignant mesothelioma. *Am J Surg Pathol* 8:277–279, 1984.

122. Loosli H, Hurlimann J: Immunohistological study of malignant diffuse mesotheliomas of the pleura. *Histopathology* 8:793–803, 1984.

123. van Muijen GNP, Ruiter DJ, Ponec M, Huiskens-van der Mey C, Warnaar SO: Monoclonal antibodies with different specificities against cytokeratins: An immunohistochemical study of normal tissues and tumors. *Am J Pathol* 114:9–17, 1984.

124. Blobel GA, Moll R, Franke WW, Kayser KW, Gould VE: The intermediate filament cytoskeleton of malignant mesotheliomas and its diagnostic significance. *Am J Pathol* 121:235–247, 1985.

125. Moll R, Dhouailly D, Sun T-T: Expression of keratin 5 as a distinctive feature of epithelial and biphasic mesotheliomas: An immunohistochemical study using monoclonal antibody AE-14. *Virchows Archiv B Cell Pathol* 58:129–145, 1989.

126. Kahn HJ, Thorner PS, Yeger H, Bailey D, Baumal R: Distinct keratin patterns demonstrated by immunoperoxidase staining of adenocarcinomas, carcinoids and mesotheliomas using polyclonal and monoclonal antikeratin antibodies. *Am J Clin Pathol* 86:566–574, 1986.

127. Montag AG, Pinkus GS, Corson JM: Keratin protein immunoreactivity of sarcomatoid and mixed types of diffuse malignant mesothelioma: An immunoperoxidase study of 30 cases. *Hum Pathol* 19:336–342, 1988.

128. Epstein JI, Budin RE: Keratin and epithelial membrane antigen immunoreactivity in nonneoplastic fibrous pleural lesions: Implications for the diagnosis of desmoplastic mesothelioma. *Hum Pathol* 17:514–519, 1986.

129. Gown AM, Boyd HC, Chang Y, Ferguson M, Reichler B, Tippens D: Smooth muscle cells can express cytokeratins of "simple" epithelium: Immunocytochemical and biochemical studies in vitro and in vivo. *Am J Pathol* 132:223–232, 1988.

130. Weiss SW, Bratthauer GL, Morris PA: Postirradiation malignant fibrous histiocytoma expressing cytokeratin. *Am J Surg Pathol* 12:554–558, 1988.

131. Cagle PT, Truong LD, Roggli VL, Greenberg SD: Immunohistochemical differentiation of sarcomatoid mesotheliomas from other spindle cell neoplasms. *Am J Clin Pathol* 92:566–571, 1989.

132. Churg A: Immunohistochemical staining for vimentin and keratin in malignant mesothelioma. *Am J Surg Pathol* 9:360–365, 1985.

133. Mullink H, Henzen-Logmans SC, Alons-van Kordelaar JJM, Tadema TM, Meijer CJLM: Simultaneous immunoenzyme staining of vimentin and cytokeratins with monoclonal antibodies as an aid in the differential diagnosis of malignant mesothelioma from pulmonary adenocarcinoma. *Virchows Arch* [Cell Pathol] 52:55–65, 1986.

134. Wang NS, Huang SN, Gold P: Absence of carcinoembryonic antigen-like material in mesothelioma. *Cancer* 44:937–943, 1979.

135. Said JW, Nash G, Tepper G, Banks-Schlegel S: Keratin proteins and carcinoembryonic antigen in lung carcinoma: An immunoperoxidase study of fifty-four cases, with ultrastructural correlations. *Hum Pathol* 14:70–76, 1983.

136. Whitaker DF, Sterett GF, Shilkin KB: Detection of tissue CEA-like substance as an aid in the differential diagnosis of malignant mesothelioma. *Pathology* 14:255–258, 1982.

137. Cibas ES, Corson JM, Pinkus GS: The distinction of adenocarcinoma from malignant mesothelioma in cell blocks of effusions: The role of

routine mucin histochemistry and immunohistochemical assessment of carcinoembryonic antigen, keratin proteins, epithelial membrane antigen, and milk fat globule-derived antigen. *Hum Pathol* 18:67–74, 1987.

138. Sheibani K, Battifora H, Burke JS: Antigenic phenotype of malignant mesotheliomas and pulmonary adenocarcinomas: An immunohistologic analysis demonstrating the value of Leu M1 antigen. *Am J Pathol* 123:212–219, 1986.

139. Singh G, Whiteside TL, Dekker A: Immunodiagnosis of mesothelioma: Use of antimesothelial cell serum in an indirect immunofluorescence assay. *Cancer* 43:2288–2296, 1979.

140. Donna A, Betta PG, Bellingeri D, Marchesini A: New marker for mesothelioma: An immunoperoxidase study. *J Clin Pathol* 39:961–968, 1986.

141. Donna A, Betta P-G, Jones JSP: Verification of the histologic diagnosis of malignant mesothelioma in relation to the binding of an antimesothelial cell antibody. *Cancer* 63:1331–1336, 1989.

142. Anderson TM, Holmes EC, Kosaka CJ, Cheng L, Saxton RE: Monoclonal antibodies to human malignant mesothelioma. *J Clin Immunol* 7:254–261, 1987.

143. Stahel RA, O'Hara CJ, Waibel R, Martin A: Monoclonal antibodies against mesothelial membrane antigen discriminate between malignant mesothelioma and lung adenocarcinoma. *Int J Cancer* 41:218–223, 1988.

144. O'Hara CJ, Corson JM, Pinkus GS, Stahel RA: ME 1: A monoclonal antibody that distinguishes epithelial-type malignant mesothelioma from pulmonary adenocarcinoma and extrapulmonary malignancies. *Am J Pathol* 136:421–428, 1990.

145. Hsu S-M, Hsu P-L, Zhao X, Kao-Shan CS, Whang-Peng J: Establishment of human mesothelioma cell lines (MS-1,-2) and production of a monoclonal antibody (Anti-MS) with diagnostic and therapeutic potential. *Cancer Res* 48:5228–5236, 1988.

146. Szpak CA, Johnston WW, Roggli V, Kolbeck J, Lottich SC, Vollmer R, Thor A, Schlom J: The diagnostic distinction between malignant mesothelioma of the pleura and adenocarcinoma of the lung as defined by a monoclonal antibody (B72.3). *Am J Pathol* 122:252–260, 1986.

147. Otis CN, Carter D, Cole S, Battifora H: Immunohistochemical evaluation of pleural mesothelioma and pulmonary adenocarcinoma: A biinstitutional study of 47 cases. *Am J Surg Pathol* 11:445–456, 1987.

148. Wick MR, Mills SE, Swanson PE: Expression of "myelomonocytic" antigens in mesotheliomas and adenocarcinomas involving the serosal surfaces. *Am J Clin Pathol* 94:18–26, 1990.

149. Warnock ML, Stoloff A, Thor A: Differentiation of adenocarcinoma of the lung from mesothelioma: Periodic acid-Schiff, monoclonal antibodies B72.3, and Leu M1. *Am J Pathol* 133:30–38, 1988.

150. Ordóñez NG: The immunohistochemical diagnosis of mesothelioma: Differentiation of mesothelioma and lung adenocarcinoma: *Am J Surg Pathol* 13:276–291, 1989.

151. Lee I, Radosevich JA, Chejfec G, Yixing MA, Warren WH, Rosen ST, Gould VE: Malignant mesotheliomas: Improved differential diagnosis from lung adenocarcinomas using monoclonal antibodies 44–3A6 and 624A12. *Am J Pathol* 123:497–507, 1986.

152. Kawai T, Greenberg SD, Truong LD, Mattioli CA, Klima M, Titus JL: Differences in lectin binding of malignant pleural mesothelioma and adenocarcinoma of the lung. *Am J Pathol* 130:401–410, 1988.

153. Noguchi M, Nakajima T, Hirohashi S, Akiba T, Shimosato Y: Immunohistochemical distinction of malignant mesothelioma from pulmonary adenocarcinoma with anti-surfactant apoprotein, anti-Lewis[a], and anti-Tn antibodies. *Hum Pathol* 20:53–57, 1989.

154. Ghosh AH, Gatter KC, Dunnill MS, Mason DY: Immunohistological staining of reactive mesothelium, mesothelioma, and lung carcinoma with a panel of monoclonal antibodies. *J Clin Pathol* 40:19–25, 1987.

155. Pinkus GS, Kurtin PJ: Epithelial membrane antigen—A diagnostic discriminant in surgical pathology: Immunohistochemical profile in epithelial, mesenchymal, and hematopoietic neoplasms using paraffin sections and monoclonal antibodies. *Hum Pathol* 16:929–940, 1985.

156. Kallianpur AR, Carstens PHB, Liotta LA, Frey KP, Siegal GP: Immunoreactivity in malignant mesotheliomas with antibodies to basement membrane components and their receptors. *Mod Pathol* 3:11–18, 1990.

157. Wick MR, Loy T, Mills SE, Legier JF, Manivel JC: Malignant epithelioid pleural mesothelioma versus peripheral pulmonary adenocarcinoma: A histochemical, ultrastructural, and immunohistologic study of 103 cases. *Hum Pathol* 21:759–766, 1990.

158. Davis JMG: Ultrastructure of human mesotheliomas. *J Natl Cancer Inst* 52:1715–1725, 1974.

159. Suzuki Y, Churg J, Kannerstein M: Ultrastructure of human malignant diffuse mesothelioma. *Am J Pathol* 85:241–262, 1976.

160. Wang NS: Electron microscopy in the diagnosis of pleural mesotheliomas. *Cancer* 31:1046–1054, 1973.

161. Warhol MJ, Hickey WF, Corson JM: Malignant mesothelioma: Ultrastructural distinction from adenocarcinoma. *Am J Surg Pathol* 6:307–314, 1982.

162. Warhol MJ, Corson JM: An ultrastructural comparison of mesotheliomas with adenocarcinomas of the lung and breast. *Hum Pathol* 16:50–55, 1985.

163. Burns TR, Greenberg SD, Mace ML, Johnson EH: Ultrastructural diagnosis of epithelial malignant mesothelioma. *Cancer* 56:2036–2040, 1985.

164. Dewar A, Valente M, Ring NP, Corrin B: Pleural mesothelioma of epithelial type and pulmonary adenocarcinoma: An ultrastructural and cytochemical comparison. *J Pathol* 152:309–316, 1987.

165. Burns TR, Johnson EH, Cartwright J, Greenberg SD: Desmosomes of epithelial malignant mesothelioma. *Ultrastruct Pathol* 12:385–388, 1988.

166. Mukherjee TM, Swift JG, Henderson DW: Freeze-fracture study of intercellular junctions in benign and malignant mesothelial cells in effusions and a comparison with those seen in pleural mesotheliomas (solid tumor). *J Submicrosc Cytol Pathol* 20:195–208, 1988.

167. Dardick I, Jabi M, McCaughey WTE, Deodhare S, van Nostrand AWP, Srigley JR: Diffuse epithelial mesothelioma: A review of the ultrastructural spectrum. *Ultrastruct Pathol* 11:503–533, 1987.

168. Klima M, Bossart MI: Sarcomatous type of malignant mesothelioma. *Ultrastruct Pathol* 4:349–358, 1983.

169. Pisani RJ, Colby TV, Williams DE: Malignant mesothelioma of the pleura. *Mayo Clin Proc* 63:1234–1244, 1988.

170. Churg A: Neoplastic asbestos-induced diseases. Ch. 8 In: *Pathology of Occupational Lung Disease* (Churg A, Green FHY, eds.), New York: Igaku-Shoin, 1988, pp. 279–325.

171. Al-Izzi M, Thurlow NP, Corrin B: Pleural mesothelioma of connective-tissue-type, localized fibrous tumour of the pleura, and reactive submesothelial hyperplasia: An immunohistochemical comparison. *J Pathol* 158:41–44, 1989.

172. Taylor DR, Page W, Hughes D, Varghese G: Metastatic renal cell carcinoma mimicking pleural mesothelioma. *Thorax* 42:901–902, 1987.

173. Said JW, Nash G, Banks-Schlegel S, Sassoon AF, Shintaku IP: Localized fibrous mesothelioma: An immunohistochemical and electron microscopic study. *Hum Pathol* 15:440–443, 1984.

174. Dervan PA, Tobin B, O'Connor M: Solitary (localized) fibrous mesothelioma: Evidence against mesothelial cell origin. *Histopathol* 10:867–875, 1986.
175. Doucet J, Dardick I, Srigley JR, van Nostrand AWP, Bell MA, Kahn HJ: Localized fibrous tumour of serosal surfaces: Immunohistochemical and ultrastructural evidence for a type of mesothelioma. *Virchows Arch* [Pathol Anat] 409:349–363, 1986.
176. Carter D, Otis CN: Three types of spindle cell tumors of the pleura: fibroma, sarcoma, and sarcomatoid mesothelioma. *Am J Surg Pathol* 12:747–753, 1988.
177. Tucker MA, Coleman CN, Cox RS, Varghese A, Rosenberg SA: Risk of second cancers after treatment for Hodgkin's disease. *N Engl J Med* 318:76–81, 1988.
178. Kannerstein M, Churg J: Peritoneal mesothelioma. *Hum Pathol* 8:83–94, 1977.
179. Winslow DJ, Taylor HB: Malignant peritoneal mesotheliomas: A clinicopathological analysis of 12 fatal cases. *Cancer* 13:127–136, 1960.
180. Piccigallo E, Jeffers LJ, Reddy KR, Caldironi MW, Parenti A, Schiff ER: Malignant peritoneal mesothelioma: A clinical and laparoscopic study of ten cases. *Dig Dis Sci* 33:633–639, 1988.
181. Mennemeyer R, Smith M: Multicystic, peritoneal mesothelioma: A report with electron microscopy of a case mimicking intra-abdominal cystic hygroma (lymphangioma). *Cancer* 44:692–698, 1979.
182. Moore JH, Crum CP, Chandler JG, Feldman PS: Benign cystic mesothelioma. *Cancer* 45:2395–2399, 1980.
183. Weiss SH, Tavassoli FA: Multicystic mesothelioma: An analysis of pathologic findings and biologic behavior in 37 cases. *Am J Surg Pathol* 12:737–746, 1988.
184. Ross MJ, Welch WR, Scully RE: Multilocular peritoneal inclusion cysts (So-called cystic mesotheliomas). *Cancer* 64:1336–1346, 1989.
185. Talerman A, Montero JR, Chilcote RR, Okagaki T: Diffuse malignant peritoneal mesothelioma in a 13-year-old girl: Report of a case and review of the literature. *Am J Surg Pathol* 9:73–80, 1985.
186. Santucci M, Biancalani M, Dini S: Multicystic peritoneal mesothelioma: A fine structure study with special reference to the spectrum of phenotypic differentiation exhibited by mesothelial cells. *J Submicrosc Cytol Pathol* 21:749–764, 1989.
187. Ackerman LV, Rosai J: *Surgical Pathology*, 5th ed. St. Louis: Mosby, 1974, p. 1172.
188. Foyle A, Al-Jabi M, McCaughey WTE: Papillary peritoneal tumors in women. *Am J Surg Pathol* 5:241–249, 1981.
189. Mills SE, Andersen WA, Fechner RE, Austin MB: Serous surface papillary carcinoma: A clinicopathologic study of 10 cases and comparison with stage III–IV ovarian serous carcinoma. *Am J Surg Pathol* 12:827–834, 1988.
190. Daya D, McCaughey WTE: Well-differentiated papillary mesothelioma of the peritoneum: A clinicopathologic study of 22 cases. *Cancer* 65:292–296, 1990.
191. Armstrong GR, Raafat F, Ingram L, Mann JR: Malignant peritoneal mesothelioma in childhood. *Arch Pathol Lab Med* 112:1159–1162, 1988.
192. Nomori H, Shimosato Y, Tsuchiya R: Diffuse malignant pericardial mesothelioma. *Acta Pathol Jpn* 35:1475–1481, 1985.
193. Llewellyn MJ, Atkinson MW, Fabri B: Pericardial constriction caused by primary mesothelioma. *Br Heart J* 57:54–57, 1987.
194. Nishikimi T, Ochi H, Hirota K, Ikuno Y, Oku H, Takeuchi K, Takeda T: Primary pericardial mesothelioma detected by gallium-67 scintigraphy. *J Nucl Med* 28:1210–1212, 1987.

195. Gössinger HD, Siostrzonek P, Zangeneh M, Neuhold A, Herold C, Schmoliner R, Laczkovics A, Tscholakoff D, Mösslacher H: Magnetic resonance imaging findings in a patient with pericardial mesothelioma. *Am Heart J* 115:1321–1322, 1988.
196. Naramoto A, Itoh N, Nakano M, Shigematsu H: An autopsy case of tuberous sclerosis associated with primary pericardial mesothelioma. *Acta Pathol Jpn* 39:400–406, 1989.
197. Hanfling SM: Metastatic cancer to the heart: Review of the literature and report of 127 cases. *Circulation* 22:474–483, 1960.
198. Smith C: Tumors of the heart. *Arch Pathol Lab Med* 110:371–374, 1986.
199. Linder J, Shelburne JD, Sorge JP, Whalen RE, Hackel DB: Congenital endodermal heterotopia of the atrioventricular node: Evidence for the endodermal origin of so-called mesotheliomas of the atrioventricular node. *Hum Pathol* 15:1093–1098, 1984.
200. Sopher IM, Spitz WU: Endodermal inclusions of the heart: So-called mesotheliomas of the atrioventricular node. *Arch Pathol* 92:180–186, 1971.
201. Fine G, Raju U: Congenital polycystic tumor of the atrioventricular node (endodermal heterotopia, mesothelioma): A histogenetic appraisal with evidence for its endodermal origin. *Hum Pathol* 18:791–795, 1987.
202. Beck B, Kowetzke G, Ludwig V, Rothig W, Sturm W: Malignant pericardial mesotheliomas and asbestos exposure. *Am J Ind Med* 3:149–159, 1982.
203. Kahn EI, Rohl A, Barnett EW, Suzuki Y: Primary pericardial mesothelioma following exposure to asbestos. *Environ Res* 23:270–281, 1980.
204. Churg A, Warnock ML, Bersch KG: Malignant mesothelioma arising after direct application of asbestos and fiberglass to the pericardium. *Am Rev Respir Dis* 118:419–424, 1978.
205. Roggli VL: Pericardial mesothelioma after exposure to asbestos. *N Engl J Med* 304:1045, 1981.
206. Japko L, Horta AA, Schreiber K, Mitsudo S, Karwa GL, Singh G, Koss LG: Malignant mesothelioma of the tunica vaginalis testis: Report of first case with preoperative diagnosis. *Cancer* 49:119–127, 1982.
207. Taxy JB, Battifora H, Ovasu R: Adenomatoid tumors: A light microscopic, histochemical and ultrastructural study. *Cancer* 34:306–316, 1974.
208. Brenner J, Sordillo PP, Magill GB, Golbey RB: Malignant mesothelioma of the pleura: Review of 123 patients. *Cancer* 49:2431–2435, 1982.
209. Chahinian AP, Pajak TF, Holland JF, Norton L, Ambinder RM, Mandel EM: Diffuse malignant mesothelioma: Prospective evaluation of 69 patients. *Ann Int Med* 96:746–755, 1982.
210. Lerner HJ, Schoenfeld DA, Martin A, Falkson G, Borden E: Malignant mesothelioma: The Eastern Cooperative Oncology Group (ECOG) experience. *Cancer* 52:1981–1985, 1983.
211. Vogelzang NJ, Schultz SM, Iannucci AM, Kennedy BJ: Malignant mesothelioma: The University of Minnesota experience. *Cancer* 53:377–383, 1984.
212. Spirtas R, Connelly RR, Tucker MA: Survival patterns for malignant mesothelioma: The SEER experience. *Int J Cancer* 41:525–530, 1988.
213. Alberts AS, Falkson G, Goedhals L, Vorobiof DA, Van Der Merwe CA: Malignant pleural mesothelioma: A disease unaffected by current therapeutic maneuvers. *J Clin Oncol* 6:527–535, 1988.
214. Ruffie P, Feld R, Minkin S, Cormier Y, Boutan-Laroze A, Ginsberg R, Ayoub J, Shepherd FA, Evans WK, Figueredo A, Pater JL, Pringle JF, Kreisman H: Diffuse malignant mesothelioma of the pleura in Ontario and Quebec: A retrospective study of 322 patients. *J Clin Oncol* 7:1157–1168, 1989.
215. Butchart EJ, Ashcroft T, Barnsley WC, Holden MP: Pleural pneumonectomy in the management of diffuse malignant mesothelioma of the pleura. *Thorax* 31:15–24, 1976.

216. Antman KH, Corson JM: Benign and malignant pleural mesothelioma. *Clin Chest Med* 6:127–140, 1985.
217. Chahinian AP: Malignant mesothelioma. In: *Clinical Interpretation and Practice of Cancer Chemotherapy* (Greenspan EM, ed.), New York: Raven Press, 1982, pp. 599–606.
218. Wanebo HJ, Martini N, Melamed MR, Hilaris B, Beattie EJ: Pleural mesothelioma. *Cancer* 38:2481–2488, 1976.
219. Martini N, McCormack PM, Bains MS, Kaiser LR, Burt ME, Hilaris BS: Current review: Pleural mesothelioma. *Ann Thorac Surg* 43:113–120, 1987.
220. Gaensler EA, McLoud TC, Carrington CB: Thoracic surgical problems in asbestos-related disorders. *Ann Thorac Surg* 40:82–96, 1985.
221. Aisner J, Wiernik PH: Malignant mesothelioma: Current status and future prospects. *Chest* 74:438–444, 1978.
222. Antman KH, Blum RH, Greenberger JS, Flowerdow G, Skarin AT, Canellos GP: Multimodality therapy for malignant mesothelioma based on a study of natural history. *Am J Med* 68:356–362, 1980.
223. Dimitrov NV, McMahon SM, Carr DT: Multidisciplinary approach to management of patients with mesothelioma. *Cancer Res* 43:3974–3976, 1983.
224. Antman KH, Klegar KL, Pomfret EA, Osteen RT, Amato DA, Larson DA, Corson JM: Early peritoneal mesothelioma: A treatable malignancy. *Lancet* II:977–981, 1985.
225. Norman PE, Whitaker D: Nine-year survival in a case of untreated peritoneal mesothelioma. *Med J Australia* 150:43–44, 1989.

6. Benign Asbestos-Related Pleural Diseases

S. DONALD GREENBERG

Benign asbestos-related pleural diseases are the most common pathologic and clinical abnormalities related to asbestos exposure. Solomon et al.[1] emphasized that the pleural manifestations of asbestos exposure include four specific entities (which form the basis for this chapter's discussion): parietal pleural plaques, diffuse pleural fibrosis, rounded atelectasis, and benign asbestos effusion. There is considerable overlap among these four disease processes (Fig. 6-1), with various combinations manifesting simultaneously or sequentially in a single individual. For example, a patient with benign asbestos effusion may subsequently be found to have diffuse pleural fibrosis, or a patient with parietal pleural plaques may develop rounded atelectasis. Benign asbestos-related pleural diseases may occur after low-level, indirect, or even environmental exposures to asbestos.

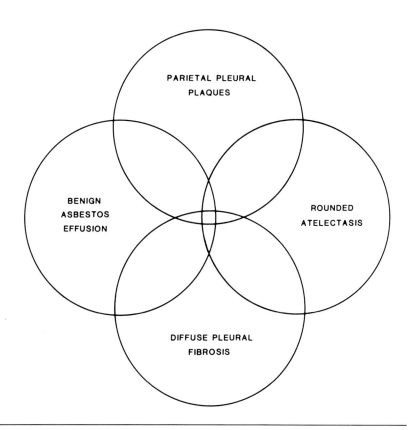

FIGURE 6-1. Venn diagram of benign asbestos-related pleural diseases showing the overlap among these four specific disorders.

However, the prevalence of these abnormalities is clearly greatest in those who are directly exposed to asbestos occupationally.

The pathogenesis of these disorders is poorly understood,[2] but it undoubtedly involves transport of asbestos fibers to the pleura, either directly through the lung parenchyma or through lymphatic pathways.[3] In the former, asbestos fibers inhaled into the lung pass into the alveoli, where they eventually work their way to the visceral pleural surface. The mechanical theory suggests that this transport occurs when the needlelike fibers work their way through the lung tissue as a result of the lung's motion during inhalation and exhalation.[4] Alternatively, fibers reach the pulmonary interstitium through a process of translocation across the alveolar epithelium.[5] Within the interstitium, the fibers would have access to pulmonary lymphatics, which in the outer third of the lung drain centripetally to the pleura. Fibers reaching the visceral pleura can then penetrate this structure and hence reach the parietal pleura, which normally is directly apposed to the visceral pleura, separated only by a potential space. The presence of fibers within the pleura elicits an inflammatory response, which may undergo organization or healing with subsequent fibrosis. In this regard, it is of interest that a recent study showed that pleural mesothelial cells in culture release a chemotactic factor for neutrophils when stimulated by asbestos fibers in vitro.[6] Clinical manifestations will then depend on the intensity of the initial inflammatory reaction and the degree and extent of any consequent pleural fibrosis.

PARIETAL PLEURAL PLAQUES

HISTORICAL BACKGROUND

Pleural plaques consist of circumscribed areas of dense, firm, greywhite fibrous tissue usually free of any inflammatory reaction. Whereas the vast majority of these pleural plaques occur on the parietal pleura, they may occur on the visceral pleura as well.[1] They most commonly occur within the parietal pleura opposite the dependent portions of the lungs.

Cartilagelike plaques on the costal pleura have long been known to pathologists. They were considered to be remnants of inflammation, similar to "sugar icing" ("*Zuckerguss*").[7] The first description of pleural plaques in connection with asbestos workers was made by Sparks, in 1931, who described irregular, small calcified plaques in the lower lung zones.[8] In 1938, Gloyne reported visceral pleural plaques that were hornlike and stiff.[9] The first description of pleural plaques in talc workers was made by Porro et al. in 1942.[10] Siegal et al. reported the initial observation of pleural plaques in tremolite talc workers.[11] In the 1950s, several reports of pleural plaques in asbestos- and talc-exposed workers appeared.[12,13]

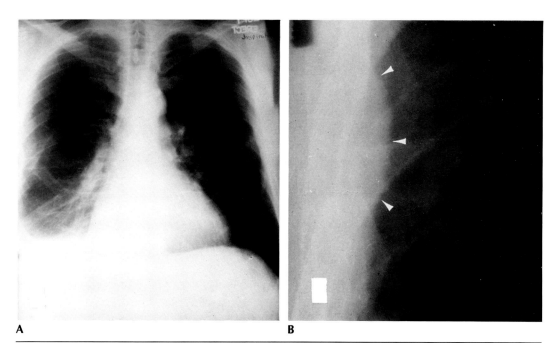

A   B

FIGURE 6-2. (A) Chest radiograph shows mild bilateral increase in interstitial markings most prominent in the lung bases, right pleural effusion, and pleural thickening with focal plaque formation. (B) The outline of this plaque viewed tangentially is seen to better advantage in this magnified view of the periphery of the right mid-lung field (arrowheads). Reprinted from Ref. 32, with permission.

Talcosis is very similar clinically and roentgenologically to asbestosis, and it is probably the asbestos found in almost all types of talc that causes the pulmonary and pleural changes.[14-16] Indeed, some of the first studies of pleural plaques were made among talc workers.[11,12] Animal experiments with "pure" talc (i.e., free of asbestos) have resulted in both pulmonary fibrosis and pleural reactions.[17] Also, talc particles have been found in pleural plaques. Therefore, it is possible that talc itself may have some effect in the formation of pleural plaques.

RADIOGRAPHIC FEATURES
Parietal pleural plaques appear on chest x-ray as discrete areas of pleural thickening, usually in the lower lung zones or on the diaphragms. They are best observed when viewed tangentially (Fig. 6-2), but may appear as a hazy density when viewed en face. The plaques often calcify, which usually does not occur until two to three decades after the initial exposure to asbestos.[18,19] Calcification greatly enhances plaque detectability with routine chest films (Fig. 6-3). In addition, oblique views are useful for detecting plaques, especially noncalcified ones.[20] Plaques generally spare the costophrenic angles;

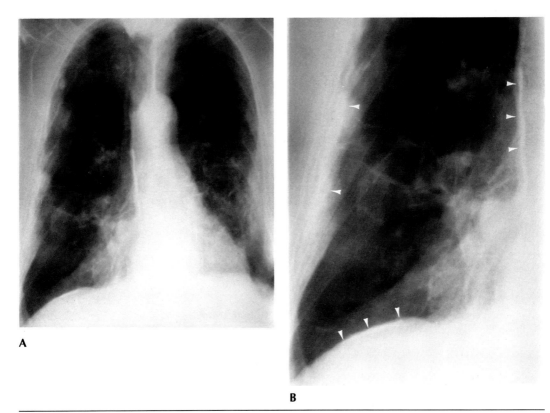

A

B

FIGURE 6-3. (A) Chest radiograph showing parietal pleural plaque formation with extensive bilateral pleural calcification. (B) The pleural calcification is seen to better advantage in this magnified view of the right hemithorax (arrowheads). Courtesy Dr. William F. Foster, Department of Radiology, Durham VA Medical Center, Durham, NC.

when blunting is observed, one should suspect the presence of pleural effusions or adhesions.[7] Pleural plaques are most often bilateral; among individuals with unilateral plaques, there is an inexplicable predominance of left-sided involvement.[21] The ILO classification of radiographs for the pneumoconioses[22] includes evaluation for pleural plaques, detailing information regarding the degree of pleural thickening, the proportion of the pleura that is thickened, and whether or not calcification is present.

Radiographic surveys of populations have shown that 1–2% of men and less than 1% of women have pleural plaques. There is, however, a high rate of false negative results, since autopsy surveys have indicated that the postmortem prevalence of plaques ranges from 4% to as high as 39% (Table 6-1).[23] In these autopsy surveys, the percentage of plaques that were detected on premortem chest films ranged from 8% to 40%. Noncalcified diaphragmatic plaques are particularly difficult to visualize on routine chest films, and were observed in none of eight cases in the series of Wain et al.[23] One must also use caution to avoid overinterpretation of films as showing pleural

TABLE 6-1. Summary of previously reported pathologic-x-ray correlation studies of patients with pleural plaques

Author	Country	Population composition	No. of autopsies*	Percent pleural plaques*	Percent detected on chest films*
Rubino et al.[18]	Italy	General population in asbestos industrial region	862	7.8%	40.3%
Hourihane et al.[24]	England	General urban population	381	4.1	13.7
Hillerdal and Lindgren[14]	Sweden	General population screen	437	6.8	12.5
Meurman[25]	Finland	General population in coastal, urban, and asbestos mining region	438	39.3	8.3
Wain et al.[23]	U.S.A.	Male veterans	434	5.8	28

SOURCE: Reprinted from Ref. 23, with permission.
*These values are calculated from published data.

plaques (i.e., false positives), which can occur secondary to shadows produced by the serratus anterior in particularly muscular individuals, or due to subpleural adipose tissue, especially in obese individuals. In this regard, computed tomography (Fig. 6-4) has been shown to improve both the specificity and sensitivity of routine chest films with respect to the identification of asbestos-related pleural disease.[26,27] However, CT of the thorax is not practical for screening of large populations.[26]

PATHOLOGIC FINDINGS

Grossly, the parietal plaques are elevated, firm, and glistening and have sharply circumscribed borders.[28] They are frequently bilateral and are usually seen within the costal pleura, where they lie parallel to the ribs. They are also seen on the domes of the diaphragm (Figs. 6-5 and 6-6). Pleural plaques vary in size from those that are just visible to the naked eye to structures that are 12 or more centimeters across.[29] They are frequently calcified. These ivory-colored structures may have either a smooth surface or a knobby appearance, consisting of multiple 5-mm nodules that create a "candle wax dripping" appearance.[29] The thickness of the plaques varies from a few millimeters to a centimeter or more. Visceral pleural plaques have been described as well but are considerably less frequent.[1] In rare instances, calcified plaques may also involve the pericardium.[30] Adhesions between the surface of parietal pleural plaques and the adjacent visceral pleura are uncommon.

Microscopically, plaques are predominantly collagenous and have but few cells (Figs. 6-7 through 6-10). This dense fibrous tissue often shows a "basket-weave" pattern[31] (see Figs. 6-8 and 6-9). However, plaques with a solid appearance lacking the "basket-weave" pattern may also be observed (see Fig. 6-10), and accounted for almost one-third of the plaques studied histologically by Wain et al.[23] Rarely,

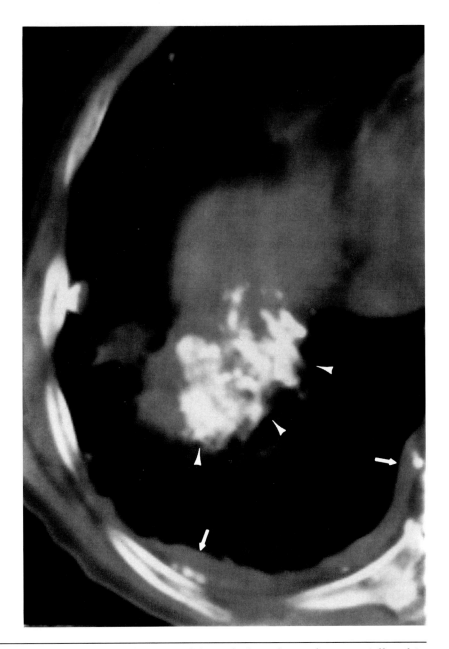

FIGURE 6-4. Computed tomographic view of the right hemithorax shows partially calcified parietal pleural plaques viewed tangentially (arrows) as well as an extensively calcified diaphragmatic plaque viewed en face (arrowheads). Courtesy Dr. William F. Foster, Department of Radiology, Durham VA Medical Center, Durham, NC.

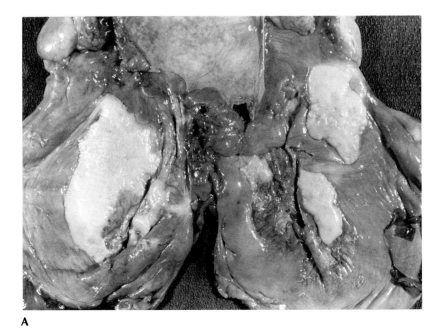

A

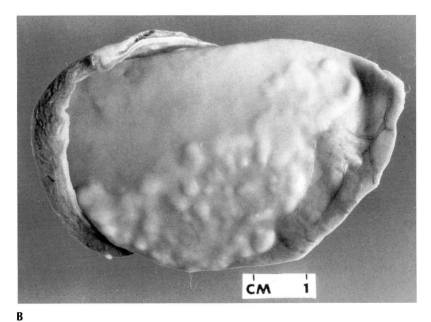

B

FIGURE 6-5. (A) Gross photograph from autopsy examination illustrates bilateral elevated white plaques on the diaphragmatic pleura. (B) Close view of a parietal diaphragmatic plaque showing smooth areas as well as knobby areas resembling "candle-wax drippings."

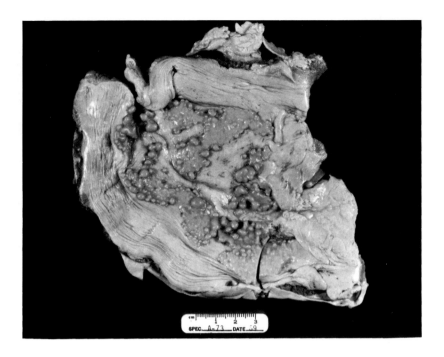

FIGURE 6-6. Gross appearance of diaphragm with parietal pleural plaque shows irregular, 10-cm plaque with smooth and nodular areas. Reprinted from Ref. 23, with permission.

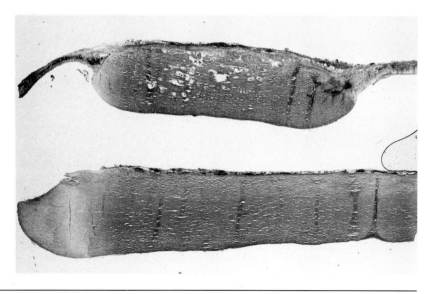

FIGURE 6-7. Low-power photomicrograph showing fibrous parietal pleural plaques as they appeared at autopsy. H&E ×10.

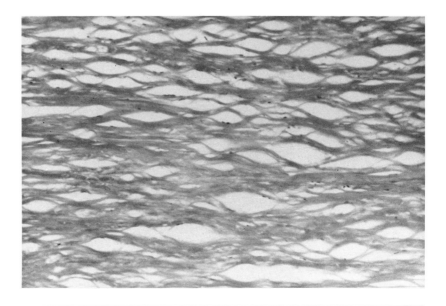

FIGURE 6-8. High magnification of a fibrous parietal pleural plaque. Note the lack of cellularity and "basket-weave" pattern of the collagen fibers. H&E ×300.

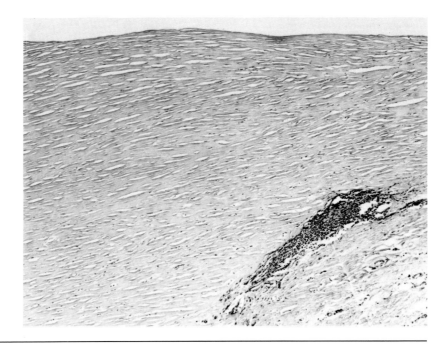

FIGURE 6-9. Low-power photomicrograph of parietal pleural plaque showing the "basket-weave" pattern of the collagen and focal collection of lymphocytes at the interface between the plaque and the underlying connective tissue of the chest wall. H&E ×68. Reprinted from Ref. 72, with permission.

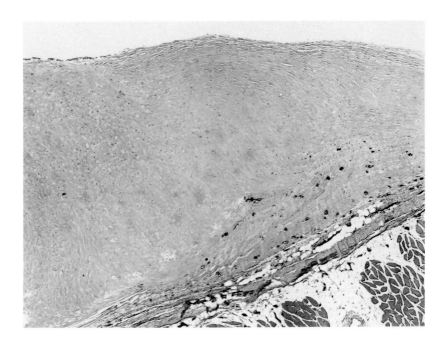

FIGURE 6-10. Parietal pleural plaque showing dense collagenous tissue without a "basket-weave" pattern (i.e., solid variant). H&E ×25.

a row of cuboidal mesothelial cells may be seen on the surface of the plaque. Although inflammatory cells are not observed within the plaque, small clusters of lymphocytes are invariably found at the edge of the plaque or at the interface between the plaque and the subjacent chest wall[32] (see Fig. 6-9). Foci of dystrophic calcification are also commonly observed within the plaque. With light microscopy, neither asbestos bodies nor fibers are seen. With electron microscopy, a few asbestos fibers may be found.[19,31]

Examination of histologic sections of lung parenchyma from patients with pleural plaques may show normal lung or a variety of pathologic features, including peribronchiolar fibrosis, visceral pleural thickening, organizing pneumonia, focal parenchymal scarring, paracicatricial emphysema, or asbestos bodies.[33] Patients with peribronchiolar fibrosis *and* asbestos bodies in histologic sections may be considered to have asbestosis[29,33] (see Chap. 4).

EPIDEMIOLOGIC CONSIDERATIONS

Various epidemiologic studies have clearly established the role of inhaled asbestos fibers in the formation of parietal pleural plaques.[19,23,24,34–40] By means of tissue digests, it has been shown that it is primarily amphibole asbestos fibers that are found in abnormal amounts in the lungs of patients with plaques.[23,36,40] The quantity of asbestos present in the lungs of patients with plaques who lack the histologic criteria for the diagnosis of asbestosis (see Chap. 4) is intermediate between that of the general population and that of individuals with asbestosis (see Chap. 11). These data agree well with the epidemiologic observations that pleural plaques often occur in individuals with brief, intermittent, or low-level asbestos exposure.[7,19,23,29] They also occur in individuals exposed to asbestos indirectly, such as family members exposed to dust brought home on an asbestos worker's clothes[37] or individuals living near an asbestos mine or production plant. Outbreaks of pleural plaques and calcification have also been observed in populations exposed to asbestos fibers from an environmental source. Examples include the high prevalence of pleural plaques among Finnish immigrants, believed to be exposed to anthophyllite asbestos in rocks used to heat sauna baths or in insulation materials for the baths,[41] or among inhabitants of the island of Cyprus[42] and in the Metsovo region of Greece,[43] where tremolite occurs naturally. In the Metsovo region of Greece, long, thin tremolite fibers are found in the whitewash materials used inside and outside the homes of the inhabitants.[43] Additional epidemics of pleural disease due to environmental asbestos exposure undoubtedly await discovery.

Fibrous zeolites found in the soil and rocks in rural areas of Turkey are also causally associated with bilateral pleural plaques. Although nonasbestiform, these zeolite fibers have length/width ratios that simulate those of asbestos fibers.[44] A detailed epidemiologic study of the fibrous zeolite (erionite) in Turkey was reported by Artvinli and Baris in 1982. In Tuzkoy, one of the villages with environmental zeolite exposure, the fibrous mineral was found in soil samples from roads and fields, as well as in building stones. Tissues of lung and pleura from the inhabitants of Tuzkoy also revealed the effects of zeolites, with 17% showing calcified pleural plaques, 10% showing fibrous pleural thickening, and 12% revealing interstitial pulmonary fibrosis.[44] These Anatolian villages also have one of the highest rates of pleural mesothelioma yet identified anywhere in the world (see Chap. 5).

In addition to the observations of pleural plaques caused by asbestos and erionite, Hillerdal lists talc as another environmental mineral that may produce bilateral pleural plaques.[19] However, talc is often contaminated with noncommercial amphiboles (anthophyllite and tremolite), so its exact role is unclear. It is of interest that cigarette smoking interacts with asbestos to greatly increase the risk for development of pleural plaques.[45,46] The proposed mechanism is that smoking impairs bronchial clearance mechanisms, thus enhancing the retention of asbestos fibers within the lungs. Finally, whereas the vast majority of cases with bilateral parietal pleural plaques are due to asbestos exposure, unilateral plaques with or without calcification may be due to other causes, including trauma with organized hemothorax, old empyema, or tuberculous pleuritis.[23,36]

CLINICAL IMPLICATIONS

The clinical implications of parietal pleural plaques are twofold: (1) the implications of plaques with regard to functional disability, and (2) the prognostic implications with regard to other asbestos-related diseases. The great majority of individuals with pleural plaques alone have no symptoms or physiologic changes.[47–49] In cases where either symptoms or clinical impairment is present, one must carefully consider contributions from cigarette smoking or from radiographically inapparent parenchymal fibrosis. Impairment from cigarette smoking is most often due to emphysema, which can be recognized radiographically.[50] Pulmonary interstitial fibrosis (i.e., asbestosis) in the presence of a negative chest x-ray occurs in 10–18% of cases.[51,52] Although Schwartz et al.[53] in a study of more than 1200 sheet metal workers found a significant correlation between radiographically detected parietal pleural plaques and restrictive ventilatory defects, these authors concede that the most probable explanation is subclinical alveolitis or interstitial fibrosis not detected by routine chest radiograms. The lack of symptoms or signs in the majority of patients with pleural plaques alone leads one to ask whether pleural plaques should be considered a disease. *Stedman's Medical Dictionary*[54] defines a disease entity as characterized by at least two of the following criteria: (1) a recognized etiologic agent (or agents); (2) an identifiable group of signs or symptoms; and (3) consistent anatomical alterations. Since pleural plaques clearly satisfy the first and third criteria, plaques, by this definition, constitute a disease entity. However, the asymptomatic nature of plaques is not necessarily applicable to other benign asbestos-related pleural disease (see later discussion).

The second issue, which is more controversial, regards the prognostic implications of plaques with respect to other potentially fatal asbestos-related diseases. Hourihane et al.[24] state that pleural mesotheliomas are more common in patients with pleural plaques, whereas Mollo et al.[39] claim that patients with bilateral plaques are more likely to develop asbestosis than those without plaques. Three different studies have independently shown a strong association between pleural plaques and laryngeal carcinoma.[23,39,55] Studies from the United Kingdom have suggested that shipyard workers with pleural plaques are at increased risk for development of carcinoma of the lung.[56,57] Others have found no increased risk of lung cancer associated with plaques alone;[23,39] and Kiviluoto et al.,[58] in a study of 700 workers with pleural plaques, found an increased risk for bronchogenic carcinoma only when there was concomitant parenchymal fibrosis (i.e., asbestosis). We agree with the position of Jarvholm et al.[48] that pleural plaques are a marker of exposure only, and that risk of subsequent asbestos-related disease correlates better with the asbestos exposure history, (i.e., dose) than with the presence or absence of plaques. There is no evidence that pleural plaques are a precursor lesion of mesothelioma.[31] Furthermore, the term *asbestosis,* which refers to pulmonary interstitial fibrosis (see Chap. 4), should not be applied to parietal pleural plaques or any of the other benign asbestos-related pleural diseases.[29,31,59,60]

DIFFUSE PLEURAL FIBROSIS

RADIOGRAPHIC FEATURES
Diffuse thickening of the visceral pleura can be detected on routine chest films. It may occur as a consequence of a connective tissue disorder, such as rheumatoid arthritis or systemic lupus erythematosus.[61] However, in the absence of clinical evidence of a connective tissue disorder, the chest x-ray showing bilateral pleural fibrosis usually indicates prior asbestos exposure.[34,35] Diffuse pleural fibrosis must be distinguished on the one hand from the more localized and often calcified parietal pleural plaque, and on the other hand from malignant pleural mesothelioma. The latter usually shows asymmetrical involvement of the hemithoraces, irregular thickening of the pleura, and invasion or destruction of portions of the chest wall. These features can often be seen to better advantage with computed tomography of the thorax.[62,63] Diffuse pleural thickening may follow benign asbestos effusion,[64] and is often unilateral (Fig. 6-11).

PATHOLOGIC FINDINGS
Diffuse pleural fibrosis is typically of varying and uneven thickness and can surround the entire lung.[65] The inferior and dorsal portions of the lung are the areas most frequently affected, and the process may extend into the major fissures (see Fig. 4-5). A constrictive pleuritis may occur and contribute to decreased vital capacity.[64,66] With time, diffuse pleural fibrosis may progress.[19] Differential diagnosis of such lesions should include infectious pleuritis, rheumatoid arthritis, and systemic lupus erythematosus. The fibrous thickening of the visceral pleura is bland and nonspecific, consisting of dense collagenous tissue and varying numbers of chronic inflammatory cells (lymphocytes, macrophages, and plasma cells) (Fig. 6-12). Fibrin deposits may be observed on the surface of the collagenous tissue. Analysis of tissue asbestos content in the lung parenchyma of patients with diffuse pleural fibrosis who lack histologic features of asbestosis shows levels intermediate between those of the general population and those of individuals with asbestosis[65] (see Chap. 11). A dose–response relationship has been demonstrated between the degree of asbestos exposure and the extent of pleural thickening.[38] With light microscopy, neither asbestos bodies nor fibers are seen within the fibrotic visceral pleura. With electron microscopy, a few asbestos fibers may be found.[19]

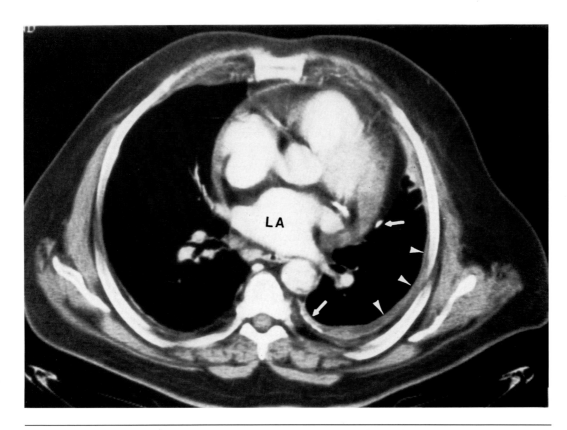

FIGURE 6-11. Computed tomography of the thorax at the level of the left atrium (LA) showing unilateral diffuse pleural thickening (arrowheads) in a 74-year-old manufacturer of asbestos cloth. Calcification is present posteriorly on the parietal pleural surface and also adjacent to the left heart border (arrows). No tumor was identified at open thoracotomy and pleural biopsy. Courtesy Dr. Caroline Chiles, Department of Radiology, Duke University Medical Center, Durham, NC.

CLINICAL IMPLICATIONS

Diffuse pleural fibrosis may be asymptomatic, but in some cases may be of sufficient extent and severity as to result in functional impairment.[53,64,66] This usually manifests as restrictive changes on pulmonary function tests, with a diminished vital capacity. Picado et al.[67] described six patients with extensive asbestos-related pleural disease who manifested diminished exercise tolerance. These investigators felt that parenchymal fibrosis was unlikely, although lung parenchyma was not available for histologic examination in any of the cases. Although some of the patients were characterized as having parietal pleural plaques, it is likely that most or all had some degree of diffuse visceral pleural fibrosis. Surgical decortication is rarely indicated in these patients, because postoperative improvement is usually only marginal.[19]

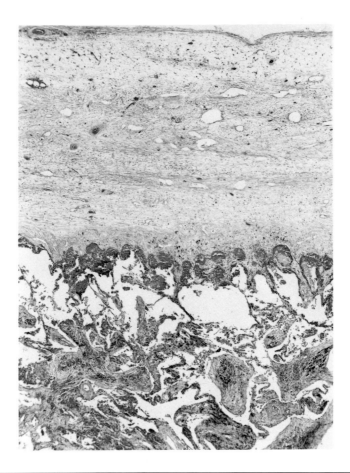

FIGURE 6-12. Diffuse fibrosis of visceral pleura in an insulator with asbestosis. Asbestos bodies in adjacent lung parenchyma are just beyond resolution at this magnification. H&E ×25.

ROUNDED ATELECTASIS

RADIOLOGIC FEATURES

Rounded atelectasis, also known as the folded lung syndrome, was originally described by Blesovsky in 1966.[68] It is characterized radiographically as a peripheral rounded mass, 2–7 cm in diameter, that is pleural based.[69] Pleural thickening that is greatest near the mass and interposition of lung parenchyma between the mass and the diaphragm are invariably present (Fig. 6-13). One of the most useful diagnostic features is the presence of curvilinear shadows extending from the mass toward the hilum.[69] The intrapulmonary location of the mass is indicated by the acute angle formed between the pleura and mass. The intralobar fissure is frequently thickened. When sequential films are available for review, the static nature of the lesion

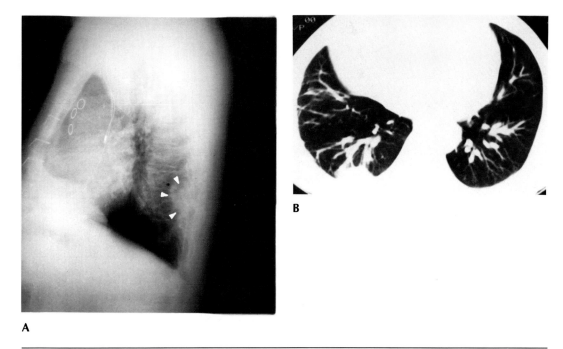

FIGURE 6-13. (A) Lateral chest radiograph showing a posterior, pleural-based mass (arrowheads). (B) Computed tomogram of the thorax shows the typical features of rounded atelectasis, with a pleural-based mass and curvilinear bronchovascular structures entering the mass. Reprinted from Ref. 72, with permission.

can be demonstrated. In cases where bronchography has been performed, bronchi have been demonstrated to curve toward the lower pole of the mass.[69] Computed tomography may assist in delineating these features in some cases, and may also detect other asbestos-related pleural changes, such as calcification[70] (Fig. 6-14). Rounded atelectasis may be bilateral in some instances, and cases with spontaneous resolution have also been reported.[71]

PATHOLOGIC FINDINGS

The pathologist must be aware of the gross and microscopic features of rounded atelectasis, since he or she may be called on to make the diagnosis at frozen section. The lesion is characterized by dense pleural fibrosis that is of greatest thickness overlying the mass (see Fig. 6-14). The pleura may be buckled or puckered and thus drawn into the underlying lung parenchyma. The lung itself may contain some fibrosis but is largely atelectatic. Because of the frequent association with asbestos exposure,[69] asbestos bodies should be searched for within the lung parenchyma.[72] Blesovsky believed that the mechanism of formation of rounded atelectasis involved localized visceral pleural thickening and fibrosis in which adhesion between

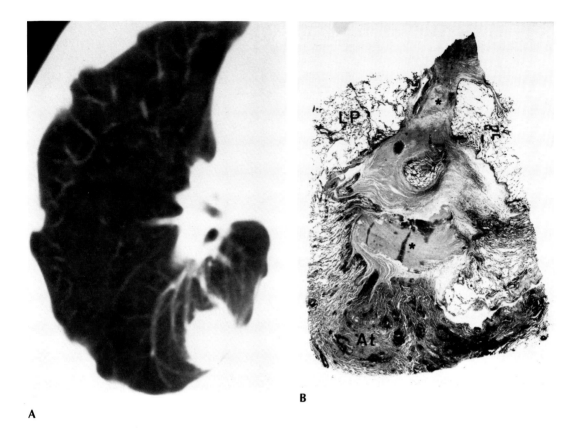

FIGURE 6-14. (A) Computed tomography of the left hemithorax in a patient with a left lower lobe mass on chest x-ray. Note the curvilinear bronchovascular structures entering the pleural-based mass, which is characteristic of rounded atelectasis. (B) Lower-power photomicrograph of the resected lesion shown in part (a), with pleural surface toward the top. There is localized thickening and fibrosis of the visceral pleura, which has buckled inwards(*). Adjacent lung parenchyma is atelectatic (At). Elsewhere, the lung parenchyma (LP) is normally expanded. H&E ×4.7.

visceral and parietal pleura was prevented from forming because of an associated pleural effusion. Contraction and buckling of the fibrotic visceral pleura then led to atelectasis and folding of the immediately adjacent lung parenchyma. In support of this pathogenetic concept, it was observed at thoracotomy that the collapsed lung reexpanded when the thickened pleura was dissected away.[68]

CLINICAL IMPLICATIONS

The strong association between rounded atelectasis and prior asbestos exposure has been emphasized.[69] Indeed, all three of the original cases described by Blesovsky had been occupationally exposed to asbestos.[69] Because of this association and the increased risk of lung cancer in asbestos workers (see Chap. 7), rounded atelectasis may be confused with lung cancer clinically and radiographically.[73] Recognition of the clinical and radiographic features of rounded atelectasis is important, since the rendering of the correct diagnosis can spare the patient a thoracotomy.[74]

BENIGN ASBESTOS PLEURAL EFFUSION

CLINICAL CRITERIA

The first case of benign asbestos-related pleural effusion was reported by Eisenstadt in 1964.[75] This was a unilateral effusion in an asbestos worker. Dr. Eisenstadt stated that a diagnosis of benign asbestos pleural effusion should only be made after biopsies of the lung and pleura were performed to rule out other disease processes. More than 250 additional cases have subsequently been reported, and it is now recognized that asbestos pleural effusion (pleurisy) is the most common asbestos-related lesion during the first decade after exposure. However, it can occur at a later date.[76] It is usually a moderate-sized effusion of up to 2000 ml that may be clear to hemorrhagic and of variable cellularity. Hillerdal lists three diagnostic criteria of an asbestos effusion: (1) tuberculosis, infection, or malignancy must be ruled out; (2) the individual must be followed for two years to verify the effusion is benign; and (3) there must be an occupational exposure to asbestos (Table 6-2). The asbestos effusion tends to recur and can last for months. Recurrence on the same or opposite side is common, and clinical symptoms are only mild to absent.[19,64] In addition to this tendency to recur, another feature characteristic of benign asbestos effusion is the presence of either rounded atelectasis or converging pleural linear structures (so-called "crow's feet") on the chest radiograph at the initial presentation.[76]

Epler et al., in 1982, reviewed chest x-rays of 1135 employees in the asbestos industry. The prevalence of asbestos effusions was 7.0%, 3.7%, and 0.2%, depending on whether the asbestos work exposure was, respectively, severe, indirect, or peripheral.[77] The latency for asbestos effusions was shorter than for asbestos plaques and was the only manifestation seen within 10 years of exposure. The incidence ranged from less than one to as many as nine cases of asbestos effusion per 1000 person-years of observation, depending on the degree of exposure. The recurrence rate was 29%; in 66% of the effusions, the workers were asymptomatic. In a related article, Gaensler et al.[74] reported on 68 patients with benign asbestos pleural effusions, the majority of whom had no symptoms. These investigators stated that benign asbestos pleural effusions were the most common asbestos-related disorder during the first 20 years after initial exposure and were seen in approximately 5% of all heavily exposed persons.[74] Robinson et al. reported on still another cohort of 22 asbestos workers

TABLE 6-2. Clinical criteria for benign asbestos pleural effusion

1. Clinically documented pleural effusion
2. History of exposure to asbestos
3. Elimination of other causes of effusion (infection, collagen vascular disease, malignancy, etc.)
4. Followup of two or three years to verify benign nature of the process

SOURCE: Modified from Refs. 19 and 74.

with asbestos pleural effusion.[78] Their mean work exposure was five years, their time between work exposure and occurrence of pleurisy was 16 years, and the mean duration of the effusion was four months.[78] The pleural fluid was blood tinged and rarely greater than 500 ml.

Hillerdal, in 1981, emphasized the benign course of these effusions even though they may be bloody and of large volume.[79] An exception was a very small group of more heavily exposed individuals who sometimes developed progressive pleural fibrosis after an initial effusion. This observation was confirmed by McLoud et al.,[80] and in some cases may result in respiratory failure.[81] Lilis et al.[82] described 20 patients in a series of 2815 insulation workers (0.7%) who had a history of symptomatic pleural effusion. Sixteen of these 20 (80%) had diffuse pleural fibrosis radiographically, whereas 5.0% of the total group had diffuse pleural fibrosis. These observations suggest that diffuse pleural fibrosis in the patients without a history of benign asbestos effusion may be the residua of asymptomatic pleural effusion in at least some of these individuals.[82] In another article, Hillerdal made the observation that asbestos workers in Finland are exposed to anthophyllite asbestos, and there is a low incidence among them of both asbestos effusion and pleural mesothelioma.[83] He indicates that these observations may be related.

PATHOLOGIC FINDINGS

The pathologic features of benign asbestos effusion have not been well defined. Core needle biopsy of the pleura in a few of the cases in the series of Robinson and Musk[78] showed pleural fibrosis with or without an inflammatory infiltrate. Decortication in four of the cases of Mattson[84] showed chronic nonspecific fibrotic pleurisy. In one of these four cases, asbestos bodies and pulmonary fibrosis were observed in the adjacent lung parenchyma. The effusion itself is characteristically an exudate, with glucose and protein levels similar to that of plasma.[85] In more than half the cases, the fluid is grossly hemorrhagic. The cell count usually is less than 6000/mm^3, with either a mononuclear or neutrophil predominance.[86] In about one-fourth of the cases, eosinophils are a prominent feature. In this regard, it should be noted that injection of asbestos fibers into the pleural cavities of experimental animals results in an exudative effusion.[2] Bilaterality of benign asbestos effusion is common, occurring in eleven of 60 patients studied by Hillerdal and Ozesmi.[85] In three cases the effusions were synchronous, whereas in the remaining eight cases they were metachronous, separated by an interval ranging from one to 15 years.

REFERENCES

1. Solomon A, Sluis-Cremer GK, Goldstein B: Visceral pleural plaque formation in asbestosis. *Environ Res* 19:258–264, 1979.
2. Sahn SA, Antony VB: Pathogenesis of pleural plaques: Relationship of early cellular response and pathology. *Am Rev Respir Dis* 130:884–887, 1984.
3. Craighead JE: Current pathogenetic concepts of diffuse malignant mesothelioma. *Hum Pathol* 18:544–557, 1987.
4. Greenberg SD: Asbestos lung disease. *Sem Respir Med* 4:130–137, 1982.
5. Brody AR, Hill LH, Adkins B, O'Connor RW: Chrysotile asbestos inhalation in rats: Deposition pattern and reaction of alveolar epithelium and pulmonary macrophages. *Am Rev Respir Dis* 123:670–679, 1981.
6. Antony VB, Owen CL, Hadley KJ: Pleural mesothelial cells stimulated by asbestos release chemotactic activity for neutrophils in vitro. *Am Rev Respir Dis* 139:199–206, 1989.
7. Hillerdal G: Pleural plaques: Occurrence, exposure to asbestos and clinical importance, Doctoral Thesis, pp. 1–227, Uppsala University #75014, Sweden, 1980.
8. Sparks JW: Pulmonary asbestosis. *Radiology* 17:1249–1257, 1931.
9. Gloyne SR: Pathology. In: *Silicosis and Asbestosis* (Lanza AJ, ed.), New York: Oxford Univ. Press, 1938.
10. Porro FW, Patten JR, Hobbs AA: Pneumoconiosis in the talc industry. *AJR* 47:507–524, 1942.
11. Siegal W, Smith AR, Greenberg L: Dust hazard in tremolite talc mining, including roentgenologic findings in talc workers. *AJR* 49:11–29, 1943.
12. Smith AR: Pleural calcification resulting from exposure to certain dusts. *AJR* 69:375–382, 1952.
13. Frost J, George J, Moller PF: Asbestosis with pleural calcification among insulation workers. *Danish Med Bull* 3:202–204, 1956.
14. Hillerdal G, Lindgren A: Pleural plaques: Correlation of autopsy findings to radiographic findings and occupational history. *Eur J Respir Dis* 61:315–319, 1980.
15. Rohl AN: Asbestos in talc. *Envir Health Persp* 9:129–132, 1974.
16. Gamble JF, Fellner W, Dimeo MJ: An epidemiologic study of a group of talc workers. *Am Rev Respir Dis* 119:741–753, 1979.
17. Wagner JC, Berry G, Cooke TJ, Hill RJ, Pooley FD, Skidmore JW: Animal experiments with talc. In: Inhaled Particles IV. Proceedings of the International Symposium, Organized by the British Occupational Hygiene Society, 1975 (Walton WH, ed.), Edinburgh: Pergamon Press, 1977, pp. 647–654.
18. Rubino GF, Scansetti G, Pira E, Piolatto G, Mollo F, Andrion A, Colombo A, Bentasso L: Pleural plaques and lung asbestos bodies in the general population: An autoptical and clinical-radiologic survey. In: *Biological Effects of Mineral Fibers* (Wagner JC, ed.) I Ann Sci Pub, 1980, pp. 545–551.
19. Hillerdal G: Nonmalignant pleural disease related to asbestos exposure. *Clin Chest Med* 6:141–152, 1985.

20. Svenes KB, Borgersen A, Haaversen O, Holten K: Parietal pleural plaques: A comparison between autopsy and x-ray findings. *Eur J Respir Dis* 69:10–15, 1986.
21. Withers BF, Ducatman AM, Yang WN: Roentgenographic evidence for predominant left-sided location of unilateral pleural plaques. *Chest* 95:1262–1264, 1989.
22. International Labour Organization: International Classification of Radiographs of the Pneumoconioses. *Occupational Safety and Health Series No. 22* (Rev). Geneva: ILO, 1980.
23. Wain SL, Roggli VL, Foster WL: Parietal pleural plaques, asbestos bodies and neoplasia: Clinical, pathologic and roentgenographic correlation of 25 consecutive cases. *Chest* 86:707–713, 1984.
24. Hourihane DO, Lessof L, Richardson PC: Hyaline and calcified pleural plaques as an index of exposure to asbestos: A study of radiological and pathological features of 100 cases with a consideration of epidemiology. *Brit Med J* 1:1069–1074, 1966.
25. Meurman L: Asbestos bodies and pleural plaques in a Finnish series of autopsy cases. *Acta Path Microbiol Scand* 181 (Suppl.):1–107, 1966.
26. Friedman AC, Fiel SB, Fisher MS, Radecki PD, Lev-Toaff AS, Caroline DF: Asbestos-related pleural disease and asbestosis: A comparison of CT and chest radiography. *Am J Roentgenol* 150:269–275, 1988.
27. Aberle DR, Gamsu G, Ray CS: High-resolution CT of benign asbestos-related diseases: Clinical and radiographic correlation. *Am J Roentgenol* 151:883–891, 1988.
28. Jones JSP: *Pathology of the Pleura*. New York: Springer-Verlag, 1988.
29. Craighead JE, Abraham JL, Churg A, et al.: The pathology of asbestos-associated diseases of the lungs and pleural cavities: Diagnostic criteria and proposed grading schema. *Arch Pathol Lab Med* 106:544–596, 1982.
30. Fischbein L, Namade M, Sachs RN, Robineau M, Lanfranchi J: Chronic constrictive pericarditis associated with asbestosis. *Chest* 94:646–647, 1988.
31. Greenberg SD: Asbestos. Ch. 22 In: *Pulmonary Pathology* (Dail DH, Hammar SP, eds.), New York: Springer-Verlag, 1988, pp. 619–635.
32. Roggli VL, Shelburne JD: New concepts in the diagnosis of mineral pneumoconioses. *Sem Respir Med* 4:138–148, 1982.
33. Sison RF, Hruban RH, Moore GW, Kuhlman JE, Wheeler PS, Hutchins GM: Pulmonary disease associated with pleural "asbestos" plaques. *Chest* 95:831–835, 1989.
34. Albelda SM, Epstein DM, Gefter WB, Miller WT: Pleural thickening: Its significance and relationship to asbestos dust exposure. *Am Rev Respir Dis* 126:621–624, 1982.
35. Andrion A, Colombo A, Dacorsi M, Mollo F: Pleural plaques at autopsy in Turen: A study on 1,019 adult subjects. *Eur J Respir Dis* 63:107–112, 1982.
36. Churg A: Asbestos fibers and pleural plaques in a general autopsy population. *Am J Pathol* 109:88–96, 1982.
37. Kilburn KH, Liles R, Anderson HA, Boylen CT, Einstein HE, Johnson SS, Warshaw R: Asbestos disease in family contacts of shipyard workers. *Am J Public Health* 75:615–617, 1985.
38. Lundorf E, Aagaard MT, Andersen J, Silberschmid M, Sabro S, Coutte A, Bolvig L: Radiological evaluation of early pleural and pulmonary changes in light asbestos exposure. *Eur J Respir Dis* 70:145–149, 1987.
39. Mollo F, Andrion A, Colombo A, Segnan N, Pira E: Pleural plaques and risk of cancer in Turin, Northwestern Italy. *Cancer* 54:1418–1422, 1984.
40. Warnock ML, Prescott RT, Kuwahara TJ: Numbers and types of asbestos fibers in subjects with pleural plaques. *Am J Pathol* 109:37–46, 1982.
41. Hillerdal G: Pleural plaques in Sweden among immigrants from Finland: With an editorial note. *Eur J Respir Dis* 64:386–390, 1983.

42. McConnochie K, Simonato L, Mavrides P, Christofides P, Pooley FD, Wagner JC: Mesothelioma in Cyprus: The role of tremolite. *Thorax* 42:342–347, 1987.

43. Langer AM, Nolan RP, Constantopoulos SH, Moutsopoulos HM: Association of Metsovo lung and pleural mesothelioma with exposure to tremolite-containing whitewash. *Lancet* 1:965–967, 1987.

44. Artvinli M, Baris YI: Environmental fiber-induced pleuro-pulmonary diseases in an Anatolian village: An epidemiologic study. *Arch Environ Health* 37:177–181, 1982.

45. Andrion A, Pira E, Mollo F: Pleural plaques at autopsy, smoking habits and asbestos exposure. *Eur J Respir Dis* 65:125–130, 1984.

46. McMillan GHG, Pethybridge RJ, Sheers G: Effect of smoking on attack rates of pulmonary and pleural lesions related to exposure to asbestos dust. *Br J Ind Med* 37:268–272, 1980.

47. Lumley KPS: Physiological changes in asbestos pleural diseases. In: *Inhaled Particles IV* (Walton WH, ed.), Oxford: Pergamon Press, 1977, pp. 781–788.

48. Jarvholm B, Arvidsson H, Bahe B, Hillerdal G, Westrin C-G: Pleural plaques—asbestos—ill-health. *Eur J Respir Dis* 68 (Suppl. 145):1–59, 1986.

49. Jarvholm B, Sanden A: Pleural plaques and respiratory function. *Am J Ind Med* 10:419–426, 1986.

50. Pratt PC: Role of conventional chest radiography in diagnosis and exclusion of emphysema. *Am J Med* 82:998–1006, 1987.

51. Epler GR, McLoud TC, Gaensler EA, Mikus JP, Carrington CB: Normal chest roentgenograms in chronic diffuse infiltrative lung disease. *N Engl J Med* 298:934–939, 1978.

52. Kipen HM, Lilis R, Suzuki Y, Valciukas JA, Selikoff IJ: Pulmonary fibrosis in asbestos insulation workers with lung cancer: A radiological and histopathological evaluation. *Br J Ind Med* 44:96–100, 1987.

53. Schwartz DA, Fuortes LJ, Galvin JR, Burmeister LF, Schmidt LE, Leistikow BN, Lamarte FP, Merchant JA: Asbestos-induced pleural fibrosis and impaired lung function. *Am Rev Respir Dis* 141:321–326, 1990.

54. *Stedman's Medical Dictionary*, 22nd ed. Baltimore: Williams & Wilkins, 1972, p. 358.

55. Hillerdal G: Pleural plaques and risks for cancer in the county of Uppsala. *Eur J Respir Dis* 61 (Suppl. 107):111–117, 1980.

56. Fletcher DE: A mortality study of shipyard workers with pleural plaques. *Br J Ind Med* 29:142–145, 1972.

57. Edge JR: Incidence of bronchial carcinoma in shipyard workers with pleural plaques. *Ann NY Acad Sci* 330:289–294, 1979.

58. Kiviluoto R, Meurman LO, Hakama M: Pleural plaques and neoplasia in Finland. *Ann NY Acad Sci* 330:31–33, 1979.

59. Churg A: Nonneoplastic diseases caused by asbestos. In: *Pathology of Occupational Lung Disease* (Churg A, Green FHY, eds.), New York: Igakushoin, 1988, pp. 213–277.

60. Murphy RL et al.: The diagnosis of non-malignant diseases related to asbestos. *Am Rev Respir Dis* 134:363–368, 1986.

61. Stanford RE: Connective tissue disease. Ch. 17 In: *Pulmonary Pathology* (Dail DH, Hammar SP, eds.), New York: Springer-Verlag, 1988, pp. 471–482.

62. Alexander E, Clark RA, Colley DP, Mitchell SE: CT of malignant pleural mesothelioma. *AJR* 137:287–291, 1981.

63. Mirvis S, Dutcher JP, Haney PJ, et al.: CT of malignant pleural mesothelioma. *AJR* 140:665–670, 1983.

64. Anonymous: Benign asbestos pleural effusions. *Lancet* I:1145–1146, 1988.

65. Stephens M, Gibbs AR, Pooley FD, Wagner JC: Asbestos-induced diffuse pleural fibrosis: Pathology and mineralogy. *Thorax* 42:583–588, 1987.

66. Britton MG: Asbestos pleural disease. *Br J Dis Chest* 76:1–10, 1982.
67. Picado C, Laporta D, Grassino A, Cosio M, Thibodeau M, Becklake MR: Mechanisms affecting exercise performance in subjects with asbestos-related pleural fibrosis. *Lung* 165:45–57, 1987.
68. Blesovsky A: The folded lung. *Br J Dis Chest* 60:19–22, 1966.
69. Mintzer RA, Cugell DW: The association of asbestos-induced pleural disease and rounded atelectasis. *Chest* 81:457–460, 1982.
70. Lynch DA, Gamsu G, Ray CS, Aberle DR: Asbestos-related focal lung masses: Manifestations on conventional and high-resolution CT scans. *Radiology* 169:603–607, 1988.
71. Hillerdal G: Rounded atelectasis: Clinical experience with 74 patients. *Chest* 95:836–841, 1989.
72. Roggli VL: Pathology of human asbestosis: A critical review. In: *Advances in Pathology* (Fenoglio-Preiser CM, ed.), Chicago: Yearbook Pub., 1989, pp. 28–47.
73. Payne CR, Jaques P, Kerr IH: Lung folding simulating peripheral pulmonary neoplasm (Blesovsky's syndrome). *Thorax* 35:936–940, 1980.
74. Gaensler EA, McLoud TC, Carrington CB: Thoracic surgical problems in asbestos related disorders. *Ann Thor Surg* 40:82–90, 1985.
75. Eisenstadt HB: Asbestos pleurisy. *Dis Chest* 46:78–81, 1964.
76. Martensson G, Hagberg S, Pettersson K, Thringer G: Asbestos pleural effusion: A clinical entity. *Thorax* 42:646–651, 1987.
77. Epler GR, McLoud TC, Gaensler EA: Prevalence and incidence of benign asbestos pleural effusion in a working population. *JAMA* 247:617–622, 1982.
78. Robinson BWS, Musk AW: Benign asbestos pleural effusion: Diagnosis and course. *Thorax* 36:896–900, 1981.
79. Hillerdal G: Non-malignant asbestos pleural disease. *Thorax* 36:669–675, 1981.
80. McLoud TC, Woods BO, Carrington CB, Epler GR, Gaensler EA: Diffuse pleural thickening in an asbestos-exposed population: Prevalence and causes. *Am J Roent* 144:9–18, 1985.
81. Miller A, Teirstein AS, Selikoff IJ: Ventilatory failure due to asbestos pleurisy. *Am J Med* 75:911–919, 1983.
82. Lilis R, Lerman Y, Selikoff IJ: Symptomatic benign pleural effusions among asbestos insulation workers: Residual radiographic abnormalities. *Br J Ind Med* 45:443–449, 1988.
83. Hillerdal G, Zitting A, van Assendelft HW, Kuusela T: Rarity of mineral fibre pleurisy among persons exposed to Finnish anthophyllite and with low risk of mesothelioma. *Thorax* 39:608–611, 1984.
84. Mattson SB: Monosymptomatic exudative pleurisy in persons exposed to asbestos dust. *Scand J Respir Dis* 56:263–272, 1975.
85. Hillerdal G, Ozesmi M: Benign asbestos pleural effusion: 73 exudates in 60 patients. *Eur J Respir Dis* 71:113–121, 1987.
86. Sahn SA: State of the Art: The pleura. *Am Rev Respir Dis* 138:184–234, 1988.

7. Carcinoma of the Lung

S. Donald Greenberg and Victor L. Roggli

During the past 50 years, the United States and other industrialized nations have witnessed a remarkable increase in mortality from carcinoma of the lung. Today, this disease is the number-one cause of cancer mortality in the United States, accounting for 130,000 deaths annually.[1] Unraveling the various causes of this increased risk has required painstaking epidemiologic studies, but it has become apparent that cigarette smoking is the single largest preventable cause of lung cancer in the world today.[2] It has been estimated that between 80% and 85% of deaths from lung cancer are directly attributable to smoking.[1,2] Cigarettes are the leading offenders; but pipe and cigar smokers are also at risk, though only if they inhale the smoke.[1-3] Asbestos workers are also at increased risk for lung cancer, particularly those who smoke tobacco products.[4,5] This chapter reviews the characteristics of asbestos-associated lung cancers and discusses the role of the pathologist in recognizing asbestos as a causative factor. As prelude, it first examines the historical context, in which asbestos was recognized to be a carcinogen for the lower respiratory tract, and discusses the epidemiologic features of asbestos-related lung cancer, including the role of asbestosis, synergism with cigarette smoking, and asbestos fiber type. (The role of cytopathology in the diagnosis of lung cancer in asbestos workers is discussed in Chap. 9, experimental models of pulmonary carcinogenesis in Chap. 10, and lung fiber burdens in asbestos workers with lung cancer in Chap. 11.)

HISTORICAL BACKGROUND

The first report of carcinoma of the lung in an asbestos worker was that of Lynch and Smith in 1935, a squamous carcinoma in a patient with asbestosis.[6] In 1943, Homburger reported three additional cases of bronchogenic carcinoma associated with asbestosis, bringing the world total reported to that date to 19 cases.[7] In his annual report for 1947 as chief inspector of factories in England and Wales, Merewether noted that among 235 deaths attributed at autopsy to asbestosis, 13% had a lung or pleural cancer.[8] During the 20 years following Lynch and Smith's initial case report, some 26 reports were published covering approximately 90 cases of carcinoma of the lung found at autopsy in asbestos workers.[9] Then in 1955, Sir Richard Doll published his classic study, the first systematic, combined epidemiologic and pathologic study of lung cancer among asbestos workers.[10] Doll concluded that carcinoma of the lung was a specific industrial hazard of asbestos workers. Also in 1955, Breslow published a case control study of asbestosis and lung cancer from California hospitals.[11] In 1968, Selikoff published data from a cohort of asbestos insulation workers that showed that insulators who smoked had a 92-fold increased risk of carcinoma of the lung over non-asbestos-exposed, nonsmoking individuals.[12] This was also the first study to suggest a multiplicative, or synergistic, effect between cigarette smoking and asbestos exposure in the production of pulmonary carcinomas. Buchanan noted that more than half of all patients with asbestosis would eventually die of respiratory tract cancer.[13] Since these pioneering studies, numerous reports have appeared confirming the association between asbestos exposure and carcinoma of the lung.[14-20]

EPIDEMIOLOGY

ASBESTOS OR ASBESTOSIS?

Epidemiologic studies have demonstrated a dose–response relationship between asbestos exposure and lung cancer risk, and there is a long latency period between initial exposure and manifestation of disease, usually beginning more than 15 years after initial exposure.[4,5,9,19] It has been suggested that the best estimate of the dose–response relationship is that it is linear[21,22] which has important implications for lung cancer risks at low levels of exposure. Such a model implies that there is a finite probability of developing lung cancer at the lowest measurable exposure levels. On the other hand, some investigators have suggested that there is a threshold level of exposure to asbestos below which no excess deaths from carcinoma of the lung will occur,[16,23] and that only those individuals with asbestosis have an excess risk of developing lung cancer.[24] Whether or not there is a threshold for asbestos-induced carcinoma of the lung and whether or not asbestosis is a prerequisite precursor lesion are issues of more than academic importance,[25] since the number of individuals exposed to low levels of asbestos greatly exceeds the numbers of individuals with asbestosis. Furthermore, lung cancers certainly occur in individuals with low-level asbestos exposure, but it is uncertain whether these are related to cigarette smoking alone or whether asbestos is also a contributing factor.

In the original study by Doll,[10] all 11 of the asbestos workers dying of carcinoma of the lung had pathologically confirmed asbestosis. Furthermore, in the review by An and Koprowska of asbestos-associated carcinoma of the lung reported from 1935 to 1962, all 41 cases occurred in individuals with asbestosis.[26] Published mortality data reveal a close correlation between relative risks of death from lung cancer and from asbestosis.[14,22,27-33] In addition, a longitudinal study of Quebec chrysotile miners indicated that most of the observed cancers occurred in subgroups of workers with prior radiographic evidence of asbestosis,[34] and a necropsy study of amphibole asbestos miners showed an increased risk for bronchial cancer only among those miners with asbestosis.[35] A number of cohort mortality studies as well as studies of populations with environmental asbestos exposure[22,29,36–42] have identified some level of exposure below which no statistical excess of lung cancers can be demonstrated.[25] These epidemiologic data support the position that there is a threshold level of asbestos exposure below which no excess mortality from lung cancer will occur.[16,23] However, investigation of the consequences of low-level exposures is the Achilles' heel of epidemiologic studies because it requires large cohorts followed for extended periods of time in order to detect statistically significant associations.[42,43] Indeed, in published cohorts with the steepest dose–response relationship, excess lung cancers were detected even in the groups with the very lowest level of exposure.[27,44] Further, asbestosis is not invariably present in all cohorts of asbestos workers with a demonstrable excess risk of lung cancer.[25,34,44,45]

Pathologic observations have also been implicated as evidence that asbestosis is a necessary prerequisite for excess lung cancer risk among asbestos workers.[24] Lung cancers among asbestos workers occur more often in the lower lobes (the site of most severe fibrosis), whereas upper lobe cancers predominate among non-asbestos-exposed smokers. Furthermore, some studies have suggested a predominance of adenocarcinomas among asbestos workers, which is the histologic pattern most frequently associated with "scar carcinomas" of the lung.[24] Also, patients with other types of diffuse pulmonary fibrosis appear to be at increased risk for the development of pulmonary adenocarcinomas.[46] Among members of the cohort of asbestos insulation workers studied by Selikoff, which has been shown to have a five-fold increase in lung cancer risk as compared to a population with similar smoking habits,[5] histologic study of lung parenchyma in the 138 cases of lung cancer with tissue available from this cohort showed asbestosis to be present in 100%.[47] Although these arguments have some merit, they must be considered in light of the fact that the vast majority of lung cancers among asbestos workers are bronchogenic carcinomas not distinguishable on the basis of their morphology or histological features from those occurring in nonexposed smokers. Furthermore, carcinoma of the lung occurs considerably more frequently among individuals with asbestosis than among individuals with other types of diffuse pulmonary fibrosis.[13,46,48] Thus the phenomenon of adenocarcinoma secondary to pulmonary fibrosis could explain only a fraction of the total cancer burden associated with asbestos exposure. In addition, the interaction between asbestos and cigarette smoking (see next section) is difficult to reconcile with the view that fibrosis is the primary preneoplastic lesion.[25]

Experimental animal studies also bear on the issue of the mechanism of asbestos-induced carcinogenesis[25] (this subject is reviewed in detail in Chap. 10). It is the authors' view that the literature in this regard indicates that fibrogenesis and carcinogenesis are separate and distinct effects of asbestos pathobiology, which have as a common denominator a dose–response relationship with respect to asbestos exposure and a dependence on fiber length.

In summary, the weight of the evidence at this time seems to indicate that, in an asbestos worker with carcinoma of the lung who also smokes cigarettes, asbestosis must be present clinically or histologically (or there should at least be a tissue asbestos content within the range of values observed in patients with asbestosis—see Chap. 11) in order to assign a substantial contributing role to asbestos in the causation of the lung cancer. The mere presence of parietal pleural plaques is not sufficient to establish causation (see Chap. 6). However, the issue of asbestos or asbestosis as the primary cause of lung cancer among asbestos workers should not be considered to be settled,[24,25,49] and more studies are needed to resolve this question with certainty.

CIGARETTE SMOKING AND SYNERGISM

Epidemiologic studies have indicated a synergistic effect between cigarette smoking and asbestos exposure in the production of lung cancer.[5,12,50,51] This concept is well illustrated in the study by Hammond et al.[5] in which cancer mortality in more than 17,000 asbestos insulators was compared with cancer death rates in the general population. In this study, it was noted that cigarette smoking increases one's risk of lung cancer approximately 11-fold, whereas asbestos exposure increases the risk about five-fold, when compared to a non-smoking, nonexposed reference population. If these two effects were merely additive, one would expect an approximately 16-fold increase in lung cancer risk among cigarette-smoking asbestos insulators. Instead, what is actually observed is a 55-fold increase in risk, indicating that the two effects are multiplicative rather than additive.[5] Other investigators have also considered that the interaction between asbestos and cigarette smoke in increasing the lung cancer risk is a synergistic or multiplicative effect.[52–56] (Possible mechanisms for this synergism are discussed in Chap. 10.)

Since most lung cancers among asbestos-exposed individuals occur in workers who also smoke, it is difficult to obtain information regarding the lung cancer risk among nonsmoking asbestos workers. Hammond et al.[5] reported four such cases among their asbestos insulators, with an expected value of 0.8; hence their calculation of a five-fold increase in risk among nonsmoking asbestos workers. Berry et al.[57] reported four additional cases of lung cancer among nonsmoking asbestos-factory workers, and concluded that, after allowance had been made for the effect of smoking on lung cancer, the relative risk due to asbestos was highest for those who had never smoked, lowest for current smokers, and intermediate for exsmokers ($p < 0.05$). Lemen[58] reported four more cases of lung cancer among nonsmoking women in a predominantly chrysotile asbestos textile plant. One of the authors (VLR) has also observed two additional cases: one in a 63-year-old asbestos worker with asbestosis, and the

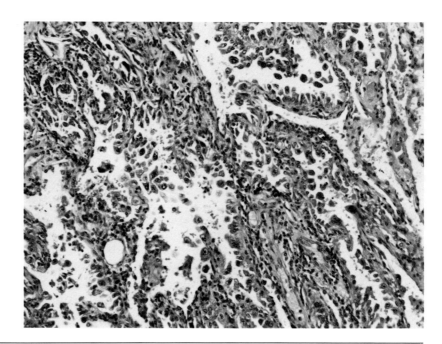

FIGURE 7-1. Bronchioloalveolar cell carcinoma of the left upper lobe in a 73-year-old housewife of an asbestos worker. Tissue asbestos analysis of nontumorous lung parenchyma indicated an elevated content of amosite and chrysotile asbestos. H&E ×130.

other in a 73-year-old housewife of an asbestos worker. Neither patient had ever smoked cigarettes, and both had a bronchioloalveolar cell carcinoma of the lung (Fig. 7-1). Tissue asbestos analysis in the second case indicated an 11-fold increase in asbestos body content above our upper limit of normal.[48] Uncoated fiber content in this latter case was also elevated, and both amosite and chrysotile fibers were identified. Asbestosis was not present histologically. It seems reasonable to hypothesize a causative role for asbestos in such cases, considering the rarity of carcinoma of the lung among lifelong nonsmokers[59] and the weak association between smoking and bronchioloalveolar cell carcinomas among women.[60] However, one must also consider other possible factors, such as the effects of passive smoking[61] and of household radon gas exposure.[62]

The U.S. Surgeon General's recent report on the effects of smoking cessation on the risk of developing carcinoma of the lung indicates that exsmokers have a risk intermediate between that of current smokers and nonsmokers.[63] The magnitude of the decrease in risk is related to a number of factors, including the age when the patient started smoking, total duration and intensity of smoking, the age at cessation of smoking, and the time elapsed since the individual quit smoking. In this regard, some studies have indicated that the risk of developing lung cancer in an exsmoker is still greater than that of a lifelong nonsmoker, even 20 or more years after cessation of smoking.[63] These factors must be considered in evaluating the role of asbestos exposure in the development of carcinoma of the lung in an exsmoker.

ROLE OF FIBER TYPE

Epidemiologic data indicate that carcinoma of the lung may develop in response to exposure to any of the types of asbestos.[4,9,14,27,54,64] However, there is considerable controversy regarding the relative potency of the various fiber types for the production of pulmonary neoplasms.[25] Individuals who believe that chrysotile is less potent as a lung carcinogen than the amphiboles, amosite and crocidolite, cite as evidence the relatively low rate of carcinoma of the lung among chrysotile miners and millers,[22,65] asbestos cement workers,[16,66] and friction-product manufacturers.[36,39] On the other hand, some chrysotile asbestos textile plants have reported extremely high lung cancer rates, with exceptionally steep dose–response curves.[27,29,67] Although it has been suggested that contamination of the asbestos fibers with mineral oil might explain the high rate of carcinoma of the lung among asbestos textile workers,[9] the steep dose–response relationship among these workers also holds for asbestosis, which is difficult to explain on the basis of contaminating oil. One major difficulty for studies trying to assess the relative potency of asbestos fiber types is the inaccuracy of historic estimates of asbestos exposure.[25,68] In this regard, Newhouse[69] noted that chrysotile textile plants were particularly dusty when compared with other types of occupational exposure to chrysotile. Furthermore, in comparing the cancer mortality for two different asbestos textile plants,[29,67] Finkelstein concluded that the risk of death from asbestos-associated cancer in factories manufacturing similar products is unrelated to the type of asbestos fiber used.[68] More work is required to resolve this issue, but the authors suspect that much of the variation in lung cancer rates among chrysotile workers can be explained on the basis of dose and relative fiber size, with longer fibers being more potent. For example, the low rate of lung cancer among automotive maintenance and brake repair workers[70,71] can be explained on the basis of relatively low dust levels, the low proportion of asbestos in the dust generated, and the preponderance of very short chrysotile fibers in brake-line dust.[72]

PATHOLOGY OF ASBESTOS-RELATED CARCINOMA OF THE LUNG

GROSS MORPHOLOGY

Lung carcinomas have been classically divided into the proximal bronchogenic carcinomas, which arise from a mainstem, segmental, or subsegmental bronchus and typically present as a hilar mass,

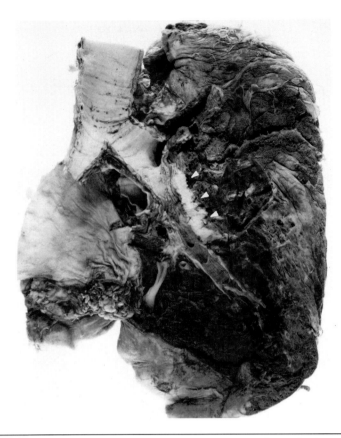

FIGURE 7-2. Gross photograph showing infiltrating carcinoma involving the bronchus intermedius of the right lung (arrowheads). The patient was a guard in a plant that manufactured amosite pipe insulation for seven years. Reprinted from Ref. 78, with permission.

and peripheral carcinomas, arising from small airways (i.e., bronchioles) and presenting as a "coin" lesion on chest roentgenogram.[73] Asbestos-related lung cancers can assume either of these gross appearances; in fact, there are no discernible differences between the macroscopic appearance of carcinomas of the lung among asbestos workers and those in individuals not exposed to asbestos.[73–76] One possible exception to this observation is the lobar distribution, with carcinomas among cigarette smokers from the general population occurring about twice as often in the upper as compared to the lower lobes, whereas the reverse is true for carcinomas among asbestos workers.[77] However, the overlap is great enough that the lobar distribution is hardly sufficient to assign attribution to asbestos exposure in the individual case.[75]

Typical examples of carcinoma of the lung in patients with asbestosis are illustrated in Figs. 7-2 through 7-4. One shows a proximal bronchogenic carcinoma (Fig. 7-2) from a Tyler asbestos plant worker

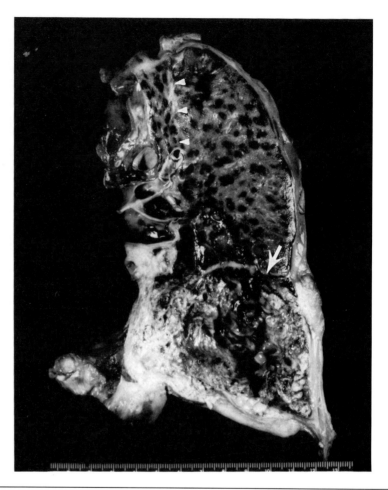

FIGURE 7-3. Gross photograph showing a cavitating carcinoma of the right lower lobe (arrow). The patient was an asbestos insulator in a shipyard for 30 years (same case as Fig. 4-4). Radiation fibrosis is present in the medial aspect of the right upper lobe (arrowheads), and a few scattered silicotic nodules were also palpable in the right upper lobe.

who was a guard at the Tyler plant for seven years and developed the neoplasm 21 years after initial exposure. This plant made pipe insulation material from amosite asbestos.[78,79] The second example is a lower-lobe cavitating cancer (Fig. 7-3) from a shipyard insulator and boilerscaler for 30 years. The third example shows a massively enlarged hilar lymph node secondary to metastatic bronchogenic carcinoma (primary tumor not visible in the section). Very fine interstitial fibrosis was just visible to the unaided eye in the lower lobes (Fig. 7-4). This patient was admitted comatose and died shortly thereafter, without providing any occupational history; asbestosis was confirmed on histologic examination. All three examples are squamous

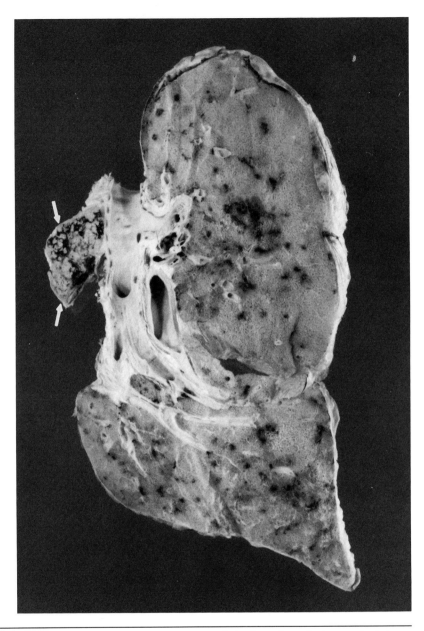

FIGURE 7-4. Metastatic bronchogenic carcinoma in a hilar lymph node (arrows). Asbestosis was present in histologic sections.

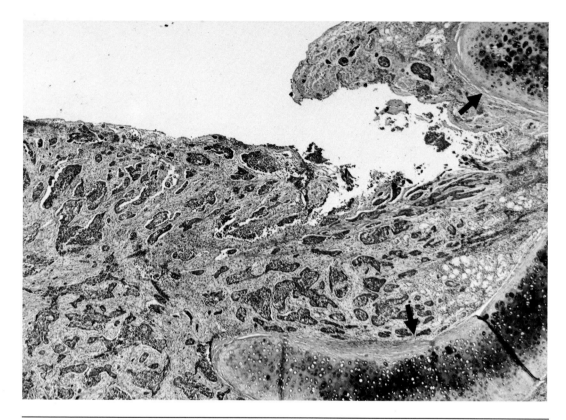

FIGURE 7-5. Squamous cell carcinoma of the right lung invading the wall of the bronchus intermedius in close proximity to the bronchial cartilages (arrows).
Same case as Fig. 7-2. H&E ×39. Reprinted from Ref. 79, with permission.

cell carcinomas (Fig. 7-5), and two of the individuals also smoked cigarettes (180 and 50 pack-years, respectively). The smoking history of
the third is unknown.

HISTOPATHOLOGY

Carcinomas of the lung have conventionally been categorized into
four histologic patterns: squamous cell carcinoma, small-cell carcinoma, adenocarcinoma, and large-cell carcinoma[73,80–82] (Table 7-1).
These patterns are illustrated in Fig. 7-6. Squamous cell carcinomas
are characterized by the presence of keratinization, or intercellular
bridges. In well-differentiated tumors, keratinization manifests in
the form of keratin pearls; in more poorly differentiated tumors, it
manifests as individual cell keratinization [see Fig. 7-6(A)]. Squamous
cell carcinomas account for about 35% of primary lung carcinomas
and usually present as proximal hilar masses. Small-cell carcinomas
have scant amounts of cytoplasm with high nuclear-to-cytoplasmic
ratios. The nuclei are often hyperchromatic or else have finely stippled
chromatin with inconspicuous nucleoli [see Fig. 7-6(B)]. Small-cell

TABLE 7-1. Histologic typing of lung cancer

    I. Squamous cell carcinoma
       A. Spindle-cell squamous cancers
   II. Small-cell carcinoma
       A. Oat-cell type
       B. Intermediate type
       C. Mixed or combined small-cell carcinomas
  III. Adenocarcinoma
       A. Acinar type
       B. Papillary type
       C. Solid pattern with mucin-production
       D. Bronchioloalveolar cell carcinoma
  IV. Large-cell carcinoma
       A. Giant-cell type
       B. Clear-cell variant
   V. Adenosquamous carcinoma

SOURCE: Modified from WHO classification of lung tumors.[80]

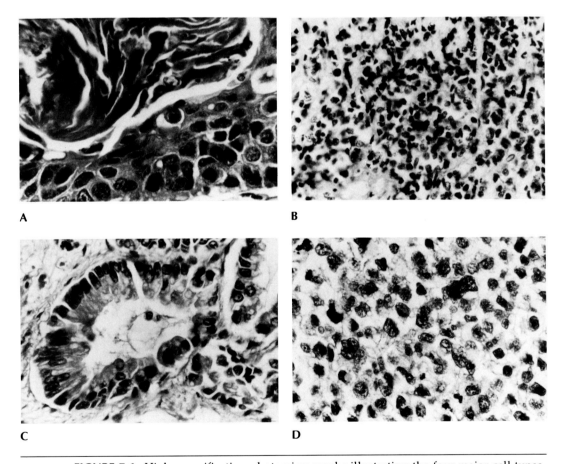

FIGURE 7-6. High-magnification photomicrographs illustrating the four major cell types of carcinoma of the lung: (A) squamous cell carcinoma, (B) small-cell carcinoma, (C) adenocarcinoma, and (D) large-cell carcinoma. H&E ×600.

carcinomas account for about 20% of primary lung carcinomas and also present as proximal tumors. Both squamous cell and small-cell carcinomas are strongly associated with a past history of cigarette smoking.[60]

Adenocarcinomas are recognized by their tendency to form glandular, acinar, or papillary structures [see Fig. 7-6(C)]. In some cases, the tumor cells form solid sheets and can only be distinguished from large-cell carcinoma by means of special stains for mucosubstances. A special variant of adenocarcinoma, known as bronchioloalveolar cell carcinoma, consists of tall columnar tumor cells that tend to grow along intact alveolar septa (see Fig. 7-1). Adenocarcinomas account for about 30% of primary lung carcinomas and usually present as peripheral nodules or masses. Large-cell carcinomas consist of sheets or nests of tumor cells with moderately abundant cytoplasm, anaplastic nuclei, and prominent nucleoli [see Fig. 7-6(D)]. They do not keratinize, form glandular or papillary structures, or produce mucosubstances. Giant-cell anaplastic carcinomas and clear-cell carcinomas are subtypes of large-cell carcinoma, which accounts for about 10% of primary lung carcinomas and more often presents as a peripheral mass. Adenocarcinomas and large-cell carcinomas are less strongly associated with cigarette smoking than are squamous cell and small-cell carcinomas.[60] Nonetheless, these tumors do have a significant association with a prior history of smoking.

Some pulmonary carcinomas may have a spindle-cell, or sarcomatoid, component, giving them a biphasic appearance.[83] We have seen examples of such carcinomas in asbestos workers presenting as superior sulcus (Pancoast) tumors (Fig. 7-7) or as proximal hilar masses (Fig. 7-8). These tumors may invade the pleura or chest wall and thus must be distinguished from malignant mesothelioma (see next section). Mixtures of adenocarcinoma and squamous cell carcinoma also occur, and these are referred to in the World Health Organization classification as adenosquamous carcinomas (see Table 7-1). It should be noted that histologic heterogeneity is frequently present in primary carcinomas of the lung, and with thorough sampling, various combinations of the four major histologic patterns can be found in almost half of the cases.[84] In addition, the authors have encountered examples of asbestos workers with synchronous primary lung neoplasms of differing histologic type (e.g., a patient with asbestosis and adenosquamous carcinoma and small-cell carcinoma in the same lung[48]).

All of the histologic patterns of lung cancer just described may occur in asbestos workers.[48,73–75,85,86] However, there is some confusion in the literature regarding the distribution of histologic types in asbestos workers as compared to nonexposed individuals. A number of earlier studies described an excess of adenocarcinomas among asbestos workers with carcinoma of the lung.[13,87–89] However, Kannerstein and Churg[90] reported in 1972 that the distribution of histologic types of lung cancer was similar for asbestos workers and members of the

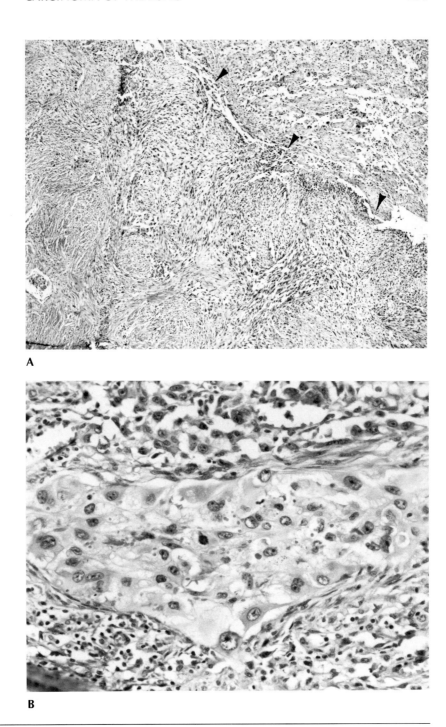

FIGURE 7-7. (A) Predominantly spindle-cell carcinoma of right upper lobe of an asbestos worker, presenting as a superior sulcus tumor. The margin of tumor invading the underlying lung parenchyma can be discerned (arrowheads). (B) Higher magnification elsewhere in the tumor shows epithelial component composed of large anaplastic cells with abundant cytoplasm. H&E: part (A) ×40, part (B) ×250.

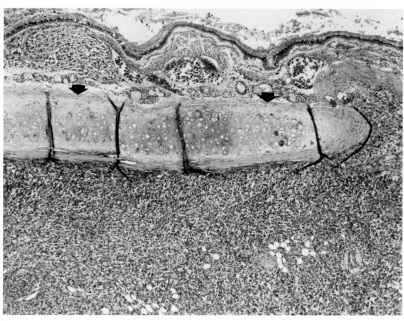

A

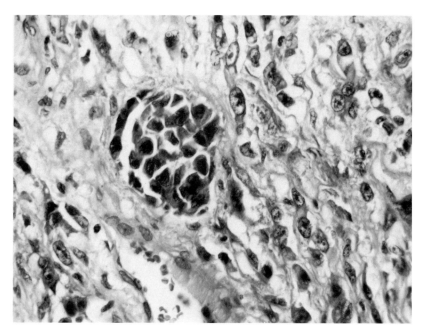

B

FIGURE 7-8. (A) Predominantly spindle-cell carcinoma invading the right mainstem bronchus in close proximity to the bronchial cartilages (arrows). Asbestosis was confirmed histologically in the pneumonectomy specimen. (B) Higher magnification elsewhere in the tumor shows epithelial component composed of a nest of loosely cohesive polygonal-shaped tumor cells that were strongly positive for cytokeratins. H&E: part (A) ×40, part (B) ×400.

general population. Since 1983, five additional studies have reported similar findings.[48,91–94] Thus the histologic features of a lung tumor are of no particular value in deciding whether or not it is an asbestos-related malignancy.[74,75] The distribution of histologic types of lung cancer in 350 patients from one of the author's series (VLR) is shown in Table 7-2. The first column includes patients with carcinoma of the lung in which asbestosis was confirmed histologically, whereas the second and third columns include patients who did not have asbestosis but had either an elevated or normal tissue asbestos-body content, respectively. The fourth column includes cases with carcinoma of the lung in which only tumor tissue was available for review, or else asbestosis could not be confirmed histologically and no lung parenchyma was available for determination of asbestos-body content. The fifth column includes 100 consecutive lung cancer resections or autopsies collected at Baylor Affiliated Hospitals, Houston, TX, from 1979–1980.[84] The percentage of adenocarcinoma cases is higher for patients with asbestosis (45%) or patients with elevated tissue asbestos-body content without asbestosis (57%) as compared to the other three groups (36–39%). Formal statistical comparison of the first three columns by partitioning of Chi-square showed no significant differences in the distribution of histologic types ($\chi^2 = 9.64$, 6 df, $p = 0.15$). These observations are consistent with the proposition that most carcinomas of the lung occurring in asbestos workers are histologically similar to those occurring in nonexposed cigarette smokers, whereas adenocarcinomas derived from the scarring process account for only a small proportion of cases, resulting in a statistically insignificant increase in the percentage of adenocarcinomas.

DIFFERENTIAL DIAGNOSIS

Primary lung carcinomas must be distinguished from pulmonary metastases and from other primary intrathoracic malignancies. Knowledge of the clinical information and radiographic findings is often useful in this regard. Primary lung carcinomas usually present as a solitary pulmonary mass or nodule, whereas metastatic disease most often manifests as multiple and bilateral nodules of similar size, most numerous in the lower lobes. A history of a primary malignancy in an extrapulmonary location is of obvious significance in this regard. The histologic appearance of the tumor is of limited use in determining whether a lung neoplasm is primary or metastatic. For example, most small-cell carcinomas are primary to the lung, whereas adenocarcinomas are common histologic patterns in a number of primary sites, and histologic features alone (especially on a small biopsy) usually are not indicative of a primary site of origin. Similarly, for tumors with a prominent clear-cell component, a renal primary source needs to be excluded.

Primary lung carcinomas must also be distinguished from other pulmonary neoplasms, most of which are distinctly uncommon.[95] Peripheral carcinomas that invade the pleura must be distinguished

TABLE 7-2. Distribution of histological types in 350 lung cancer cases with and without asbestosis[a]

	Asbestosis	AB's increased[b]	Normal AB's[b]	Other[c]	Reference population[d]
Squamous cell carcinoma	19 (26.0%)	18 (24.0%)	7 (25.9%)	28 (33.7%)	31 (31.0%)
Small-cell carcinoma	15 (20.5)	12 (16.0)	5 (18.5)	10 (12.0)	11 (11.0)
Adenocarcinoma	33 (45.2)	43 (57.3)	10 (37.0)	30 (36.1)	39 (39.0)
Large-cell carcinoma	2 (2.7)	2 (2.7)	4 (14.8)	13 (15.7)	19 (19.0)
Adenosquamous carcinoma	4 (5.5)	0 0.0	1 (3.7)	2 (2.4)	—
TOTAL	73	75	27	83	100

[a]More than one primary lung cancer in eight cases.
[b]No histologic evidence of asbestosis. AB's = Asbestos bodies.
[c]No lung parenchyma available for assessment of asbestosis or asbestos bodies.
[d]100 consecutive lung cancer cases collected at Baylor Affiliated Hospitals, 1979–1980.[84]

from malignant mesothelioma (see Chap. 5). The gross features of the tumor may be of limited utility in this regard,[96] and the pathologist must rely on histological, histochemical, immunohistochemical, or ultrastructural features of the tumor to make this distinction. Uncommonly, a pulmonary carcinoma with a prominent spindle-cell component may occur in the lung periphery and invade the pleura, mimicking a biphasic pleural mesothelioma (see Figs. 7-7 and 7-8). The localized nature of the tumor with a prominent pulmonary parenchymal component or the presence of a hilar mass with prominent involvement of a proximal bronchus are useful differentiating features in this regard.

THE PATHOLOGIST'S ROLE IN IDENTIFYING ASBESTOS-ASSOCIATED CARCINOMAS OF THE LUNG

It has been estimated that in the 25 years from 1985–2009, there will be 76,700 deaths from asbestos-related carcinomas of the lung in the United States alone.[97] In consideration of the occurrence of 130,000 lung cancer deaths annually (or 3.25 million from 1985–2009), the great majority of which are related to cigarette smoking,[1,2] it is clear that a major challenge for the medical profession and society in general will be to determine which lung cancers are related to asbestos exposure in order that appropriate compensation may be provided where indicated. This will require careful consideration of clinical, radiographic, and pathologic data in the individual case, as well as epidemiologic and relevant experimental animal studies. As noted in the previous discussion, there are no pathologic features of carcinoma of the lung in asbestos workers that permit their distinction in the individual case from the much more common tobacco-related cancers in non-asbestos-exposed individuals. Therefore, the primary role of the pathologist is to render an accurate and precise diagnosis of carcinoma of the lung based on available pathological materials and to help exclude other differential diagnostic considerations.

Another important aspect of the pathologist's role has been referred to as "the second diagnosis,"[98] that is, the identification of other abnormalities that are related to inhalation of asbestos fibers. These include the identification of benign asbestos-related pleural diseases, such as parietal pleural plaques or diffuse pleural fibrosis (see Chap. 6), asbestosis (see Chap. 4), and asbestos bodies in histologic sections. Similarly, the pathologist should search for evidence of tissue injury related to inhalation of tobacco smoke, including centrilobular emphysema, chronic bronchitis, and small-airways disease.[99] This requires adequate sampling of lung parenchyma at a distance well removed from the primary tumor and its effects on immediately adjacent tissues.[75,100] These changes are best observed with lungs that have been fixed by intratracheal instillation of formalin,[74,99] which procedure should be employed, when feasible, on lobectomy or pneumonectomy specimens. In addition, lung cancer cases for which a role for asbestos is suspected should have portions of formalin-fixed lung tissue uninvolved by tumor preserved for possible tissue asbestos analysis at some subsequent time if indicated (see Chap. 11). Such analyses should be performed preferably at specialized centers with experience with these procedures, since proper interpretation of results requires determination of a normal range of expected values.

REFERENCES

1. Fielding JE: Smoking: Health effects and control. *N Engl J Med* 313:555–561, 1985.
2. Department of Health and Human Services. The health consequences of smoking: Cancer: A report of the surgeon general. Rockville, MD, 1982.
3. Rodenstein DO, Stänescu DC: Pattern of inhalation of tobacco smoke in pipe, cigarette, and never smokers. *Am Rev Respir Dis* 132:628–632, 1985.
4. Selikoff IJ, Lee DHK: *Asbestos and Disease.* New York: Academic Press, 1978.
5. Hammond EC, Selikoff IJ, Seidman H: Asbestos exposure, cigarette smoking, and death rates. In: Health Hazards of Asbestos Exposure (Selikoff IJ, Hammond EC, eds.), *Ann NY Acad Sci* 330:473–490, 1979.
6. Lynch KM, Smith WA: Pulmonary asbestosis. Carcinoma of lung in asbestos silicosis. *Am J Cancer* 24:56–64, 1935.
7. Homburger F: The coincidence of primary carcinoma of the lungs and pulmonary asbestosis. Analysis of literature and report of three cases. *Am J Pathol* 19:797–807, 1943.
8. Merewether ERA: *Annual report to the chief inspector of factories for the year 1947.* London: Her Majesty's Stationery Office, 1949, pp. 79–87.
9. McDonald JC, McDonald AD: Epidemiology of asbestos-related lung cancer. In: *Asbestos-Related Malignancy* (Antman K, Aisner J, eds.), Orlando, FL: Grune and Stratton, 1987, pp. 57–79.
10. Doll R: Mortality from lung cancer in asbestos workers. *Br J Ind Med* 12:81–86, 1955.
11. Breslow L: Industrial aspects of bronchogenic neoplasms. *Dis Chest* 28:421–430, 1955.
12. Selikoff IJ, Churg J, Hammond EC: Asbestos exposure, smoking and neoplasia. *JAMA* 204:104–110, 1968.
13. Buchanan WD: Asbestosis and primary intrathoracic neoplasms. *Ann NY Acad Sci* 132:507–518, 1965.
14. Acheson ED, Gardner MJ, Winter PD, Bennett C: Cancer in a factory using amosite asbestos. *Int J Epidemiol* 13:3–10, 1984.
15. Finkelstein MM: Mortality among employees of an Ontario asbestos-cement factory. *Am Rev Respir Dis* 129:754–761, 1984.
16. Ohlson C-G, Hogstedt C: Lung cancer among asbestos cement workers: A Swedish cohort study and a review. *Br J Ind Med* 42:397–402, 1985.
17. Botha JL, Irwig LM, Strebel PM: Excess mortality from stomach cancer, lung cancer, and asbestosis and/or mesothelioma in crocidolite mining districts in South Africa. *Am J Epidemiol* 123:30–40, 1986.
18. Hughes JM, Weill H, Hammad YY: Mortality of workers employed in two asbestos cement manufacturing plants. *Br J Ind Med* 44:161–174, 1987.
19. Enterline PE, Hartley J, Henderson V: Asbestos and cancer: A cohort followed up to death. *Br J Ind Med* 44:396–401, 1987.

20. Raffn E, Lynge E, Juel K, Korsgaard B: Incidence of cancer and mortality among employees in the asbestos cement industry in Denmark. *Br J Ind Med* 46:90–96, 1989.

21. Peto J: Dose–response relationships for asbestos-related disease: Implications for hygiene standards. Part II. Mortality. *Ann NY Acad Sci* 330:195–203, 1979.

22. McDonald JC, Liddell FDK, Gibbs GW, Eyssen GE, McDonald AD: Dust exposure and mortality in chrysotile mining, 1910–1975. *Br J Ind Med* 37:11–24, 1980.

23. Browne K: A threshold for asbestos related lung cancer. *Br J Ind Med* 43:556–558, 1986.

24. Browne K: Is asbestos or asbestosis the cause of the increased risk of lung cancer in asbestos workers? *Br J Ind Med* 43:145–149, 1986.

25. Cullen MR: Controversies in asbestos-related lung cancer. *Occup Med: State Art Revs* 2:259–272, 1987.

26. An SH, Koprowska I: Primary cytologic diagnosis of asbestosis associated with bronchogenic carcinoma: Case report and review of literature. *Acta Cytolog* 6:391–398, 1962.

27. Dement JM, Harns RL, Symons MJ, Shy CM: Exposures and mortality among chrysotile asbestos workers. Part II: Mortality. *Am J Ind Med* 4:421–434, 1983.

28. Hodgson JT, Jones RD: Mortality of asbestos workers in England and Wales 1971–81. *Br J Ind Med* 43:158–164, 1986.

29. McDonald AD, Fry JS, Woolley AJ, McDonald JC: Dust exposure and mortality in an American factory using chrysotile, amosite and crocidolite in mainly textile manufacture. *Br J Ind Med* 40:368–374, 1983.

30. Newhouse ML, Berry G, Wagner JC: Mortality of factory workers in East London 1933–80. *Br J Ind Med* 42:4–11, 1985.

31. Puntoni R, Vercelli M, Merlo F, Valerio F, Santi L: Mortality among shipyard workers in Genoa, Italy. *Ann NY Acad Sci* 330:353–377, 1979.

32. Rubino GF, Piolatto G, Newhouse ML, Scansetti G, Aresini GA, Murray R: Mortality of chrysotile asbestos miners at the Balangero Mine, Northern Italy. *Br J Ind Med* 36:187–194, 1979.

33. Selikoff IJ, Hammond EC, Seidman H: Mortality experience of insulation workers in the United States and Canada 1943–1976. *Ann NY Acad Sci* 330:91–116, 1979.

34. Liddell FDK, McDonald JC: Radiologic findings as predictors of mortality in Quebec asbestos workers. *Br J Ind Med* 37:257–267, 1980.

35. Sluis-Cremer GK, Bezuidenhout BN: Relation between asbestosis and bronchial cancer in amphibole asbestos miners. *Br J Ind Med* 46:537–540, 1989.

36. Berry G, Newhouse ML: Mortality of workers manufacturing friction materials using asbestos. *Br J Ind Med* 40:1–7, 1983.

37. Enterline P, DeCoufle P, Henderson V: Respiratory cancer in relation to occupational exposures among retired asbestos workers. *Br J Ind Med* 30:162–166, 1973.

38. Hughes J, Weill H: Lung cancer risk associated with manufacture of asbestos-cement products. In: *Biological Effects of Mineral Fibers* (Wagner JC, ed.), Lyon: International Agency for Research on Cancer, 1980, pp. 627–635.

39. McDonald AD, Fry JS, Woolley AJ, McDonald JC: Dust exposure and mortality in an American chrysotile asbestos friction products plant. *Br J Ind Med* 41:151–157, 1984.

40. Peto J, Doll R, Herman G, Binns R, Goffe T, Clayton R: Relationship of mortality to measures of environmental pollution in an asbestos textile factory. *Ann Occup Hyg* 29:305–355, 1985.

41. Pampalon R, Siemiatycki J, Blanchet M: Environmental asbestos pollution and public health in Quebec. *Union Med Can* 111:475–489, 1982.

42. McDonald JC: Health implications of environmental exposure to asbestos. *Environ Health Persp* 62:319–328, 1985.

43. Mossman BT, Gee JBL: Asbestos-related diseases. *N Engl J Med* 320:1721–1730, 1989.

44. Seidman H, Selikoff IJ, Hammond EC: Short-term asbestos work exposure and long-term observations. *Ann NY Acad Sci* 330:61–89, 1979.

45. Becklake MR: Asbestos-related diseases of the lung and other organs: Their epidemiology and implications for clinical practice. *Am Rev Respir Dis* 114:187–227, 1976.

46. Fraire AE, Greenberg SD: Carcinoma and diffuse interstitial fibrosis of lung. *Cancer* 31:1078–1086, 1973.

47. Kipen HM, Lilis R, Suzuki Y, Valciukas JA, Selikoff IJ: Pulmonary fibrosis in asbestos insulation workers with lung cancer: A radiological and histopathological evaluation. *Br J Ind Med* 44:96–100, 1987.

48. Roggli VL, Pratt PC, Brody AR: Asbestos content of lung tissue in asbestos-associated diseases: A study of 110 cases. *Br J Ind Med* 43:18–28, 1986.

49. Edelman DA: Does asbestosis increase the risk of lung cancer? *Int Arch Occup Environ Health* 62:345–349, 1990.

50. Selikoff IJ, Hammond EC: Asbestos and smoking. *JAMA* 242:458, 1979.

51. Selikoff IJ, Seidman H, Hammond EC: Mortality effects of cigarette smoking among amosite asbestos factory workers. *J Natl Cancer Inst* 65:507–513, 1980.

52. Berry G, Newhouse ML, Turok M: Combined effect of asbestos exposure and smoking on mortality from lung cancer in factory workers. *Lancet* 2:476–479, 1972.

53. Saracci R: Asbestos and lung cancer: An analysis of the epidemiological evidence on the asbestos-smoking interaction. *Int J Cancer* 20:323–331, 1977.

54. Meurman LO, Kiviluoto R, Hakama M: Combined effect of asbestos exposure and tobacco smoking on Finnish anthophyllite miners and millers. *Ann NY Acad Sci* 330:491–495, 1979.

55. Newhouse M: Epidemiology of asbestos-related tumors. *Sem Oncol* 8:250–257, 1981.

56. Huuskonen MS: Asbestos and cancer. *Eur J Respir Dis* 63 (Suppl. 123):145–152, 1982.

57. Berry G, Newhouse ML, Antonis P: Combined effect of asbestos and smoking on mortality from lung cancer and mesothelioma in factory workers. *Br J Ind Med* 42:12–18, 1985.

58. Lemen RA: Occupationally induced lung cancer epidemiology. In: *Occupational Respiratory Diseases* (Merchant JA, ed.), U.S. Dept. of Health and Human Services (NIOSH) Pub. No. 86–102, 1986, pp. 629–656.

59. Kabat GC, Wynder EL: Lung cancer in nonsmokers. *Cancer* 53:1214–1221, 1984.

60. Rosenow EC, Carr DT: Bronchogenic carcinoma. *CA-A J for Clin* 29:233–245, 1979.

61. Lefcoe NM, Ashley MJ, Pederson LL, Keays JJ: The health risks of passive smoking: The growing case for control measures in enclosed environments. *Chest* 84:90–95, 1983.

62. Samet JM, Marbury MC, Spengler JD: Health effects and sources of indoor air pollution. Part II. *Am Rev Respir Dis* 137:221–242, 1988.

63. Surgeon General. Smoking Cessation and Respiratory Cancers. Ch. 4 In: *The Health Benefits of Smoking Cessation.* U.S. Dept. of Health and Human Services, Publication No. 90-8416, Rockville, MD, 1990, pp. 107–141.

64. Roggli VL, Greenberg SD, Seitzman LH, McGavran MH, Hurst GA, Spivey CG, Nelson KG, Hieger LR: Pulmonary fibrosis, carcinoma, and ferruginous body counts in amosite asbestos workers: A study of six cases. *Am J Clin Pathol* 73:496–503, 1980.

65. McDonald JC, Becklake MR, Gibbs GW, McDonald A, Rossiter CE: The health of chrysotile asbestos mine and mill workers of Quebec. *Arch Environ Health* 26:61–68, 1974.

66. Weiss W: Mortality of a cohort exposed to chrysotile asbestos. *J Occup Med* 19:737–740, 1977.

67. McDonald AD, Fry JS, Woolley AJ, McDonald J: Dust exposure and mortality in an American chrysotile textile plant. *Br J Ind Med* 40:361–367, 1983.

68. Finkelstein M: On the relative toxicity of asbestos fibres. *Br J Ind Med* 42:69–72, 1985.

69. Newhouse ML: Cancer among workers in the asbestos textile industry. In: *Biological Effects of Asbestos* (Bogovski P, Gilson JC, Timbrell V, Wagner JC, eds.), Lyon: IARC Scientific Pubs. No. 8, 1973, pp. 203–208.

70. Rushton L, Alderson MR, Nagarajah CR: Epidemiological survey of maintenance workers in London Transport Executive bus garages and Chiswick Works. *Br J Ind Med* 40:340–345, 1983.

71. Cheng VKI, O'Kelly FJ: Asbestos exposure in the motor vehicle repair and servicing industry in Hong Kong. *J Soc Occup Med* 36:104–106, 1986.

72. Williams RL, Muhlbaier JL: Asbestos brake emissions. *Environ Res* 29:70–82, 1982.

73. Green FHY, Vallyathan V: Pathology of occupational lung cancer, In: *Occupational Respiratory Diseases* (Merchant JA, ed.), U.S. Dept. of Health and Human Services (NIOSH) Pub. No. 86-102, 1986, pp. 657–668.

74. Craighead JE, Abraham JL, Churg A, Green FHY, Kleinerman J, Pratt PC, Seemayer TA, Vallyathan V, Weill H: The pathology of asbestos-associated diseases of the lungs and pleural cavities: Diagnostic criteria and proposed grading schema. *Arch Pathol Lab Med* 106:544–596, 1982.

75. Churg A, Golden J: Current problems in the pathology of asbestos-related disease. *Pathol Annu* 17(2):33–66, 1982.

76. Churg A: Neoplastic asbestos-induced diseases. Ch. 8 In: *Pathology of Occupational Lung Disease* (Churg A, Green FHY, eds.), New York: Igaku-Shoin, 1988, pp. 279–325.

77. Weiss W: Lobe of origin in the attribution of lung cancer to asbestos. *Br J Ind Med* 45:544–547, 1988.

78. Greenberg SD, Hurst GA, Matlage WT, Christianson CS, Hurst IJ, Mabry LC: Sputum cytopathological findings in former asbestos workers. *Tex Med* 72:1–5, 1976.

79. Greenberg SD, Hurst GA, Matlage WT, Miller JM, Hurst IJ, Mabry LC: Tyler asbestos workers program. *Ann NY Acad Sci* 271:353–364, 1976.

80. World Health Organization: The World Health Organization histologic typing of lung tumors, ed. 2. *Am J Clin Pathol* 77:123–136, 1982.

81. Carter D, Eggleston JC: Tumors of the Lower Respiratory Tract. Atlas of Tumor Pathology, ser. 2, fasc. 17. Washington, DC: Armed Forces Institute of Pathology, 1980.

82. Hammar SP: Common Neoplasms. Ch. 28 In: *Pulmonary Pathology* (Dail DH, Hammar SP, eds.), New York: Springer-Verlag, 1988, pp. 727–845.

83. Humphrey PA, Scroggs MS, Roggli VL, Shelburne JD: Pulmonary carcinomas with a sarcomatoid element: An immunocytochemical and ultrastructural analysis. *Hum Pathol* 19:155–165, 1988.

84. Roggli VL, Vollmer RT, Greenberg SD, McGavran MH, Spjut HJ, Yesner R: Lung cancer heterogeneity: A blinded and randomized study of 100 consecutive cases. *Hum Pathol* 16:569–579, 1985.

85. Greenberg SD: Asbestos lung disease. *Sem Respir Med* 4:130–137, 1982.

86. Greenberg SD: Asbestos. Ch. 22 In: *Pulmonary Pathology* (Dail DH, Hammar SP, eds.), New York: Springer-Verlag, 1988, pp. 619–636.

87. Whitwell F, Newhouse ML, Bennett DR: A study of the histologic cell types of lung cancer in workers suffering from asbestosis in the United Kingdom. *Br J Ind Med* 31:298–303, 1974.

88. Hourihane DO'B, McCaughey WTE: Pathological aspects of asbestosis. *Postgrad Med J* 42:613–622, 1966.
89. Hasan FM, Nash G, Kazemi H: Asbestos exposure and related neoplasia: The 28-year experience of a major urban hospital. *Am J Med* 65:649–654, 1978.
90. Kannerstein M, Churg J: Pathology of carcinoma of the lung associated with asbestos exposure. *Cancer* 30:14–21, 1972.
91. Ives JC, Buffler PA, Greenberg SD: Environmental associations and histopathologic patterns of carcinoma of the lung: The challenge and dilemma in epidemiologic studies. *Am Rev Respir Dis* 128:195–209, 1983.
92. Auerbach O, Garfinkel L, Parks VR, Conston AS, Galdi VA, Joubert L: Histologic type of lung cancer and asbestos exposure. *Cancer* 54:3017–3021, 1984.
93. Vena JE, Byers TE, Cookfair D, Swanson M: Occupation and lung cancer risk: An analysis of histologic subtypes. *Cancer* 56:910–917, 1985.
94. Churg A: Lung cancer cell type and asbestos exposure. *JAMA* 253:2984–2985, 1985.
95. Dail DH: Uncommon Tumors. Ch. 29 In: *Pulmonary Pathology* (Dail DH, Hammar SP, eds.), New York: Springer-Verlag, 1988, pp. 847–972.
96. Harwood TR, Gracey DR, Yokoo H: Pseudomesotheliomatous carcinoma of the lung: A variant of peripheral lung cancer. *Am J Clin Pathol* 65:159–167, 1976.
97. Lilienfeld DE, Mandel JS, Coin P, Schuman LM: Projection of asbestos-related diseases in the United States, 1985–2009. I. Cancer. *Br J Ind Med* 45:283–291, 1988.
98. Mark EJ: The second diagnosis: The role of the pathologist in identifying pneumoconioses in lungs excised for tumor. *Hum Pathol* 12:585–587, 1981.
99. Pratt PC: Emphysema and chronic airways disease. Ch. 24 In: *Pulmonary Pathology* (Dail DH, Hammar SP, eds.), New York: Springer-Verlag, 1988, pp. 651–669.
100. Churg A: Current issues in the pathologic and mineralogic diagnosis of asbestos-induced disease. *Chest* 84:275–280, 1983.

8. Other Neoplasia

S. Donald Greenberg and Victor L. Roggli

As noted in Chaps. 5 and 7, asbestos exposure is related to carcinoma of the lung and malignant mesothelioma of the pleural and peritoneal cavities. In addition, epidemiologic studies have suggested a relationship between asbestos exposure and malignancies of other sites, including the gastrointestinal tract, larynx, kidney, liver, pancreas, ovary, and hematopoietic systems.[1,2] The pathologic features of these malignant neoplasms do not differ from those occurring in individuals not exposed to asbestos. Therefore, the role of the pathologist includes the accurate diagnosis of these diseases and also the examination of the lungs and pleural cavities for evidence of other asbestos-related tissue injury (see Chaps. 4 and 6). This chapter reviews the evidence for the association of these various malignancies with exposure to asbestos, including relevant experimental studies where the data are available. Pathologic features will also be noted when they are of relevance to the interpretation of the available epidemiologic studies. Possible mechanisms of asbestos-induced carcinogenesis (reviewed in detail in Chap. 10) are not included in this review.

GASTROINTESTINAL CANCER

HISTORICAL BACKGROUND

Selikoff et al.,[3] in 1964, were the first to suggest there was an excess of cancers of the digestive tract among individuals exposed to asbestos. This observation was based on an epidemiologic study of asbestos insulation workers, and the association was maintained in subsequent follow-up studies involving larger numbers of workers followed for longer periods of time.[1] The rationale for this observation relates to the fact that many asbestos fibers deposited in the airways are removed by the mucociliary escalator and can be recovered from the sputum of exposed workers (see Chap. 9). If this sputum is subsequently swallowed, then fibers may be transported to various sites in the gastrointestinal tract. Direct contact of asbestos with epithelial cells of the gastrointestinal tract could then result in malignant transformation, similar to that believed to occur from interaction of asbestos fibers with bronchial epithelial cells or mesothelial cells. These considerations have generated concern regarding possible risks not only among asbestos workers but also among populations exposed to asbestos in food, beverages, and drinking water.[4]

ANIMAL STUDIES

Relatively few studies have examined the occurrence of gastrointestinal neoplasms in experimental animals exposed to asbestos. In the classic inhalational studies of Wagner et al.[5] and Davis et al.,[6] no excess numbers of neoplasms were observed at sites other than the lung and serous cavities. Animal studies involving the ingestion of chrysotile[7,8] or amosite[7] asbestos in Fisher 344 rats resulted in an increased incidence of intestinal tumors, but the increase did not reach statistical significance. Asbestos fibers were recovered from ashed colon specimens, and the colonic tissue level of cyclic AMP was significantly decreased in animals fed asbestos as compared to control diets.[8] In a study of hamsters fed amosite asbestos in their drinking water, two squamous cell carcinomas of the forestomach were identified, though these could not be specifically attributed to asbestos.[9] It is of interest that studies have demonstrated penetration of the intestinal mucosa by asbestos fibers,[10,11] and this migration of fibers to the peritoneal serosal tissues may be relevant to the pathogenesis of peritoneal mesothelioma.[10-12] However, in a study of a baboon gavaged with chrysotile and crocidolite asbestos, no significant intestinal penetration or migration of fibers to other tissue sites was demonstrated.[13] All in all, experimental animal studies do not support a role for inhaled or ingested asbestos fibers in the production of gastrointestinal neoplasms.[14]

EPIDEMIOLOGIC STUDIES

A number of studies have demonstrated an excess of gastrointestinal carcinomas among asbestos workers,[1,3,15-19] and projections for the next 25 years have resulted in estimates of 33,000 excess deaths from gastrointestinal cancers among asbestos-exposed individuals.[20] However, a number of investigators have challenged the hypothesis that asbestos exposure is causally related to gastrointestinal carcinomas.[21-24] In a recent review of 32 independent cohorts of asbestos workers, Edelman[23] found no consistent evidence to indicate that exposure to asbestos increases the risk of gastrointestinal cancer. Furthermore, there was no apparent dose–response relationship between accumulated asbestos dose and the risk of gastrointestinal cancer.[23] On the other hand, not all of the cohorts in Edelman's review showed an increased standardized mortality ratio (SMR) for lung cancer, which is universally accepted as causally related to asbestos exposure (see Chap. 7). In this regard, a review of 18 studies by Doll and Peto[2] showed a statistically strong correlation between SMR's for lung cancer and SMR's for gastrointestinal cancer. These results imply that when sufficient asbestos exposure in a population has occurred to result in a detectable increase in lung cancer risk, then it is likely that that population will also demonstrate an increased risk of gastrointestinal cancers.

One of the difficulties in these epidemiologic studies is the uncertainty regarding the diagnosis of gastrointestinal carcinomas.[25,26] Doll and Peto[2] believe that the excess risk of gastrointestinal carcinomas reported in some cohorts of asbestos workers could be explained on the basis of carcinomas of the lung or pleural or peritoneal mesotheliomas being misdiagnosed as gastrointestinal carcinomas. Although this could be the explanation for excess cases of carcinoma of the stomach, colon, or rectum, it seems considerably less likely to be the case for esophageal carcinomas (Fig. 8-1). Indeed, these authors state that the evidence relating esophageal cancer to asbestos exposure is suggestive of a causal relationship, but not conclusive.[2] This conclusion is tempered by the observation of Acheson and Gardner[21] that social factors are particularly important in regard to cancers of the upper alimentary tract, and differences between the workforces studied and the standard population with which they have been compared must be taken into account. The present authors believe there is sufficient evidence to indicate that in individuals with esophageal carcinoma and substantial exposure to asbestos as well as evidence of other asbestos-related tissue injury, asbestos is a probable contributing factor to the carcinoma. However, for the reasons just noted, the relationship between asbestos exposure and colorectal or gastric carcinoma remains unconvincing.

Despite a number of epidemiologic studies investigating the association between asbestos ingestion and gastrointestinal cancer,[27-33] the existence of such an association has not been definitively established.[4] Only one study, which involved the population in the San Francisco Bay area, suggested a positive correlation, and that was weak.[28] The types of fibers present in drinking water are generally short, ultramicroscopic fibers of questionable carcinogenic potential (see Chap. 10). Overall, the evidence fails to indicate any increased risk of alimentary tract tumors following the direct ingestion of asbestos.[34]

LARYNGEAL CANCER

A number of investigators have reported an association between asbestos exposure and laryngeal carcinoma.[19,35-40] The rationale for such an association involves contact of the laryngeal mucosa both with aerosolized fibers breathed into the lung and with fibers in sputum cleared from the lung by the mucociliary escalator. Digestion studies of laryngeal tissues obtained from asbestos workers have demonstrated the presence of asbestos bodies[41] as well as uncoated asbestos fibers.[42] No information is available concerning the dose–response relationship with respect to asbestos and cancer of the larynx, nor is there clear evidence with regard to variation in risk by fiber type.[43]

Some investigators have challenged the relationship between asbestos exposure and laryngeal carcinoma.[24,44-46] Experimental studies with rats exposed to aerosolized asbestos have not shown an excess of laryngeal tumors.[5,6] In a recent review of 13 cohort and eight case-control studies, Edelman[46] concluded that an increased risk of laryngeal cancer for asbestos workers has not been established. Other

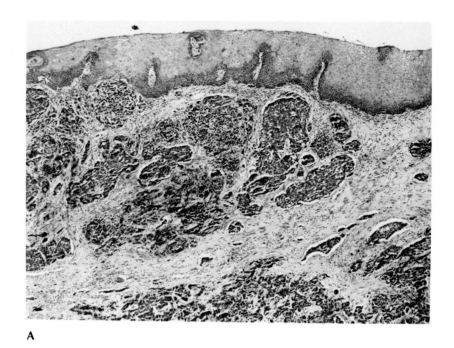

A

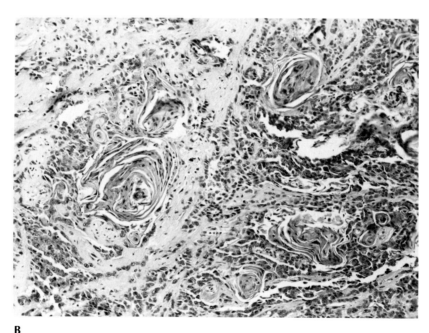

B

FIGURE 8-1. (A) Low-power view of esophageal carcinoma in a 63-year-old construction worker with bilateral parietal pleural plaques, showing esophageal mucosa (*above*) and infiltrating nests of carcinoma (*below*). (B) High-power view showing detail of squamous cell carcinoma with keratin pearls. H&E, part (A) ×40, part (B) ×100.

risk factors, such as cigarette smoking and alcohol consumption, have not been adequately accounted for in most of the reported studies. On the other hand, not all of the studies included in Edelman's review showed an increased SMR for lung cancer, either. Furthermore, the SMR's for laryngeal carcinoma exceeded 1.0 in at least some subgroups of workers examined in 10 of 13 cohort studies.[46] Edelman's review does not include references to three separate pathologic studies showing a strong relationship between laryngeal carcinoma and parietal pleural plaques.[47–49] Finally, Doll and Peto[2] and Smith et al.,[50] reviewing essentially the same cohort and case-control studies, concluded that asbestos should be regarded as one of the causes of laryngeal cancer. However, the relative risk is less than that for lung cancer and the absolute risk is much less.[2] The present authors agree with the position that asbestos, along with cigarette smoking and alcohol consumption, is a risk factor for laryngeal carcinoma, particularly in individuals with a substantial exposure to asbestos and evidence of other asbestos-related tissue injury.

The pathologic features of laryngeal carcinomas in asbestos workers are not different from those occurring in individuals with no known exposure to asbestos. Among the half dozen or so cases reviewed by one of the authors (VLR), all have been squamous cell carcinomas (Fig. 8-2). Asbestos bodies have never been described in histologic sections of laryngeal tissues, and normal ranges of asbestos fiber content have not been established for larynges from the general population. Thus there is at present no indication for performing digestion analyses of laryngeal tissues in an individual case. In the presence of neoplastic processes, uncontrolled replication of malignant cells will result in a dilutional effect on whatever fibers may have been present in the tissues prior to the initiation of the malignant process.

RENAL CELL CARCINOMA

Selikoff et al.[1] were the first to report an association between asbestos exposure and renal cell carcinoma. This observation was supported by the cohort study of Enterline et al.[18,51] and the case-control study of Maclure.[52] Smith et al.[53] reviewed the cohort study of Enterline et al.[18] and two other large cohort studies of asbestos workers (including the study of Selikoff et al.[1]) and concluded that the available evidence supports a causal association between asbestos exposure and renal cell carcinoma. The rationale for this association involves the penetration of asbestos fibers into the lumen of capillaries, where they may then be transported to other organs, such as the kidneys.[54,55] Studies have identified the presence of asbestos fibers in human urine samples,[56,57] and both amphibole and chrysotile fibers have been observed.

On the other hand, Acheson et al.[58] and Peto et al.[59] were unable to confirm an association between asbestos exposure and renal carci-

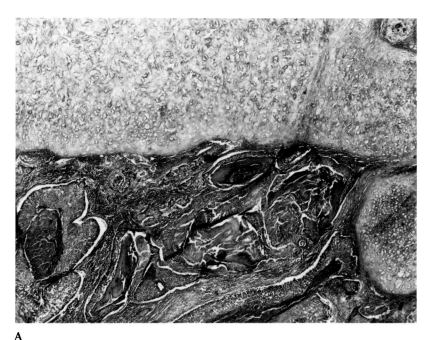

A

B

FIGURE 8-2. (A) Low-power view of laryngeal carcinoma in a 65-year-old patient with bilateral calcified parietal pleural plaques, showing laryngeal cartilages (*above and right*) and adjacent invasive carcinoma (*below*). (B) High-power view showing detail of squamous cell carcinoma with keratin pearls. H&E, part (A) ×25, part (B) ×100.

noma in humans. In this regard, Smith et al.[53] argued that with the exception of the three large cohort studies noted earlier, none of the other studies in the literature had sufficient statistical power to detect an excess mortality from kidney cancer among workers exposed to asbestos. Experimental animal studies in which rats were chronically exposed to aerosolized asbestos fibers have failed to produce an excess of renal tumors,[5,6] although one study, in which rats were fed 50 mg/kg body weight/day of a powdered filter material composed of 53% chrysotile, reported a statistically significant excess of renal malignancies.[60] Studies of urine samples from populations drinking water contaminated with asbestos[61] or from chrysotile asbestos cement workers[62] failed to show a significant elevation of urinary asbestos fibers. In the latter study,[62] considerable precautions were taken to avoid sample contamination, a problem that has plagued some of the earlier studies.[57] In a study of a baboon gavaged with chrysotile and crocidolite asbestos, none of the urine samples from the test animal exceeded the level of background contamination for chrysotile, and only one crocidolite bundle was observed in a test sample.[13] Furthermore, virtually all fibers found in urine samples are shorter than 2.0–2.5 μm,[62] and the carcinogenic potential of such fibers is questionable (see Chap. 10). Overall, in the authors' opinion, the balance of the evidence available at present does not support an association between asbestos exposure and renal cell carcinoma.

LYMPHOMA/LEUKEMIA

Ross et al.[63] reported in 1982 an excess of large-cell lymphomas primary to the gastrointestinal tract and oral cavity in a case-control study of male patients with a substantial exposure to asbestos. Kagan and Jacobson[64] reported six cases of multiple myeloma, six cases of chronic lymphocytic leukemia, and one case of primary large-cell lymphoma of the lung in patients with a history of asbestos exposure ranging from 3–37 years. Roggli et al.[65] referred to three patients with hematopoietic malignancies and parietal pleural plaques, including one patient with nodular poorly differentiated lymphocytic lymphoma, one with chronic granulocytic leukemia, and one with acute myelomonocytic leukemia. None had asbestosis histologically. Kishimoto et al.[66] reported two additional cases of acute myelocytic leukemia in individuals with a long history of exposure to asbestos. Asbestos bodies and crocidolite asbestos fibers were recovered from the bone marrow in both instances. The rationale for the association between asbestos exposure and lymphoid neoplasms relates to the occurrence of asbestos bodies and fibers in lymph nodes[67] and to the variety of perturbations of the immune system observed in patients with exposure to asbestos.[68]

Other studies have failed to identify an increased incidence of leukemia or lymphoma among asbestos workers. These include two reports from Sweden[69,70] as well as the long-term follow-up of a large cohort of U.S-Canadian insulation workers by Selikoff et al.[1] In a study of 412 tumors other than lung tumors or mesotheliomas occurring in rats exposed to aerosolized asbestos or room air (controls), Wagner et al.[5] observed eight lymphomas/leukemias in asbestos-exposed rats versus two in controls. Davis et al.[6] also noted a single example of lymphoma/leukemia in a rat exposed to aerosolized chrysotile asbestos. None of these observations was considered to be statistically significant.[5,6] Overall, in the authors' opinion, the balance of the evidence available at present does not support an association between asbestos exposure and lymphoma or leukemia.

OVARIAN CANCER

Several studies have reported an increased mortality from ovarian cancer among women exposed occupationally to amphibole asbestos.[71–73] Some peritoneal mesotheliomas were reported among women asbestos workers in each of these studies. In contrast, no increased mortality from ovarian cancer was reported among women working only with chrysotile asbestos[71] or among women involved with friction products manufacture.[74] In these two latter studies, no peritoneal mesotheliomas were reported either. In a case-control study of ovarian cancer, Cramer et al.[75] reported that women with ovarian cancer were about three times more likely to have used talcum powder for perineal dusting or sanitary napkins containing talc than matched control patients without ovarian neoplasms. Cosmetic talc is known to be contaminated with the noncommercial amphibole fibers, tremolite and anthophyllite (see Chap. 1). Wagner et al.[5] reported 10 examples of ovarian cancer among more than 350 rats at risk that were exposed to aerosolized asbestos and none in controls. However, this difference did not reach statistical significance.

As noted by Doll and Peto,[2] peritoneal mesothelioma and ovarian carcinoma may have similar clinical presentations, and there is some overlap in histologic appearances as well (see Chap. 5). It seems at least as likely that the epidemiologic association of asbestos exposure and ovarian cancer is due to the misdiagnosis of peritoneal mesothelioma as that occupational asbestos exposure actually causes ovarian cancer.[2]

PANCREATIC CARCINOMA

Selikoff et al.[1] initially reported an excess of pancreatic carcinoma among asbestos insulation workers. However, their subsequent review of death certificate diagnoses of pancreatic cancer based on the best medical evidence available in individual cases led to the reclassification of 26 of 49 cases as peritoneal mesothelioma, metastatic lung cancer, metastatic colon cancer, or peritoneal carcinomatosis with unknown primary site.[76] This left 23 cases of pancreatic cancer with an expected number of 17.5, a difference that was not statistically significant. Hence, the available information does not support an association between pancreatic carcinoma and occupational exposure to asbestos.

Additional associations between asbestos exposure and cancer that have been reported include an association with cancer of the eye[18] and with cancer of the penis.[77] More information is needed before definitive conclusions regarding these sites can be made.

REFERENCES

1. Selikoff IJ, Hammond EC, Seidman H: Mortality experience of insulation workers in the United States and Canada, 1943–1976. *Ann NY Acad Sci* 330:91–116, 1979.
2. Doll R, Peto J: Other asbestos-related neoplasms. Ch. 4 In: *Asbestos-Related Malignancy* (Antman K, Aisner J, eds.), Orlando, FL: Grune & Stratton, 1987, pp. 81–96.
3. Selikoff IJ, Churg J, Hammond EC: Asbestos exposure and neoplasia. *J Am Med Assoc* 188:22–26, 1964.
4. Working Group for the DHHS Committee to Coordinate Environmental and Related Programs: Report on cancer risks associated with the ingestion of asbestos. *Environ Hlth Persp* 72:253–265, 1987.
5. Wagner JC, Berry G, Skidmore JW, Timbrell V: The effects of the inhalation of asbestos in rats. *Br J Cancer* 29:252–269, 1974.
6. Davis JMG, Beckett ST, Bolton RE, Collings P, Middleton AP: Mass and number of fibers in the pathogenesis of asbestos-related lung disease in rats. *Br J Cancer* 37:673–688, 1978.
7. Ward JM, Frank AL, Wenk M, Devor D, Tarone RE: Ingested asbestos and intestinal carcinogenesis in F344 rats. *J Environ Pathol Toxicol* 3:301–312, 1980.
8. Donham KJ, Berg JW, Will LA, Leininger JR: The effects of long-term ingestion of asbestos on the colon of F344 rats. *Cancer* 45:1073–1084, 1980.
9. Smith WE, Hubert DD, Sobel HJ, Peters ET, Doerfler TE: Health of experimental animals drinking water with and without amosite asbestos and other mineral particles. *J Environ Pathol Toxicol* 3:277–300, 1980.
10. Storeygard AR, Brown AL: Penetration of the small intestinal mucosa by asbestos fibers. *Mayo Clin Proc* 52:809–812, 1977.
11. Westlake GE, Spjut HJ, Smith MN: Penetration of colonic mucosa by asbestos particles: An electron microscopic study in rats fed asbestos dust. *Lab Invest* 14:2029–2033, 1965.
12. Winkler GC, Rüttner JR: Penetration of asbestos fibers in the visceral peritoneum of mice: A scanning electron microscopic study. *Expl Cell Biol* 50:187–194, 1982.
13. Hallenbeck WH, Markey DR, Dolan DG: Analyses of tissue, blood, and urine samples from a baboon gavaged with chrysotile and crocidolite asbestos. *Environ Res* 25:349–360, 1981.
14. Condie LW: Review of published studies of orally administered asbestos. *Environ Hlth Persp* 53:3–9, 1983.
15. McDonald JC, Liddell FDK, Gibbs GW, Eyssen GE, McDonald AD: Dust exposure and mortality in chrysotile mining, 1910–1975. *Br J Ind Med* 37:11–24, 1980.
16. Finkelstein MM: Mortality among employees of an Ontario asbestos-cement factory. *Am Rev Respir Dis* 129:754–761, 1984.

17. Botha JL, Irwig LM, Strebel PM: Excess mortality from stomach cancer, lung cancer, and asbestosis and/or mesothelioma in crocidolite mining districts in South Africa. *Am J Epidemiol* 123:30–40, 1986.
18. Enterline PE, Hartley J, Henderson V: Asbestos and cancer: A cohort followed up to death. *Br J Ind Med* 44:396–401, 1987.
19. Raffn E, Lynge E, Juel K, Korsgaard B: Incidence of cancer and mortality among employees in the asbestos cement industry in Denmark. *Br J Ind Med* 46:90–96, 1989.
20. Lilienfeld, DE, Mandel JS, Coin P, Schuman LM: Projection of asbestos-related diseases in the United States, 1985–2009. I. Cancer. *Br J Ind Med* 45:283–291, 1988.
21. Acheson ED, Gardner MJ: Asbestos: The control limit for asbestos. London: Health and Safety Commission, HMSO, 1983.
22. Levine DS: Does asbestos exposure cause gastrointestinal cancer? *Dig Dis Sci* 30:1189–1198, 1985.
23. Edelman DA: Exposure to asbestos and the risk of gastrointestinal cancer: A reassessment. *Br J Ind Med* 45:75–82, 1988.
24. Mossman BT, Gee JBL: Asbestos-related diseases. *N Eng J Med* 320:1721–1730, 1989.
25. Heasman MA, Lipworth L: Accuracy of certification of cause of death. GRO Studies on Medical and Population Subjects, No. 20, London: HMSO, 1966.
26. Newhouse ML, Wagner JC: Validation of death certificates in asbestos workers. *Br J Ind Med* 26:302–307, 1969.
27. Meigs JW, Walter S, Hestbon J, Millette JR, Craun GG, Woodhall RS, Flannery JT: Asbestos-cement pipe and cancer in Connecticut, 1955–1974. *Environ Res* 42:187–197, 1980.
28. Conforti PM, Kanarek M, Jackson L, Cooper RC, Murchio JC: Asbestos in drinking water and cancer in the San Francisco Bay Area: 1969–1974 incidence. *J Chronic Dis* 34:211–224, 1981.
29. Sadler TD, Rom WN, Lyon JL, Mason JO: The use of asbestos-cement pipe for public water supply and the incidence of cancer in selected communities in Utah, 1967–1976. Master's thesis, University of Utah, Salt Lake City, Utah, 1981.
30. Sigurdson EE: Observations of cancer incidence in Duluth, Minnesota. *Environ Hlth Persp* 53:61–67, 1983.
31. Millette JR, Craun GF, Stober JA, Kraemer DF, Tousignant HG, Hildago E, Duboise RL, Benedict J: Epidemiology study of the use of asbestos-cement pipe for the distribution of drinking water in Escambia County, Florida. *Environ Hlth Persp* 53:91–98, 1983.
32. Siemiatycki J: Health effects on the general population (mortality in the general population in asbestos mining areas), In: Proceedings of the World Symposium on Asbestos, Montreal, 25–27 May 1982, Asbestos Information Centre, Quebec, pp. 337–348, 1983.
33. Polissar L, Severson RK, Boatman ES: A case-control study of asbestos in drinking water and cancer risk. *Am J Epidemiol* 119:456–471, 1984.
34. Royal Commission on Matters of Health and Safety Arising from the Use of Asbestos in Ontario: Report of the Royal Commission on Matters of Health and Safety Arising from the Use of Asbestos in Ontario. Toronto: Ontario Ministry of the Attorney General, 1984.
35. Stell PM, McGill T: Asbestos and laryngeal carcinoma. *Lancet* 2:416–417, 1973.
36. Newhouse ML, Berry G: Asbestos and laryngeal carcinoma. *Lancet* 2:615, 1973.
37. Libshitz HI, Wershba MS, Atkinson GW, Southard ME: Asbestosis and carcinoma of the larynx: A possible association. *J Am Med Assoc* 228:1571–1572, 1974.

38. Stell PM, McGill T: Exposure to asbestos and laryngeal carcinoma. *J Laryngol Otol* 89:513–517, 1975.
39. Morgan RW, Shettigara PT: Occupational asbestos exposure, smoking and laryngeal carcinoma. *Ann NY Acad Sci* 271:309–310, 1976.
40. Becklake MD: Asbestos-related diseases of the lung and other organs: Their epidemiology and implications for clinical practice. *Am Rev Respir Dis* 114:187–227, 1976.
41. Roggli VL, Greenberg SD, McLarty JL, Hurst GA, Spivey CG, Hieger LR: Asbestos body content of the larynx in asbestos workers: A study of five cases. *Arch Otolaryngol* 106:533–535, 1980.
42. Hirsch A, Bignon J, Sebastien P, Gaudichet A: Asbestos fibers in laryngeal tissues: Findings in two patients with asbestosis associated with laryngeal tumors. *Chest* 76:697–699, 1979.
43. Huuskonen MS: Asbestos and cancer. *Eur J Respir Dis* 63 (Suppl 123): 145–152, 1982.
44. Hinds MW, Thomas DB, O'Reilly HP: Asbestos, dental x-rays, tobacco, and alcohol in the epidemiology of laryngeal cancer. *Cancer* 44:1114–1120, 1979.
45. Chan CK, Gee JB: Asbestos exposure and laryngeal cancer: An analysis of the epidemiologic evidence. *J Occup Med* 30:23–27, 1988.
46. Edelman DA: Laryngeal cancer and occupational exposure to asbestos. *Int Arch Occup Environ Health* 61:223–227, 1989.
47. Hillerdal G: Pleural plaques and risks for cancer in the county of Uppsala. *Eur J Respir Dis* 61 (Suppl 107):111–117, 1980.
48. Mollo F, Andrion A, Colombo A, Segnan N, Pira E: Pleural plaques and risk of cancer in Turin, Northwestern Italy: An autopsy study. *Cancer* 54:1418–1422, 1984.
49. Wain SL, Roggli VL, Foster WL: Parietal pleural plaques, asbestos bodies, and neoplasia: A clinical, pathologic, and roentgenographic correlation of 25 consecutive cases. *Chest* 86:707–713, 1984.
50. Smith AH, Handley MA, Wood R: Epidemiological evidence indicates asbestos causes laryngeal cancer. *J Occup Med* 32:499–506, 1990.
51. Enterline PE, Henderson V: Asbestos and kidney cancer. *Am J Ind Med* 17:645–646, 1990.
52. Maclure M: Asbestos and renal adenocarcinoma: A case-control study. *Environ Res* 42:353–361, 1987.
53. Smith AH, Shearn VI, Wood R: Asbestos and kidney cancer: The evidence supports a causal association. *Am J Ind Med* 16:159–166, 1989.
54. Holt PF: Transport of inhaled dust to extrapulmonary sites. *J Pathol* 133:123–129, 1981.
55. Brody AR, Hill LH, Adkins B, O'Connor RW: Chrysotile asbestos inhalation in rats: Deposition pattern and reaction of alveolar epithelium and pulmonary macrophages. *Am Rev Respir Dis* 123:670–679, 1981.
56. Cook PM, Olson GF: Ingested mineral fibers: Elimination in human urine. *Science* 204:195–198, 1979.
57. Finn MB, Hallenbeck WH: Detection of chrysotile in workers' urine. *Ann Ind Hyg Assoc J* 46:162–169, 1985.
58. Acheson ED, Gardner MJ, Winter PD, Bennett C: Cancer in a factory using amosite asbestos. *Internat J Epidemiol* 13:3–10, 1984.
59. Peto J, Doll R, Hermon C, Binns W, Clayton R, Goffe T: Relationship of mortality to measures of environmental asbestos pollution in an asbestos textile factory. *Ann Occup Hyg* 29:305–335, 1985.
60. Gibel W, Lohs K, Horn K, Wildner G, Hoffman F: Animal experiments concerning cancerogenic effects of asbestos fiber material following oral administration. *Arch Geschwulstforsch* 46:437–442, 1976.
61. Boatman ES, Merrill T, O'Neill A, Polissar L, Millette JR: Use of quantitative analysis of urine to assess exposure to asbestos fibers in drinking water in the Puget Sound Region. *Environ Hlth Persp* 53:131–141, 1983.

62. Guillemin MP, Litzistorf G, Buffat PA: Urinary fibres in occupational exposure to asbestos. *Ann Occup Hyg* 33:219–233, 1989.
63. Ross R, Nichols P, Wright W, Lukes R, Dworsky R, Paganini-Hill A, Koss M, Henderson B: Asbestos exposure and lymphomas of the gastrointestinal tract and oral cavity. *Lancet* 2:1118–1120, 1982.
64. Kagan E, Jacobson RJ: Lymphoid and plasma cell malignancies: Asbestos-related disorders of long latency. *Am J Clin Pathol* 80:14–20, 1983.
65. Roggli VL, Pratt PC, Brody AR: Asbestos content of lung tissue in asbestos-associated diseases: A study of 110 cases. *Br J Ind Med* 43:18–28, 1986.
66. Kishimoto T, Ono T, Okada K: Acute myelocytic leukemia after exposure to asbestos. *Cancer* 62:787–790, 1988.
67. Roggli VL, Benning TL: Asbestos bodies in pulmonary hilar lymph nodes. *Mod Pathol* 3:513–517, 1990.
68. Kagan E: Current perspectives in asbestosis. *Ann Allerg* 54:464–474, 1985.
69. Bengsston NO, Hardell L, Eriksson M: Asbestos exposure and malignant lymphoma. *Lancet* 2:1463, 1982.
70. Olsson H, Brandt L: Asbestos exposure and non-Hodgkin's lymphoma. *Lancet* 1:588, 1983.
71. Acheson ED, Gardner MJ, Pippard EC, Grime LP: Mortality of two groups of women who manufactured gas masks from chrysotile and crocidolite asbestos: A 40-year follow-up. *Br J Ind Med* 39:344–348, 1982.
72. Newhouse ML, Berry G, Wagner JC: Mortality of factory workers in East London, 1933–1980. *Br J Ind Med* 42:4–11, 1985.
73. Wignall BK, Fox AJ: Mortality of female gas-mask assemblers. *Br J Ind Med* 39:34-38, 1982.
74. Berry G, Newhouse ML: Mortality of workers manufacturing friction materials using asbestos. *Br J Ind Med* 40:1–7, 1983.
75. Cramer DW, Welch DR, Scully RE, Wojciechowski CA: Ovarian cancer and talc: A case-control study. *Cancer* 50:372–376, 1982.
76. Selikoff IJ, Seidman H: Cancer of the pancreas among asbestos insulation workers. *Cancer* 47:1469–1473, 1981.
77. Raffn E, Korsgaard B: Asbestos exposure and carcinoma of penis. *Lancet* 2:1394, 1987.

9. Cytopathology and Asbestos-Associated Diseases

S. DONALD GREENBERG

Asbestos is a tremendous health hazard. Commercial use of asbestos in the United States rose from 120,000 tons in 1930 to 857,000 tons in 1973.[1] In the United States alone about 500 factories employ 31,000 workers to manufacture 3000 different articles of asbestos. An additional 5 million workers in the construction industry have had greater than two asbestos fibers/cc exposure in the workplace.

Asbestos is a fibrous silicate commercially obtained from crushed asbestos rock.[2] These asbestos rocks are superficial within the earth's crust and are obtained by open pit mining. During the mining of asbestos or the manufacture of asbestos-containing products, respirable-sized asbestos fibers are suspended within the ambient air. These fibers enter the lungs, where some are phagocytized and coated by free alveolar macrophages, forming asbestos bodies[3] (Fig. 9-1). The uncoated fibers are noxious to the lungs and may produce interstitial fibrosis (i.e., asbestosis, see Chap. 4) with or without associated lung carcinoma (see Chap. 7) and malignant mesothelioma (see Chap. 5).[2] This chapter discusses in detail the cytopathology of these asbestos-associated diseases.

The inhaled asbestos fibers are of varying lengths and widths. For the most part, those greater than 100 microns in length are trapped within the nasal vibrissae and do not enter into the lungs. Asbestos fibers longer than 40 microns tend to impinge on the walls of the trachea and main bronchi, and rarely enter into the small peripheral airways and gas-exchanging regions of the lung. Thus, most asbestos bodies are approximately 35 microns in length and approximately 1–2 microns in diameter[4] (Fig. 9-2). Nonetheless, the respirability of asbestos fibers is largely determined by fiber diameter, so that some very long fibers ($>100\,\mu$) may reach the most peripheral regions of the lung. The time for the in vivo formation of an asbestos body can be estimated from experimental observations in guinea pigs, in which implanted asbestos fibers form bodies in four to six months.

HISTORICAL BACKGROUND

In 1929, asbestos bodies (then called "curious bodies") were first reported in the sputa of asbestos miners.[5] From 1929 to 1962, cytopathology of asbestos-associated diseases was largely ignored as a diagnostic tool. In 1962, An and Koprowska published the first case of a concurrent cytologic diagnosis of asbestos bodies and squamous carcinoma of the lung, in a cigarette smoker of 150 pack-years.[6] Further medical work-up showed the patient also to have asbestosis. These authors' review of the medical literature disclosed 41 previous

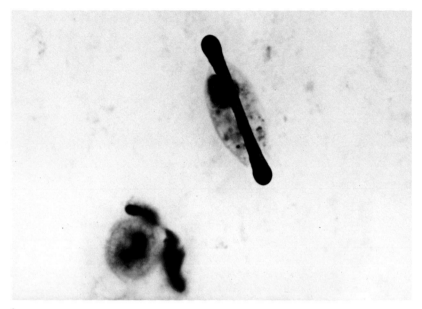

A

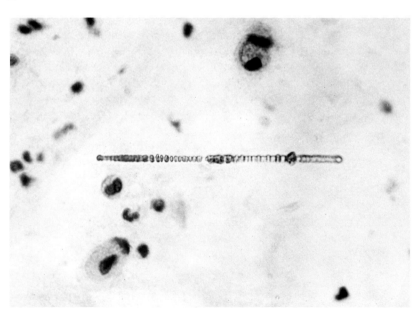

B

FIGURE 9-1. (A)–(D) Close view of single asbestos bodies in sputum. Several are partly within free alveolar macrophages. Papanicolaou, ×700. Reprinted from Ref. 15, with permission.

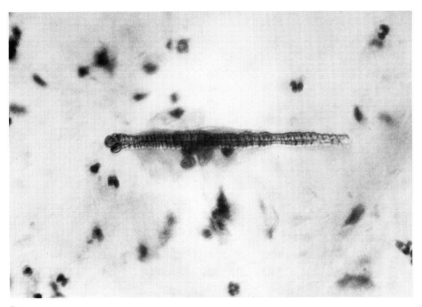

C

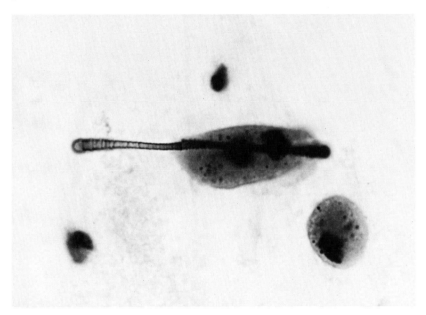

D

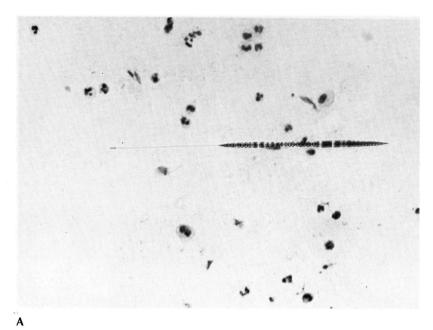

A

B

FIGURE 9-2. (A)–(D) Close view of single asbestos bodies in sputum. Note the variation in the heads of the bodies. Papanicolaou, ×700. Reprinted from Ref. 3, with permission.

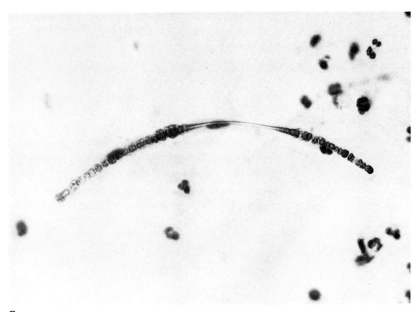

C

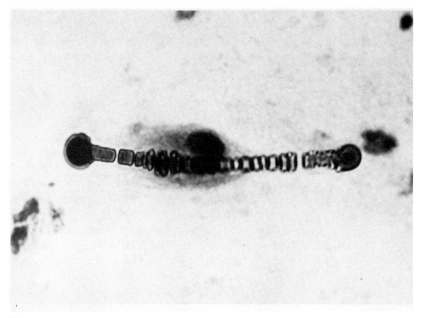

D

cases of concurrent asbestosis and lung cancer; however, there was no description of sputum cytology positive for asbestos bodies in any of these 41 earlier cases.

In a study of sputum cytology of asbestos workers, Huuskonen et al., in 1978, reported 114 asbestosis patients, 59% of whom were chronic cigarette smokers.[7] Sputum cytology showed 36 workers (31.6%) with squamous metaplasia, 20 (17.5%) with columnar cell atypia, and 5 (4.4%) with benign dysplasia. There were two patients with suspicious cells for carcinoma and one with anaplastic carcinoma. It was concluded that the results did not answer the question of whether bronchial cancer of patients with asbestosis is curable if detected early with cytological methods. Gupta and Frost, in 1981, reported that respiratory tract asbestos exposure is manifested in sputum and bronchoscopy cytology by one or more of the following findings: asbestos bodies, chronic inflammation, and epithelial cell alterations.[8] They concluded that asbestos bodies may be seen in the sputum but cannot be readily associated with asbestos exposure, since many with known exposure do not demonstrate these bodies while some smokers without known asbestos exposure do have asbestos bodies in their sputum. However, they acknowledge that these latter subjects may have had an unknown exposure to asbestos.

In 1982, Kotin and Paul reported on the results of a lung cancer detection program in an asbestos industry.[9] They concluded that there was no evidence that early diagnosis will significantly improve the prognosis of lung cancer. Also in 1982, Simard et al. reported on sputum cytology and asbestos exposure from Montreal, Quebec, Canada.[10] Their preliminary results showed no indication of any significant increase in the rate of neoplastic or dysplastic lesions in smoking asbestos workers.

Dodson et al., in 1983, reported on an ultrastructural study of sputum from former asbestos workers.[11] Their results were the first to confirm the presence of uncoated asbestos fibers, diatomaceous earth, and aluminosilicates in sputum. In 1984, Kobusch et al. reported a follow-up to their ongoing sputum cytology study from Montreal, Quebec, Canada, concerning pulmonary cytology in chrysotile asbestos workers.[12] They found that 74 (8.5%) had mild atypia, and 10 (1.2%) had moderate atypia. In four of their 867 workers, carcinoma of the lung was detected. They concluded that sputum cellular atypia increased with age and asbestos exposure. This sputum study apparently did not include a diligent search for asbestos bodies, for no mention of this is reported. Certainly, this would have been a golden opportunity to clarify the role of chrysotile asbestos in the formation of asbestos bodies and to determine whether chrysotile exposure is associated with asbestos bodies in sputum.

TYLER ASBESTOS WORKERS PROGRAM

The Tyler Asbestos Workers Program was developed for former asbestos workers in order to provide them with the most up-to-date care for the early detection and treatment of pulmonary diseases, particularly carcinoma.[3] Approximately 90% of these men were also cigarette smokers, rendering them more likely to develop carcinoma of the lung. The cohort for the program is composed of 900 former amosite asbestos workers, most of whom still live within a 150-mile radius of Tyler, Texas. The Tyler asbestos insulation plant operated between 1954 and 1972. Amosite asbestos from South Africa was used as a covering to insulate pipes. The program began in July 1974, and was funded by a contract from the National Cancer Institute, Division of Cancer Control and Rehabilitation. The program continues today through funding from a National Cancer Institute grant that began in 1985.

Serial sputum cytology specimens collected at four-month intervals provide a means of studying both cytologic atypias and quantitation of asbestos bodies. Control groups matched for age and cigarette smoking but without an asbestos work history were also examined.[3] Sputum is collected by both aerosol inhalation in the clinic and early morning cough at home. All sputa are collected directly into Saccomanno's fixative. Three sequential early-morning home-collected sputa are pooled into one. Sputum induction is carried out by transoral inhalation of an ultrasonic aerosol mist of an 8% solution of sodium chloride in water. After inhaling for three minutes, the individual coughs and expectorates directly into the Saccomanno's fixative. Four Papanicolaou-stained smears are prepared from each specimen.

Screening of the Papanicolaou-stained sputum smears averages five to seven minutes per slide. Black ink dots are placed by atypical cells and green ink dots by asbestos bodies. The sputum specimens are reported as unsatisfactory (saliva), no atypia, mild atypia, severe atypia, or positive for carcinoma. The total number of ferruginous bodies/specimen (four slides) is reported as few (1–14), moderate (15–29), or many (more than 30) (Fig. 9-3). For purposes of statistical analysis, the worker is classified as to the highest number of asbestos bodies found in any one specimen. The asbestos bodies in the Papanicolaou-stained smears are often within clusters of debris (Fig. 9-4). Staining of one or two slides for iron improves the sensitivity of the search for asbestos bodies.[13]

BRONCHIAL EPITHELIAL ATYPIAS

Sputum cytopathology can be used to study the various atypias of the bronchial epithelium. In so doing, sputum cytopathology serves as the diagnostic yardstick of bronchial epithelial dysplasia. The classic cytopathology of bronchial dysplasia is much the same as that of the cervix uteri from which it was patterned. The normal respiratory epithelium is columnar ciliated, with approximately 250 cilia/cell. The initial change following inflammation and/or irritation is squamous metaplasia. Squamous metaplasia implies that the lining columnar epithelial cells have been replaced by flattened squamous

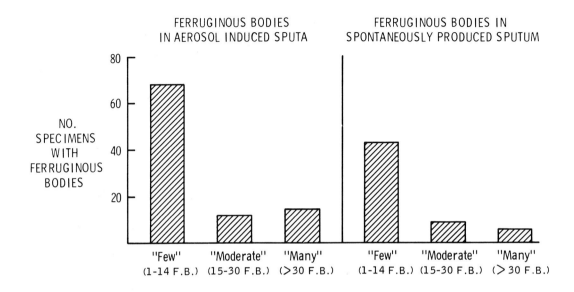

FIGURE 9-3. Histogram demonstrating the quantitation of asbestos bodies into categories of "few," "moderate," and "many" in aerosol-induced and spontaneous sputum specimens. Reprinted from Ref. 3, with permission.

cells that lack cilia. The nuclei within these cells of squamous metaplasia show no atypia; therefore, this change is often referred to as "benign metaplasia."

Following squamous metaplasia, the progressive degrees of bronchial dysplasia are mild, moderate, and severe. In the practice of cytopathology, one looks to the nucleus to determine the degree of atypia. Mild dysplasia (atypia) is recognized by a slight increase and margination of the nuclear chromatin (DNA) with a slight increase in the cell's nuclear/cytoplasmic ratio. Most chronic cigarette smokers have squamous metaplasia and/or mild atypia. These two changes are not particularly worrisome and are certainly reversible on cessation of smoking. The next two, moderate and severe dysplasia, have some overlap in diagnostic features. For this reason, the cytopathologic diagnosis may be moderate to severe. In both, the nuclear chromatin is significantly increased and irregularly dispersed,

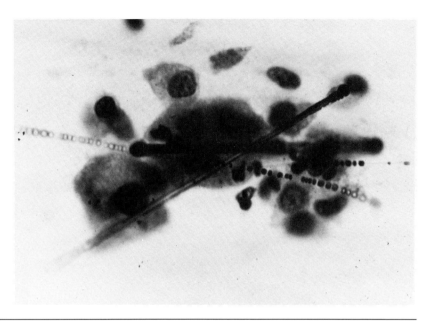

FIGURE 9-4. Photomicrograph showing numerous asbestos bodies within a thick covering of free alveolar macrophages. Papanicolaou, ×600. Reprinted from Ref. 55, with permission.

forming "hills and valleys." Also, the nuclear membrane shows subtle irregular infoldings, and the nuclear/cytoplasmic ratio is further increased. Squamous cell carcinoma is recognized by large single cells with very hyperchromatic nuclei and markedly irregular nuclear membranes. A cytoplasmic extension, or "tail," indicates that the malignant cell is invasive. If the cell's cytoplasm is orangiophilic, it is a well-differentiated squamous cancer cell. If it is amphophilic, it signifies a poorly differentiated squamous cancer cell.

Epidemiologic studies and reviews have demonstrated a significant cause-and-effect relationship between asbestosis and carcinoma of the lung.[1] However, this association is almost always found in cigarette-smoking asbestos workers in whom the cigarette smoke is the initiator, while the asbestos fibers are the promoter of the carcinoma[14] (Fig. 9-5). Sputum cytopathology is a simple, noninvasive, painless, and inexpensive means of early detection of premalignant and malignant pulmonary lesions.[15]

CELL-IMAGE-ANALYSIS STUDY OF PREMALIGNANT ATYPIAS
In the routine practice of cytopathology the atypical cells within a Papanicolaou-stained smear are evaluated subjectively. Inherent to this type of examination are the intraobserver and interobserver differences in grading the degree of atypia of the bronchial epithelial cells in sputum. Cell image analysis was undertaken to study the atypical cells and to render more precise, objective diagnoses.[16]

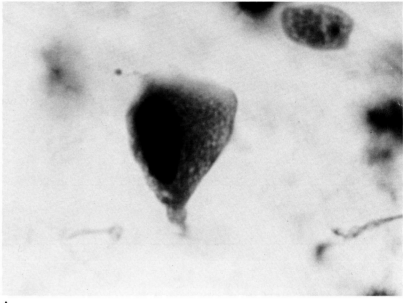

A

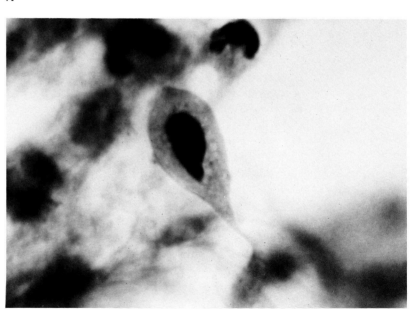

B

FIGURE 9-5. (A) and (B) Two atypical cells in sputum, illustrating the irregularity and hyperchromasia of malignant cells of squamous carcinoma. Papanicolaou, ×900. Reprinted from Ref. 3, with permission.

Because of its fine degree of diagnostic objectivity and reproducibility, cell-image-analysis cytology is considered to be the future state of the art.[17-32]

Atypical bronchial epithelial cells from the sputum of male cigarette smokers were digitized via scanning microphotometry and analyzed by computerized image analysis (Fig. 9-6). A set of specific analytic features based on cell morphology was extracted and combined mathematically to be expressed as a single number (Atypia Status Index, or ASI). This index represents the stages of the cellular atypia (i.e., squamous metaplasia; mild, moderate or severe atypia; or carcinoma) as a single number varying between 0.0 and 5.5 (Figs. 9-7 and 9-8). The ASI for each cell correlated highly (94–99%) with visual cytopathologic classifications. The distributions of cells according to their indices were profiled for patients at various stages of carcinogenesis and used to classify patients relative to their degree of cell atypia.[20] These results compared favorably to those of the clinical evaluation.

Atypical bronchial squamous epithelial cells from cigarette smokers were digitized using a high-resolution microphotometric scanning system operating at a wavelength of 530 nm. All cells used for the purpose of developing a computer training set, as well as those used as a test set, were classified by a team of three cytopathologists. Reduction in the dimensionality of the feature space and cell classification were performed using the Atypia Status Index. The distribution of cellular ASI values was arranged from lowest to highest and plotted for each subject as a profile. Subjects at different stages of carcinogenesis were found to have significantly different profiles ($p < 0.01$).

The incidence of carcinoma of the lung continues to rise steadily, and attempts at early diagnosis to improve prognosis have not yet been rewarding. The goal of cell-image-analysis research has been to decrease the incidence of lung cancer by detecting premalignant bronchial dysplasias in individuals in whom development of lung cancer is potentially preventable.[28] To achieve this, a cell atypia profile (CAP) is generated by assigning ASI's to 200 bronchial epithelial cells in a single sputum specimen. Computerized cell-image-analysis and statistical data analysis are used to generate ASI's and CAP's for each subject. This study was a step toward the development of automated cell image analysis for mass screening of premalignant atypias in sputum of those considered at high risk for lung cancer (i.e., men and women of 40 years of age and older, with more than 20 pack-years of cigarette smoking).

PLEURAL EFFUSIONS

Pleural effusions are an important clinical problem in individuals with a prior history of asbestos exposure. They may be of benign

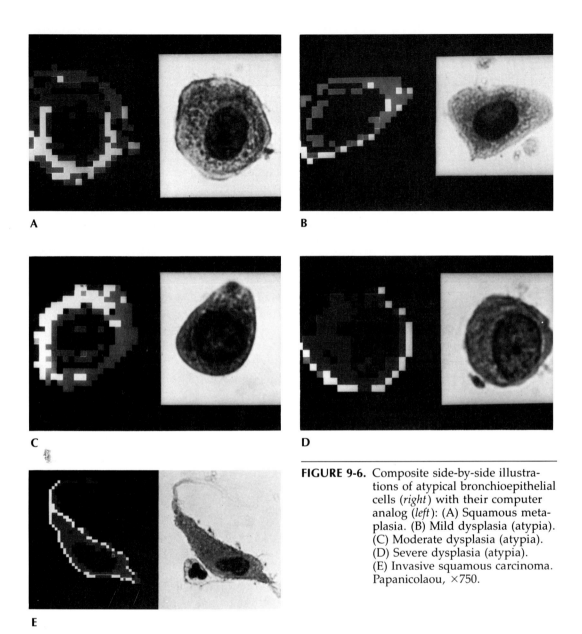

FIGURE 9-6. Composite side-by-side illustrations of atypical bronchioepithelial cells (*right*) with their computer analog (*left*): (A) Squamous metaplasia. (B) Mild dysplasia (atypia). (C) Moderate dysplasia (atypia). (D) Severe dysplasia (atypia). (E) Invasive squamous carcinoma. Papanicolaou, ×750.

inflammatory origin, as in the case of benign asbestos effusion (discussed in detail in Chap. 6), or they may be secondary to malignancy. Asbestos workers are at increased risk for malignant mesothelioma and carcinoma of the lung, either of which may give rise to a pleural effusion. In addition, asbestos workers are not exempt from non-asbestos-related causes of effusions that occur in the general popu-

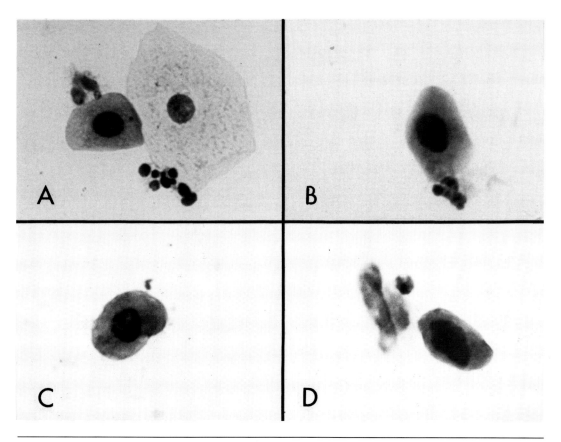

FIGURE 9-7. Composite high-magnification photomicrographs showing examples of: (A) Squamous metaplasia; (B) mild dysplasia (atypia); (C) moderate dysplasia (atypia); (D) severe dysplasia (atypia). Papanicolaou, ×650. Reprinted from Ref. 28, with permission.

lation, such as tuberculosis, congestive heart failure, and viral and bacterial infections. Cytopathologic examination of pleural fluid plays an important role in sorting through these differential diagnostic considerations.

Malignant pleural effusions are most often due to metastatic adenocarcinoma. Adenocarcinoma of the lung continues to be the leading cause of malignant effusions, followed by carcinoma of the breast.[33] By cytologic examination alone, it is extremely difficult to differentiate between a malignant pleural effusion of metastatic adenocarcinoma and that of a malignant epithelial mesothelioma. Indeed, mesothelial cells in effusions are often problematic in that, when sufficiently atypical to be recognizably malignant, they are difficult to distinguish from cells of adenocarcinoma. And when they are sufficiently well differentiated to be recognizable as mesothelial cells, it is difficult to distinguish between a well-differentiated

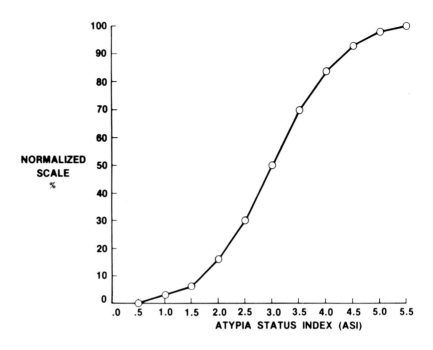

FIGURE 9-8. Graph illustrating the development of the Atypia Status Index. Sputum cells of squamous metaplasia are to the left (between 0.5 and 1.5). Squamous carcinoma cells are to the right (between 4.5 and 5.5). Progressive mild-to-severe atypical cells are between 1.5 and 4.5. Reprinted from Ref. 16, with permission.

mesothelioma and reactive mesothelial hyperplasia.[34] Although some investigators have advocated the use of cytopathology of pleural effusions and/or needle biopsy of the pleura for the diagnosis of mesothelioma,[35,36] the author prefers to render a diagnosis of malignant pleural effusion and suggest an open lung and pleural biopsy. It is helpful if neutral mucin can be identified histochemically in tumor cells, a finding limited to adenocarcinomas. If a cell block is available, one can perform electron microscopy to determine if the microvilli of the tumor cells are long and slender (mesothelioma) versus short and broad (adenocarcinoma).[37,38]

More recently, immunohistochemistry has been investigated as a means of distinguishing between malignant mesothelioma and adenocarcinoma in pleural effusions. Both mesotheliomas and adenocarcinomas stain immunohistochemically for cytokeratins, particularly when antibodies to both low- and high-molecular weight keratins are employed. However, adenocarcinomas stain for carcinoembryonic antigen, whereas mesotheliomas are generally negative.[38–40] Mesothelial cells in effusions are often positive for vimentin as well, but the utility of this finding in distinguishing between mesothelioma and metastatic adenocarcinoma is controversial.[40] Investigations of monoclonal antibody B72.3, which reacts with an oncofetal tumor-associated glycoprotein, has shown some promise in distinguishing between adenocarcinoma cells and mesothelial cells in pleural effusions.[41–43] This antibody reacts positively with adenocarcinoma cells, using the avidin-biotinylated-complex immunoperoxidase technique on paraffin-embedded cell blocks, but fails to react with mesothelial cells. Similar results have been reported for Leu-M1, antibodies to which stain adenocarcinoma cells but not mesothelioma cells in pleural effusions.[44] In addition, mesothelioma cells react immunohistochemically with the monocyte/macrophage marker My4, whereas adenocarcinoma cells do not.[44] However, immunohistochemical techniques have not provided a means for distinguishing between reactive and malignant mesothelial cells in pleural effusions.[40,44]

Analysis of pleural lymphocyte subpopulations in patients with pleural mesothelioma show that the majority of the lymphocytes that are present are T-cells, with a helper/inducer to suppressor/cytotoxic T-cell ratio that is higher than the normal peripheral blood ratio. This observation is not specific for mesothelioma, and has also been observed in tuberculous pleurisy, pleurisy following radiotherapy for malignancies, and effusions secondary to congestive heart failure.[44]

FLOW CYTOMETRY

Flow cytometry is a valuable technique for measuring the DNA content of normal (e.g., reactive) and neoplastic cells, and advances in this technology have been rapid in the past several years.[45] Frierson et al.[46] used flow cytometry to measure the DNA content of proliferating mesothelial cells in 28 benign effusions in comparison to that of 19 malignant pleural mesotheliomas retrieved from paraffin blocks. These investigators found that 53% of the mesotheliomas were DNA aneuploid (as compared to 0% of benign effusions), and suggested that the finding of DNA aneuploidy in an effusion specimen containing atypical mesothelial cells would strongly support a diagnosis of mesothelioma.[46] In contrast, Burmer et al.,[47] in a larger study of 46 malignant mesotheliomas, found that only 35% were DNA aneuploid by flow cytometry, and most showed intermediate to low proliferation rates. An analysis of 28 malignancies likely to be confused with malignant mesothelioma showed that 85% were aneuploid, and most showed intermediate to high proliferation rates.[47] Together these results indicate that diploid DNA content in a pleural effusion does not exclude mesothelioma, and the presence of DNA aneuploidy does not exclude some malignancy other than mesothelioma. In the future, a combination of flow cytometric DNA content measurement with mesothelial-specific markers (see Chap. 5) could prove useful as an adjunct in the diagnosis of mesothelioma from effusions, sparing the patient the morbidity of an open biopsy in cases that are positive.

OCCURRENCE AND SIGNIFICANCE OF ASBESTOS BODIES IN CYTOPATHOLOGY SPECIMENS

Inhaled asbestos fibers are physical irritants to the lungs.[48] When inhaled, they fall upon alveolar ducts and alveoli. It is the sharp ends of these fibers that irritate the lung, penetrate the alveolar walls, and enter into adjacent alveolar spaces.[48] Free alveolar macrophages phagocytize the fibers and coat them with ferritin and proteins, forming the innocuous asbestos bodies (Fig. 9-9). Continuous exposure to asbestos fibers is a major health problem, because only about 20% of the inhaled fibers can be coated by the alveolar macrophages. It is the uncoated asbestos fibers that produce disease.

Asbestos bodies represent the product of the free alveolar macrophages' attempt to detoxify inhaled asbestos fibers.[48] Asbestos-body maturation has been studied via scanning electron microscopy, using material isolated from the lungs of former asbestos workers. These results have demonstrated that the progression from a membrane-bound, smoothly coated fiber to the typically beaded form may result from the cracking and erosion associated with the inspiratory and expiratory forces of the lung[49] (see also Chap. 3).

In a study of asbestos-body phagocytosis by human free alveolar macrophages, phagocytosis was initially documented via light microscopy.[50] The process was then studied more carefully via scanning electron microscopy, which demonstrated morphologic and surface membrane changes in free alveolar macrophages. Free alveolar macrophage viability was also evaluated following 24–72 hours of incubation with asbestos bodies. Slight cytotoxicity was observed following the initial 24-hour culture period, but no further toxicity was observed in the 48-hour and 72-hour incubations. These studies demonstrated that asbestos bodies are readily phagocytized in culture by free alveolar macrophages and are only minimally cytotoxic to human lung cells.[50]

In histologic sections, asbestos bodies may be observed embedded within fibrotic pulmonary interstitium or free within alveolar spaces. It is apparently the latter that are mobilized onto the mucociliary escalator to be expectorated or swallowed in sputum. These intra-alveolar asbestos bodies are likewise accessible to bronchoalveolar lavage fluid or fine-needle aspiration, so the bodies (and uncoated fibers) may be recovered in these specimens as well.

SPUTUM

Asbestos bodies are the hallmark of exposure to asbestos fibers and may be found in the lungs of more than 90% of the general population when digestion-concentration techniques are employed.[51] However, asbestos bodies in sputum are an uncommon finding. They are seen much less often than are asbestos bodies and fibers within the lung. In Houston, Texas, a search was made for asbestos bodies in the sputum and bronchial washings of 31,353 cytology specimens for the years 1974–1979, involving 11,000 patients from the outpatient clinics of a 600-bed general hospital.[52] Asbestos bodies were found in only five patients; and in retrospect, each of them was discovered to have had significant occupational exposure to asbestos dust. Also, asbestosis was subsequently proven in four of the five patients. Furthermore, no asbestos bodies were found in 12,000 sputum specimens from 1972–1975 in the cytopathology laboratory of the Harris County Hospital District in Houston, Texas.[52] From these studies, it was concluded that asbestos bodies in sputum and bronchial-washing specimens are highly specific markers for past asbestos exposure and reflect a significant asbestos load within the lung.

On the other hand, 35% of the Tyler asbestos workers had asbestos bodies in their sputum (Fig. 9-10). The occurrence of asbestos bodies was related to two factors—the worker's age and the length of the worker's occupational exposure. At only five days' exposure, approximately 10% of the workers showed asbestos bodies. This increased to 50% at one year and 80% at five years (Fig. 9-11). None of the controls showed asbestos bodies in their sputum.[13] The aerosol-induced specimens produced more asbestos bodies than did the spontaneous sputa.

Chrysotile asbestos fibers do not readily form asbestos bodies, for often they are short, usually five microns or less, and, in addition, they tend to undergo leaching of their magnesium content within the lung. This leaching of the magnesium causes the chrysotile fibers to break up into individual fibrils, which phenomenon then allows them to be cleared more readily from the lungs. This is important in considering a study of sputum cytology for asbestos bodies, because chrysotile asbestos bodies are found in only limited numbers. However, chrysotile asbestos bodies are readily identified in lung tissue from chrysotile miners,[53] so it would be of considerable interest to know if they also have chrysotile asbestos bodies in their sputa. Amphiboles such as crocidolite and amosite yield significant numbers of asbestos bodies, depending on the pulmonary concentration of these fibers and the length of time over which they were inhaled. The Tyler Asbestos Workers Study yielded large numbers of asbestos bodies in sputum, probably because the level of amphibole asbestos fibers in the workplace was often greater than 100 amosite fibers/cc.

Correlative studies of sputum and lung asbestos-body content have demonstrated that asbestos bodies do not appear in sputum until there is a substantial lung burden of asbestos bodies. Bignon et al.[54] showed that the presence of sputum asbestos bodies correlated with a lung asbestos burden of 1000 or more asbestos bodies per cm^3 of lung parenchyma (approximately 1000 asbestos bodies per gram of wet lung tissue). Roggli et al.[55] subsequently showed that asbestos bodies appear in sputum when the lung asbestos burden is 900 or more asbestos bodies per gram of wet lung. In the latter study, weighed samples of 4–5 gm of lung from the upper and lower lobes were digested. The findings are consistent with the fact that asbestos

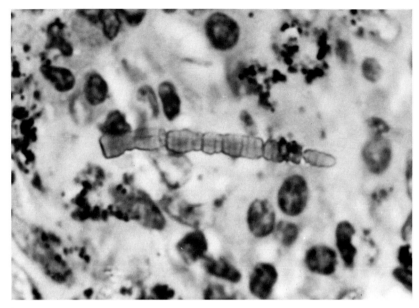

A

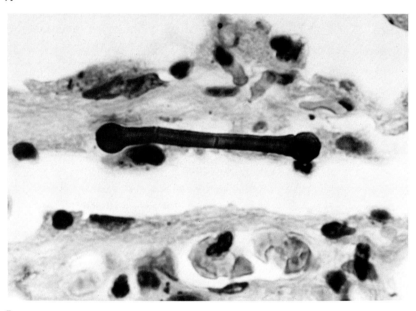

B

FIGURE 9-9. (A)–(D) Close view of asbestos bodies within lung tissues. Their overall shape is similar to those seen in sputum. Parts (A)–(C), H&E ×850; part (D), Perl's iron, ×700. Reprinted from Refs. 3 and 15, with permission.

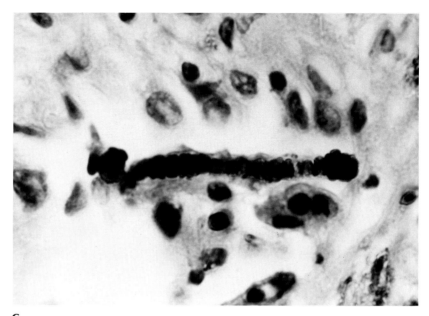

C

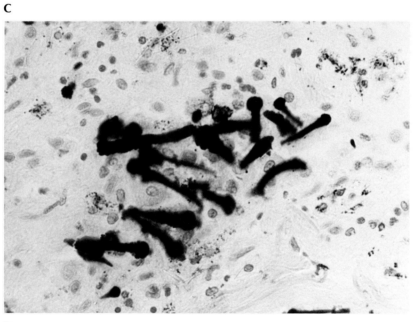

D

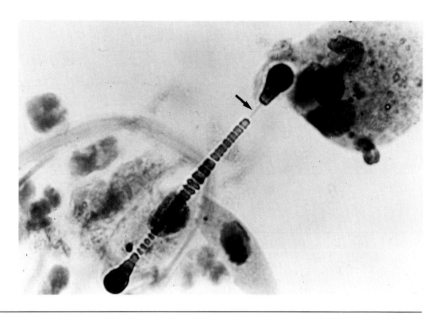

FIGURE 9-10. Unique photomicrograph showing an asbestos body with an incomplete coat of iron (ferritin) and protein. The arrow points to the fiber forming the core of the body. Papanicolaou, ×700. Reprinted from Ref. 56, with permission.

bodies appear in sputum only after considerable increase in lung asbestos body load. Furthermore, asbestos bodies may be identified in the sputum of occupationally exposed persons before there are clinical changes (e.g., chest x-rays). Lack of better correlations between the sputum and lung tissue digests may have been due to the fibrosis and restriction of the lungs with severe asbestosis, preventing coughing and clearance of the asbestos bodies.

In the Tyler Asbestos Workers Program, the clinical significance of ferruginous bodies in sputa was examined in 674 former asbestos workers. Data from occupational histories, smoking behavior questionnaires, chest radiographs, and pulmonary function tests were correlated with counts of asbestos bodies in the sputa.[56] Over a five-year study period, statistical analysis revealed that asbestos bodies in the sputum were significantly related to radiographic findings of interstitial pulmonary disease and pleural fibrosis, as well as to spirometric findings of restrictive lung disease. Age and cigarette smoking were also found to be related to the presence of asbestos bodies in sputum. In addition, there was a significant relationship between sputum asbestos bodies and the presence of atypical cells ($p < 0.001$).[56] Thus, asbestos bodies in sputum may be a marker not only for occupational exposure but also for possible bronchial epithelial atypia. Others have reported that the presence of asbestos bodies

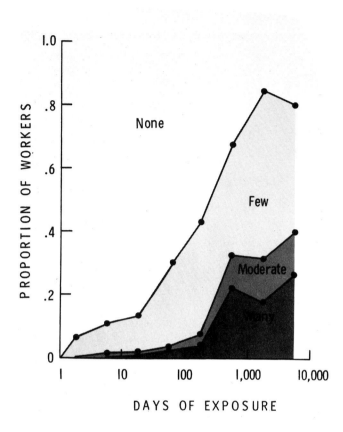

FIGURE 9-11. Graph demonstrating the proportion of asbestos workers with asbestos bodies in their sputum compared to the length of their employment (in days). Reprinted from Ref. 13, with permission.

does not always act as a marker for epithelial atypias.[9,10] These latter investigators found that atypias appeared to be equally distributed between cigarette smoking workers who did and did not have sputum asbestos bodies. Interestingly, the yield of atypical cells in the Tyler study was approximately the same by either the spontaneous or aerosolized method, whereas the latter method yielded about three times as many asbestos bodies as the former.[57]

Thus, it appears that the detection of asbestos bodies in sputum is a rather insensitive marker of exposure, with only 35% of a cohort heavily exposed to amphibole asbestos having positive sputum specimens. However, sputum asbestos bodies are an exquisitely specific marker of occupational exposure, with no false positive cases identified in more than 11,000 subjects screened. Sputum asbestos bodies are therefore an irrefutable marker of substantial asbestos exposure, with a specificity approaching 100%.[58] Periodic observation of sputum specimens from individuals working with asbestos remains the best method of determining their level of exposure.[2] A recent study suggests that detection of uncoated asbestos fibers in digests of sputum via transmission electron microscopy is a more sensitive way of confirming such exposure.[59] Of course, this increase in sensitivity would be likely to occur at the expense of specificity, as is the case for asbestos bodies in bronchoalveolar lavage fluid (see next subsection). It should be remembered that identification of asbestos bodies (or fibers) in cytological specimens is a marker of *exposure*, and not necessarily of disease.

BRONCHOALVEOLAR LAVAGE
Several studies of asbestos bodies in bronchoalveolar lavage have been reported by Dr. P. DeVuyst, a pioneer in this field.[60–63] A number of asbestos-related pulmonary diseases have been studied by means of this technique: interstitial lung fibrosis, pleural fibrosis and calcification, pleural effusions, and lung and pleural malignancy. The assessment of asbestos exposure in these diseases is often difficult because of the numerous jobs and hobbies in which asbestos is used and because the patient is often unaware of any exposure. Attempting to find a more objective and reliable indicator of exposure, DeVuyst et al. analyzed bronchoalveolar lavages for their asbestos-body content in patients with obvious or suspected occupational contact with asbestos in comparison with unexposed control subjects. The relationship between the presence of asbestos bodies and the different types of disease was also examined.

Asbestos bodies were counted by light microscopy in bronchoalveolar lavage fluid obtained from 563 subjects.[63] The presence of asbestos bodies was found to reflect occupational exposure to asbestos and was rarely found in unexposed control subjects at concentrations above 1/ml of fluid (6.0% of white collar workers and 17.8% of blue collar workers). The overlap of results observed between subjects with definite exposure and those without underlines the difficulty in assessing exposure by questioning alone, which can lead to underestimate or even overestimate of the risk.

The highest counts (log mean, 120.5 AB/ml; range, 0 to 42,600) were found in patients with radiologic evidence of asbestosis, most likely reflecting the known association of this disease with retention of large amounts of long amphibole fibers, rather than in patients with pleural disease. Although there is considerable overlap, the mean asbestos-body recovery is significantly higher in asbestos workers with asbestosis than in workers with benign pleural disease ($n = 131$) (mean = 4.9 AB/ml) or in workers without chest x-ray changes ($n = 82$) (mean = 4 AB/ml).[62] Bronchoalveolar lavage fluids were positive for asbestos bodies in 98% of asbestosis cases and in 95% of benign pleural disease cases. Asbestos bodies, however, can be recovered in bronchoalveolar fluids from control subjects without asbestos-related disease and with a negative occupational history for asbestos exposure. This finding is more frequent in blue collar workers (n = 85) (nearly 45% positive results) than in white collar workers (n = 82) (nearly 20% positive results). In these control subjects, asbestos bodies are generally found in low concentrations (less than 5 AB/ml of bronchoalveolar fluid).

A considerable overlap of results was observed between groups with different diseases or without any apparent disease. Apart from uncertainties in the radiologic diagnosis, this may be explained by differences in latency since first exposure, in individual response to asbestos inhalation, or in pathogenic properties of different asbestos types. Whether individuals with asbestos bodies in their lavage fluid but without any apparent disease are at increased risk to develop bronchogenic carcinoma or mesothelioma is not known.

An interesting observation from this study is that asbestos bodies were found in bronchoalveolar lavage fluid in 65 of 78 patients presenting with asbestos-related disease but in whom exposure was not confirmed by the occupational history. Thus, the finding of asbestos bodies in bronchoalveolar lavage fluid correlates with the occupational risk and can disclose unknown exposure better than a questionnaire, but a positive lavage is not proof of disease.[62-64] Quantitative differences in asbestos-body counts suggest a different pathogenesis for pleural and parenchymal disease.

Roggli et al. studied the asbestos-body content of bronchoalveolar lavage fluid from 20 patients with a history of occupational asbestos exposure, 31 patients with sarcoidosis, and five patients with idiopathic pulmonary fibrosis.[65] The cellular lavage pellet was digested in sodium hypochlorite and filtered onto Nuclepore filters for asbestos-body quantification by light microscopy (Figs. 9-12 and 9-13). Asbestos bodies were found in 15 of 20 asbestos-exposed individuals, nine of 31 sarcoidosis cases, and two of five patients with idiopathic pulmonary fibrosis. There was a statistically significant difference in the number of asbestos bodies per million cells recovered (or per milliliter of recovered lavage fluid) in the asbestos-exposed group as compared to the other categories of chronic interstitial lung disease (Fig. 9-14). Indeed, the highest levels occurred in patients with asbestosis. Large numbers of asbestos bodies in the lavage fluid (> 1 AB/10^6 cells or > 0.2 AB/ml bronchoalveolar lavage fluid) were indicative of considerable occupational asbestos exposure, whereas occasional asbestos bodies were a nonspecific finding.

Sebastien et al. recently compared the asbestos-body content of bronchoalveolar lavage fluid with the asbestos-body concentration of lung parenchyma in 69 asbestos-exposed individuals.[66] Values of asbestos bodies recovered ranged over six orders of magnitude for both bronchoalveolar lavage fluid and lung parenchyma, and the correlation between the two was highly significant (r = 0.74, $p < 0.0001$). Asbestos bodies were found in bronchoalveolar lavage fluid at a concentration of one or more per milliliter bronchoalveolar lavage fluid

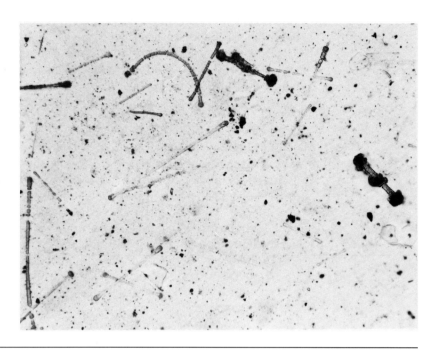

FIGURE 9-12. Asbestos bodies on Nuclepore filter isolated by digesting bronchoalveolar lavage-fluid cellular pellet in hypochlorite solution. Unstained, ×400. Reprinted from Ref. 65, with permission.

when the asbestos-body concentration in lung parenchyma exceeded 1000 AB/gm dry weight (approximately 100 AB/cc lung parenchyma). Similar results were reported in a study of 100 consecutive patients by DeVuyst et al.[67] These data indicate that bronchoalveolar lavage fluid is a more sensitive indicator of asbestos exposure than sputum, but is less specific.

In addition to the potentially useful information regarding asbestos-body content, and hence an objective marker of exposure, analysis of bronchoalveolar lavage fluid allows for observation of pathogenetic mechanisms occurring at the alveolar level. Jaurand et al. found an inverse correlation between the number of asbestos fibers (as detected by electron microscopy) and the number of alveolar macrophages recovered in lavage fluid.[68] However, there was no correlation between numbers of fibers recovered and enzymatic lysosomal activities in lavage fluid. Gellert et al. measured albumin-to-globulin ratio in serum and bronchoalveolar lavage fluid and clearance of ^{99m}Tc-DTPA.[69] They concluded that asbestos-exposed individuals have increased bronchial epithelial permeability compared to controls. Rebuck and Braude drew attention to the cascade of inflammatory changes induced by asbestos fibers.[70] They stated that, in asbestosis, like the other forms of diffuse interstitial lung disease, it is the alveolitis that precedes and predicts eventual fibrosis.

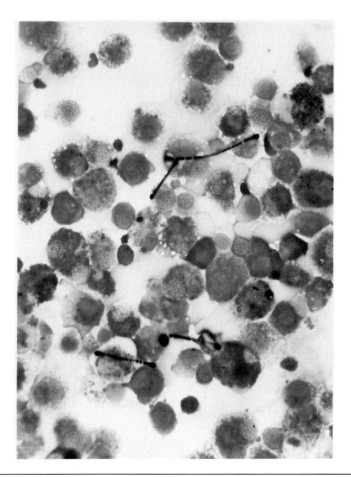

FIGURE 9-13. Cytocentrifuge preparation of bronchoalveolar lavage fluid in an individual with asbestosis. Typical asbestos bodies are present. Wright stain, ×400. Reprinted from Ref. 65, with permission.

FINE-NEEDLE ASPIRATES OF THE LUNG

As reported by Roggli et al., asbestos bodies were identified in cytologic preparations from fine-needle aspirates of the lung in two individuals, one with considerable occupational exposure to asbestos and one for whom no source of asbestos exposure could be identified[71] (Figs. 9-15–9-17). In each case, large numbers of asbestos bodies were subsequently recovered from samples of lung parenchyma by use of a quantitative hypochlorite-digestion concentration technique. Scanning electron microscopy and energy-dispersive x-ray analysis demonstrated that the main types of asbestos present were the commercial amphiboles, amosite and crocidolite. This was the first report of asbestos bodies in fine-needle aspirates of the lung. It was concluded that the identification of asbestos bodies in fine-needle

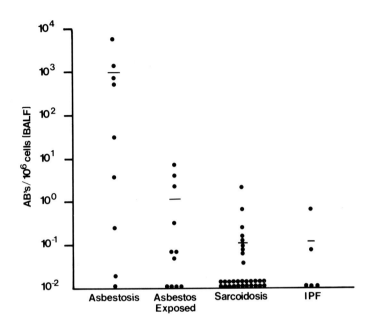

FIGURE 9-14. Distribution of asbestos-body content per million cells recovered for 56 cases. Each dot represents one case; mean value for each group is indicated by a horizontal line. Note the logarithmic scale. IPF = Idiopathic pulmonary fibrosis. Reprinted from Ref. 65, with permission.

aspirates of the lung indicates considerable occupational exposure to asbestos.[71] Subsequently, Leiman[71a] has reported finding asbestos bodies in fine-needle aspirates in 57 out of a series of 1256 transthoracic needle aspirates (4.5%) from a center serving a large mining population in South Africa. More than half of the masses undergoing aspiration were malignancies and about one-third were infectious processes.

PLEURAL FLUID

The author knows of no reports of asbestos bodies in pleural fluid.[72,73] Asbestos bodies have, however, been recovered from tissue digests of the parietal pleura. It is possible that the pleural asbestos bodies arrived via the circulation; however, a direct passage across the pleural space would seem more likely. Such asbestos bodies and fibers reside within the subpleural connective tissues that are thought to be the site of origin of malignant mesotheliomas.

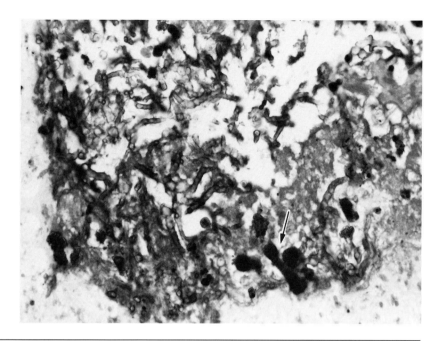

FIGURE 9-15. Hematoxylin- and eosin-stained fine-needle aspirate cell block shows a clump of branching septate hyphae, compatible with *Aspergillus* sp., and a nearby dumbbell-shaped asbestos body (arrow), one of many identified in the aspirated material. ×400.

ROLE OF CYTOPATHOLOGY IN DIAGNOSIS AND PREVENTION

The National Cancer Institute Cooperative Early Lung Cancer Detection Program was a collaborative study divided amongst the Johns Hopkins, Mayo Clinic, and Memorial Sloan-Kettering institutions.[74-77] The study was conducted over a five-year period during which time sputum cytology and chest x-rays, done at 4–6 month intervals, were performed to screen 15,000 men at high risk for lung cancer (45 years of age or older who smoked at least 1 pack of cigarettes/day). The two goals of the study were: (1) to determine if such screening could detect occult or early (Stage 1) lung cancer, and (2) to determine if the surgical treatment of such occult or early lung cancer would lead to decreased patient mortality. The first goal was achieved—occult lung cancers were detected by sputum cytology and chest x-rays. The sputum cytology was most useful in the detection of central carcinomas, while the chest x-ray was most valuable in detecting peripheral carcinomas. The second overall goal of showing decreased mortality was not reached. Nevertheless, a subgroup of Stage 1 squamous cell carcinomas of the lung did show five-year survivals of 50–70%. However, this subgroup represented only

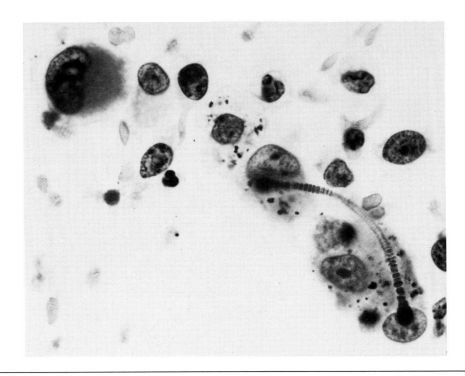

FIGURE 9-16. Papanicolaou-stained fine-needle aspirate smear demonstrates an asbestos body associated with several macrophages. Numerous asbestos bodies were identified in the specimen. A malignant cell is present at upper left. ×1000. Reprinted from Ref. 71, with permission.

5–10% of the total lung cancers. These findings indicate that it is doubtful whether chest roentgenographic surveys or examination of sputum cytology for malignant cells will reduce the mortality of asbestos workers from lung cancer. Thus, programs for the identification of premalignant atypias in sputum (see earlier section on "Bronchial Epithelial Atypias"), cessation of smoking, and chemoprevention (see next subsection) are the best current strategies for reducing lung cancer mortality among asbestos workers.

RETINOIDS AND BETA-CAROTENES
Human cancer risks are inversely correlated with (a) blood retinol and (b) dietary beta-carotene. Although retinol in the blood might well be protective, this would be of little immediate value without discovery of the external determinants of blood retinol. If dietary beta-carotene is truly protective, there are a number of mechanisms whereby it might act.[78–81]

A current extension of the on-going Tyler Asbestos Workers Program is the administration of capsules of beta-carotene.[82] These are given to the workers in a double-blind fashion. Dietary beta-carotene is an analogue of retinoid. It is proposed that the beta-carotene will

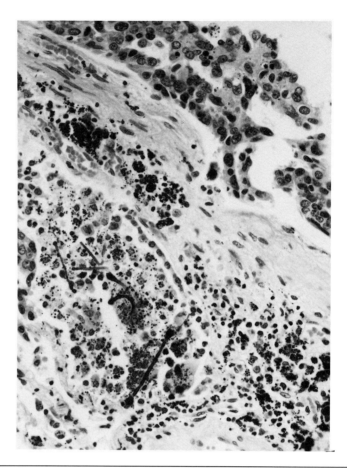

FIGURE 9-17. Sections of a primary lung tumor at autopsy (same case as Fig. 9-16) demonstrate sheets of malignant cells with ill-defined lumen formation and adjacent desmoplastic stroma. Several asbestos bodies are visible adjacent to the tumor at lower left. H&E, ×400. Reprinted from Ref. 71, with permission.

act to arrest progressive bronchial atypia, as seen by sputum cytology, by blocking the DNA within the bronchial epithelial cells. This study uses beta-carotene, which does not have the liver cytotoxicity of retinoids.[83] To date, 637 workers have been enrolled in the study, and preliminary data indicate a highly significant ($p < 0.001$) inverse relationship between cigarette smoking and serum beta-carotene levels. Furthermore, workers with the lowest levels of serum beta-carotene also have significantly high levels ($p < 0.05$) of sputum atypia.[84]

SUMMARY AND CONCLUSIONS

Cigarette smokers with asbestos exposure may show bronchial atypia. Such atypia would support the likelihood of an increase in lung cancer amongst cigarette-smoking asbestos workers with asbestosis.[14]

Sputum cytology presents a unique means of studying the lung's reaction to the inhalation of asbestos fibers. Since the 1970s, with workplace safety levels of < 2 asbestos fibers/cc, the finding of asbestos bodies in sputum of asbestos workers is no longer a common occurrence.[85] However, many patients with asbestos-associated diseases presenting to health care facilities today were first exposed to asbestos prior to 1970 and hence before the current workplace safety levels were established. Cytopathology is likely to play an important role in the diagnosis and management of these patients in the decades to come.

REFERENCES

1. Greenberg SD: Asbestos. Ch. 22 In: *Pulmonary Pathology* (Dail DH, Hammar SP, eds.), New York: Springer-Verlag, 1988, pp. 619–636.
2. Greenberg SD, Hurst GA, Christianson SC, Matlage WJ, Hurst IJ, Mabry LC: Pulmonary cytopathology of former asbestos workers. *Am J Clin Pathol* 66:815–822, 1976.
3. Greenberg SD, Hurst GA, Matlage WT, Miller JM, Hurst IJ, Mabry LC: Tyler asbestos workers program. *Ann NY Acad Sci* 271:353–364, 1976.
4. Roggli VL, Greenberg SD, Seitzman LH, McGavran MH, Hurst GA, Spivey CG, Nelson KG, Hieger LR: Pulmonary fibrosis, carcinoma and ferruginous body counts in amosite asbestos workers. *Am J Clin Pathol* 73:496–503, 1980.
5. Stewart MJ, Haddow AC: Demonstration of the peculiar bodies of pulmonary asbestosis in material obtained by lung puncture and in the sputum. *J Pathol Bacteriol* 32:172, 1929.
6. An SH, Koprowska I: Primary cytologic diagnosis of asbestosis associated with bronchogenic carcinoma: Case report and review of literature. *Acta Cytolog* 6:391–398, 1962.
7. Huuskonen MS, Taskinen E, Vaaranen V: Sputum cytology of asbestosis patients. *Scand J Work Environ Health* 4:284–294, 1978.
8. Gupta PK, Frost JK: Cytologic changes associated with asbestos exposure. *Sem Oncol* 8:283–289, 1981.
9. Kotin P, Paul W: Results of a lung cancer detection program in an asbestos industry. *Recent Results in Cancer Research* 82:131–137, 1982.
10. Simard A, Vauclair R, Feldstein M, Bergeron F, Morissette N, Band P: Sputum cytology and asbestos exposure: A preliminary report. *Recent Results in Cancer Research* 82:147–152, 1982.
11. Dodson RF, Williams MG, McLarty JW, Hurst GA: Asbestos bodies and particulate matter in sputum from former asbestos workers: An ultrastructural study. *Acta Cytolog* 27:635–640, 1983.
12. Kobusch AB, Simard A, Feldstein M, Vauclair R, Gibbs GW, Bergeron F, Morissette N, Davis R: Pulmonary cytology in chrysotile asbestos workers. *J Chron Dis* 37:599–607, 1984.
13. Farley ML, Greenberg SD, Shuford EH, Hurst GA, Spivey CG: Ferruginous bodies in sputa of former asbestos workers. *Acta Cytolog* 21:693–700, 1977.
14. Brown K: Is asbestos or asbestosis the cause of the increased risk of lung cancer in asbestos workers? *Br J Ind Med* 43:145–149, 1986.
15. Greenberg SD, Hurst GA, Matlage WT, Christianson CS, Hurst IJ, Mabry LC: Sputum cytopathological findings in former asbestos workers. *Tex Med* 72:39–43, 1976.

16. Kimzey SL, Greenberg SD, Baky AA, Winkler DG: Cell atypia profiles for bronchial epithelial cells: Mathematical evaluation of sputum cellular atypia in squamous cell carcinogenesis of the lung. *Analyt Quant Cytol* 2:186–194, 1980.

17. Baky AA, Winkler DG, Hunter NR, Subach JA, Greenberg SD, Spjut HJ, Estrada R, Kimzey SL: Atypia status index of respiratory cells—A measurement for the detection and monitoring of neoplastic changes in squamous cell carcinogenesis. *Analyt Quant Cytol* 2:175–185, 1980.

18. Engvall J, Greenberg SD, Spjut HJ, Estrada R, Subach J, Kimzey SL, King JF, DiTrapani PM: Development of a mathematical model to analyze color and density as discriminant features for pulmonary squamous epithelial cells. *Pattern Recognition* 13:37–47, 1981.

19. Baky AA, Winkler DG, Hunter NR, Greenberg SD, Hodapp CJ, Kimzey SL: Nuclear boundary detection algorithm based on a minimax derivative statistic for atypical bronchial squamous epithelial cells. *Analyt Quant Cytol* 3:33–38, 1981.

20. Winkler DG, Baky AA, Hunter NR, Greenberg SD, Rogers TD, Spjut HJ, Estrada R: Image analysis of atypical bronchial epithelial cells—A qualitative examination of squamous cell carcinogenesis. *Analyt Quant Cytol* 3:295–298, 1981.

21. Swank PR, Greenberg SD, Winkler DG, Hunter NR, Smith S, Spjut HJ, Estrada R, Taylor GR: Nuclear segmentation of bronchial epithelial cells by minimax and thresholding techniques—A comparison. *Analyt Quant Cytol* 5:153–158, 1983.

22. Greenberg SD: Recent advances in diagnostic pulmonary cytology. *Hum Pathol* 14:901–912, 1983.

23. Greenberg SD: Diagnosis of sputum atypias by cell image analysis: A review. *Survey and Synthesis of Pathology Research* 2:229–234, 1983.

24. Swank PR, Greenberg SD, Montalvo J, Hunter NR, Thompson JL, Winkler DG, Spjut HJ, Estrada R, Taylor GR: The classification of bronchial epithelial atypias by the atypia status index. *Analyt Quant Cytol* 5:255–262, 1983.

25. Hunter NR, Taylor GR, Swank PR, Winkler DG, Thompson JL, Montalvo J, Greenberg SD, McFadyen GM, Estrada R: Precision cell location and relocation techniques: An application for cell image analysis. *Analyt Quant Cytol* 6:139–143, 1984.

26. Greenberg SD (ed.): Computer-assisted image analysis cytology. In *Monographs in Clinical Cytology* (Vol. 9), Basel: S. Karger, 1984, pp. 1–201.

27. Swank PR, Greenberg SD, Montalvo J, Hunter NR, Spjut HJ, Estrada R, Winkler DG, Taylor GR: The application of visual cell profiles in the study of premalignant atypias in sputum. *Acta Cytolog* 29:373–378, 1985.

28. Greenberg SD, Hunter BA, Taylor GR, Swank PR, Winkler BA, Spjut HJ, Estrada RG, Grenia C, Clark M, Herson J: Application of cell image analysis to the diagnosis of cell atypias in sputum: A review. *Diag Cytopathol* 2:168–174, 1986.

29. Swank PR, Greenberg SD, Winkler DG, Taylor GR, Hunter NR, Montalvo J, Thompson BA, Spjut HJ, Estrada R: Cell atypia profiles for monitoring preneoplastic changes in pulmonary squamous cell carcinogenesis. *Pathol Immunopathol Res* 5:47–53, 1986.

30. Greenberg SD, Spjut HJ, Estrada RG, Hunter NR, Grenia C: Morphometric markers for evaluation of preneoplastic lesions in the lung. *Analyt Quant Cytol* 9:49–54, 1987.

31. Swank PR, Greenberg SD: Optical automation for sputum cytology. *Applied Optics* 26:3373–3378, 1987.

32. Swank PR, Greenberg SD, Hunter NR, Spjut HJ, Estrada R, Trahan EB, Montalvo JG, Taylor GR: The reliability of cytopathologists' classifications of bronchial epithelial atypias from kodachrome slides. *Pathol Immunopathol Res* 6:234–240, 1987.

33. Irani DR, Underwood RD, Johnson EH, Greenberg SD: Malignant pleural effusions. A clinical cytopathologic study. *Arch Intern Med* 147: 1133–1136, 1987.
34. Roberts GH, Campbell GM: Exfoliative cytology of diffuse mesothelioma. *J Clin Pathol* 25:577–582, 1972.
35. Whitaker D, Shilkin KB: Diagnosis of pleural malignant mesothelioma in life: A practical approach. *J Pathol* 143:147–175, 1984.
36. Sherman ME, Mark EJ: Effusion cytology in the diagnosis of malignant epithelioid and biphasic pleural mesothelioma. *Arch Pathol Lab Med* 114:845–851, 1990.
37. Burns TR, Greenberg SD, Mace ML, Johnson EH: Ultrastructural diagnosis of epithelial malignant mesothelioma. *Cancer* 56:2036–2040, 1985.
38. Hammar SP, Bolen JW: Pleural neoplasms. Ch. 30 In: *Pulmonary Pathology* (Dail DH, Hammar SP, eds.), New York: Springer-Verlag, 1988, pp. 973–1028.
39. Cibas ES, Corson JM, Pinkus GS: The distinction of adenocarcinoma from malignant mesothelioma in cell blocks of effusions: The role of routine mucin histochemistry and immunohistochemical assessment of carcinoembryonic antigen, keratin proteins, epithelial membrane antigen, and milk fat globule-derived antigen. *Hum Pathol* 18:67–74, 1987.
40. Duggen MA, Masters CB, Alexander F: Immunohistochemical differentiation of malignant mesothelioma, mesothelial hyperplasia and metastatic adenocarcinoma in serous effusions, utilizing staining for carcinoembryonic antigen, keratin, and vimentin. *Acta Cytolog* 31:807–814, 1987.
41. Martin SE, Moshiri S, Thor A, Vilasi V, Chu EW, Schlom J: Identification of adenocarcinoma in cytospin preparations of effusions using monoclonal antibody B72.3. *Am J Clin Pathol* 86:10–18, 1986.
42. Szpak CA, Johnston WW, Lottich SC, Kufe D, Thor A, Schlom J: Patterns of reactivity of four novel monoclonal antibodies (B72.3, DF3, B1.1, and B6.2) with cells in human malignant and benign effusions. *Acta Cytolog* 28:356–367, 1984.
43. Johnston WW: Cytologic correlations. Ch. 31 In: *Pulmonary Pathology* (Dail DH, Hammar SP, eds.), New York: Springer-Verlag, 1988, pp. 1029–1094.
44. Guzman J, Bross KJ, Würtemberger G, Costabel U: Immunocytology in malignant pleural mesothelioma: Expression of tumor markers and distribution of lymphocyte subsets. *Chest* 95:590–595, 1989.
45. Coon JS, Landay AL, Weinstein RS: Advances in flow cytometry for diagnostic pathology. *Lab Invest* 57:453–479, 1987.
46. Frierson HF, Jr., Mills SE, Legier JF: Flow cytometric analysis of ploidy in immunohistochemically confirmed examples of malignant epithelial mesothelioma. *Am J Clin Pathol* 90:240–243, 1988.
47. Burmer GC, Rabinovitch PS, Kulander BG, Rusch V, McNutt MA: Flow cytometric analysis of malignant pleural mesotheliomas. *Hum Pathol* 20:777–783, 1989.
48. Greenberg SD: Asbestos lung disease. *Sem Resp Med* 4:130–136, 1982.
49. Mace ML, McLemore TL, Roggli V, Brinkley BR, Greenberg SD: Scanning electron microscopic examination of human asbestos bodies. *Cancer Letters* 9:95–104, 1980.
50. McLemore TL, Mace ML, Roggli V, Marshall MV, Lawrence EC, Wilson RK, Martin RR, Brinkley BR, Greenberg SD: Asbestos body phagocytosis by human free alveolar macrophages. *Cancer Letters* 9:85–93, 1980.
51. Roggli VL, McGavran MH, Subach J, Sybers HD, Greenberg SD: Pulmonary asbestos body counts and electron probe analysis of asbestos body cores in patients with mesothelioma: A study of 25 cases. *Cancer* 50:2423–2432, 1982.

52. Modin BE, Greenberg SD, Buffler PA, Lockhart JA, Seitzman LH, Awe RJ: Asbestos bodies in a general hospital/clinic. *Acta Cytolog* 26:667–670, 1982.
53. Holden J, Churg A: Asbestos bodies and the diagnosis of asbestosis in chrysotile workers. *Environ Res* 39:232–236, 1986.
54. Bignon J, Sebastien P, Jaurand MC, Hem B: Microfiltration method for quantitative study of fibrous particles in biological specimens. *Environ Health Persp* 9:155–160, 1974.
55. Roggli VL, Greenberg SD, McLarty JW, Hurst GA, Hieger LR, Farley ML, Mabry LC: Comparison of sputum and lung asbestos body counts in former asbestos workers. *Am Rev Respir Dis* 122:941–945, 1980.
56. McLarty JW, Greenberg SD, Hurst GA, Spivey CG, Seitzman LH, Hieger LR, Farley ML, Mabry LC: The clinical significance of ferruginous bodies in sputa. *J Occ Med* 22:92–96, 1980.
57. McLarty JW, Greenberg SD, Hurst GA, Spivey CG, Farley ML, Mabry LC: Statistical comparison of aerosolized induced and spontaneous sputum specimens in the Tyler Asbestos Workers Program. *Acta Cytolog* 24:70–75, 1980.
58. Roggli VL, McLarty JW, Greenberg SD: Asbestos bodies in sputum: A clinical marker of exposure. *J Occ Med* 25:508, 1983.
59. Dodson RF, Williams MG, Corn CJ, Idell S, McLarty JW: Usefulness of combined light and electron microscopy: Evaluation of sputum samples for asbestos to determine past occupational exposure. *Modern Pathol* 2:320–322, 1989.
60. DeVuyst PD, Jedwab J, Dumortier P, Vandermoten G, Van de Weyer R, Yernault JC: Asbestos bodies in bronchoalveolar lavage. *Am Rev Respir Dis* 126:972–976, 1982.
61. DeVuyst PD, Mairesse M, Gaudichet A, Dumortier P, Jedwab J, Yernault JC: Mineralogical analysis of bronchoalveolar lavage fluid as an aid to diagnosis of "imported" pleural asbestosis. *Thorax* 38:628–629, 1983.
62. Yernault JC, DeVuyst P, Dumortier P: Correlation of bronchoalveolar lavage and clinical and functional findings in asbestosis. *Am Rev Respir Dis* 134:1335, 1986.
63. DeVuyst P, Dumortier P, Moulin E, Yourassowsky N, Yernault JC: Diagnostic value of asbestos bodies in bronchoalveolar lavage fluid. *Am Rev Respir Dis* 136:1219–1224, 1987.
64. Barbers RG, Abraham JL: Asbestosis occurring after brief inhalational exposure: Usefulness of bronchoalveolar lavage in diagnosis. *Br J Ind Med* 46:106–110, 1989.
65. Roggli VL, Piantadosi CA, Bell DY: Asbestos bodies in bronchoalveolar lavage fluid: A study of 20 asbestos exposed individuals and comparison to patients with other chronic interstitial lung diseases. *Acta Cytolog* 30:470–476, 1986.
66. Sebastien P, Armstrong B, Monchaux G, Bignon J: Asbestos bodies in bronchoalveolar lavage fluid and in lung parenchyma. *Am Rev Respir Dis* 137:75–78, 1988.
67. DeVuyst P, Dumortier P, Moulin E, Yourassowsky N, Roomans P, de Francquen P, Yernault JC: Asbestos bodies in bronchoalveolar lavage reflect lung asbestos body concentration. *Eur Resp J* 1:362–367, 1988.
68. Jaurand MC, Gaudichet A, Atassi K, Sebastien P, Bignon J: Relationship between the number of asbestos fibres and the cellular and enzymatic content of bronchoalveolar fluid in asbestos-exposed subjects. *Bull Europ Physiopath Respir* 16:595–606, 1980.
69. Gellert AR, Perry D, Langford JA, Riches PG, Rudd RM: Asbestosis: Bronchoalveolar lavage fluid proteins and their relationship to pulmonary epithelial permeability. *Chest* 88:730–735, 1985.

70. Rebuck AS, Braude AC: Bronchoalveolar lavage in asbestosis. *Arch Intern Med* 143:950–952, 1983.
71. Roggli VL, Johnston WW, Kaminsky DB: Asbestos bodies in fine needle aspirates of the lung. *Acta Cytolog* 28:493–498, 1984.
71a. Leiman G: Asbestos bodies in fine needle aspirates of lung masses: Markers of underlying pathology. *Acta Cytolog* 35:171–174, 1991.
72. Greenberg SD: The cytopathology of asbestos associated pulmonary disease. *Diag Cytopathol* 1:177–182, 1985.
73. Auerbach O, Conston AS, Garfinkel L, Parks VR, Kaslow HD, Hammond EC: Presence of asbestos bodies in organs other than the lung. *Chest* 77:133–137, 1980.
74. Berlin NI, Buncher R, Fontana RS, Frost JK, Melamed MR: Early lung cancer detection: Introduction. *Am Rev Respir Dis* 130:545–549, 1984.
75. Frost JK, Ball WC Jr., Levin ML, Tockman MMS, Baker RR, Carter D, Eggleston JC, Erozan YS, Gupta PK, Khouri NF, Marsh BR, Stitik FP: Results of the initial (prevalence) radiologic and cytologic screening in the Johns Hopkins Study. *Am Rev Respir Dis* 130:549–554, 1984.
76. Flehinger BJ, Melamed MR, Zaman MB, Heelan RT, Perchick WB, Martini N: Results of the initial (prevalence) radiologic and cytologic screening in the Memorial Sloan-Kettering Study. *Am Rev Respir Dis* 130:555–560, 1984.
77. Fontana RS, Sanderson DR, Taylor WF, Woolner LB, Miller WE, Muhm JR, Uhlenhopp MA: Results of the initial (prevalence) radiologic and cytologic sceening in the Mayo Clinic Study. *Am Rev Respir Dis* 130:561–565, 1984.
78. Sporn MB, Newton DL: Chemoprevention of cancer with retinoids. *Federation Proc* 38:2528–2534, 1979.
79. Editorial, Vitamin A, retinol, carotene, and cancer prevention. *Br Med J* 281:957–958, 1980.
80. Newberne PM, Rogers AE: Vitamin A, retinoids, and cancer. In: *Nutrition and Cancer: Etiology and Treatment* (Newell GR, Ellison NM, eds.), New York: Raven Press, 1981.
81. Peto R, Doll R, Buckley JD, Sporn MB: Can dietary beta-carotene materially reduce human cancer rates? *Nature* 290:201–208, 1981.
82. Mossman BT, Marsh JP, Hill S, Gilbert R, Shatos M, Doherty J, Hemenway D: Mineral dust alveolar disease: Asbestos and silica - I. (Abst.) *Chest* 91:301, 1987.
83. McLarty JW (Personal communication).
84. McLarty JW, Yanagihara R, Riley L: Beta-carotene, retinol, and lung cancer chemoprevention. Pathology of Occupational Lung Disease: An Update. Dept. of Pathol., Baylor Coll of Med., Houston, TX, May 19, 1989.
85. Key MM (Personal communication).

10. Experimental Models of Asbestos-Related Diseases

VICTOR L. ROGGLI AND ARNOLD R. BRODY

Much of our understanding of the mechanisms by which asbestos injures the lung has derived from experimental animal studies. Such studies have confirmed the fibrogenic and carcinogenic properties of asbestos fibers that have been surmised from human observations, and have provided insights into the ways in which asbestos fibers interact with biological systems. This information has been obtained by means of inhalational exposures, intratracheal instillation studies, and in vitro studies of various cellular systems. Each of these techniques has its own particular advantages and limitations. Inhalational studies, being more physiologic, more closely approximate the actual human situation; but they are time consuming and expensive, and relatively few facilities have the capabilities for such studies. Intratracheal instillation is simpler to perform and less expensive, but has the disadvantages that the normal defense mechanisms of the respiratory tract are bypassed and the distribution is nonuniform; hence the results are not directly comparable to inhalational exposures. In vitro studies of cellular systems permit one to investigate the direct effects of asbestos and other particulates on cellular function under carefully controlled conditions. However, it is not always clear how the results apply to the more complex in vivo conditions or whether the particular mechanism under investigation contributes significantly to the overall pathogenesis of asbestos-induced tissue injury. Notwithstanding these limitations, each of these approaches has contributed substantially to our understanding of the mechanisms underlying asbestos-related diseases.

This chapter reviews our understanding of the pathogenesis of asbestos-related diseases as derived from experimental models. In order to understand asbestos-related tissue injury, it is first necessary to understand the patterns of deposition of asbestos fibers within the lung parenchyma, and the subsequent clearance of fibers from the lung via the mucociliary escalator, the macrophage defense system, and the pulmonary lymphatics. Next, the factors influencing the production of pulmonary fibrosis and thoracic neoplasms in inhalational models will be reviewed. Finally, in vitro studies suggesting particular mechanisms by which asbestos produces its effects will be examined. Although asbestos-induced fibrogenesis and carcinogenesis share many common features and may involve similar molecular mechanisms of tissue injury, these two processes will be reviewed separately for the sake of clarity.

HISTORICAL BACKGROUND

Experimental models of asbestos-induced tissue injury were established in the 1930s and '40s by the pioneering work of L. U. Gardner[1] and E. J. King et al.[2] In 1951, Vorwald et al.[3] published the results of the classic inhalational studies performed at Saranac Lake in New York. These investigators showed that inhalation (or intratracheal instillation) of chrysotile, crocidolite, and amosite asbestos produced in most (but not all) animal species a bronchiolocentric pattern of interstitial fibrosis similar to that observed in human asbestosis. Long asbestos fibers were found to be more injurious than short fibers, and the duration of exposure required to develop disease varied inversely with the concentration of long fibers in the atmosphere.[3] The development of a dependable and reproducible fiber aerosolization system by Timbrell[4] paved the way for the inhalational studies of Wagner et al.[5] reported in 1974. These studies performed with SPF Wistar rats showed that both amphibole and chrysotile forms of asbestos produced asbestosis in a dose-dependent fashion, and that the fibrosis continued to progress after removal from exposure. Furthermore, inhalational exposure to all forms of asbestos tested resulted in the production of thoracic neoplasms, including adenomas, carcinomas, and mesotheliomas.[5] There was a positive correlation between the severity of asbestosis and the development of pulmonary neoplasms. These early studies paved the way for subsequent investigations and provided the basis for more detailed analysis of pathogenetic mechanisms at the cellular level.[6]

DEPOSITION AND CLEARANCE OF ASBESTOS FIBERS

The mammalian respiratory system is equipped with a variety of defense mechanisms for protection against foreign matter, and these mechanisms in turn effect the size, shape, and numbers of particles that are deposited and that ultimately accumulate in the lower respiratory tract. These defense mechanisms include four major components: (1) the fine hairs, or vibrissae, in the nasal cavity that filter out most of the larger particles [$>10 \mu$ aerodynamic equivalent diameter (AED)] that are inhaled; (2) the mucociliary escalator of the tracheobronchial tree, which carries upwards toward the mouth any particles that impact on the surface of the airways; (3) the alveolar macrophages, which phagocytize particles that make their way past the first two levels of defenses and are deposited in the gas-exchange regions of the lung; and (4) the pulmonary lymphatics, through which many particles deposited in the lung are transported to regional lymph nodes.[7]

Particles that have the greatest probability of deposition and retention in the gas-exchange regions of the lung are in the size range of 1–5 μ AED. Particles less than 0.5 μ in maximum dimension are deposited by Brownian motion or diffusion. Deposition patterns may be influenced by such factors as tidal volume, respiratory rate, and pattern of breathing (nose versus mouth). Similarly, subsequent clearance of particles deposited in the lung is dependent on a number of factors, including the anatomic site of deposition, particle solubility, and the efficiency of the host's phagocytic system. In addition, cigarette smoking has been shown to interfere with particle clearance from the lower respiratory tract.[8]

A unique feature of fibrous dusts is that fibers of considerable length can be deposited in the lower respiratory tract, even though most particles 5 μ or greater in size are excluded. This is due to the tendency for fibrous dusts to line up along the direction of laminar airflow, so that the diameter of a fiber rather than its length is the primary determinant of respirability.[9,10] As a result, most fibers deposited in the lungs of humans or experimental animals are 1 μ or less in diameter, but may exceed 200 μ in length (see Chap. 3). In this respect, there are some important differences between the amphibole fibers and the serpentine, chrysotile. Very long fibers of chrysotile tend to be curly and are thus more likely to impact in the upper respiratory tract, where they are subsequently removed on the mucociliary escalator.[9,10] Even very long amphibole fibers tend to be straight, and thus they have a greater likelihood of penetrating into the gas-exchange regions of the lung. Differences between the accumulation of amphibole versus chrysotile fibers within the lungs of experimental animals following long-term inhalational exposure were noted by Wagner et al.,[5] and these observations have stimulated the investigation of the pulmonary deposition and clearance of asbestos fibers, with particular attention to differences between chrysotile and the amphiboles.

FIBER DEPOSITION

The development of methods for producing radio-labeled asbestos fibers[11] has greatly facilitated the determination of the patterns of fiber deposition in the respiratory tract. Early studies using these techniques demonstrated a tendency for fiber deposition and concentration at bifurcation points in the conducting airways, with a relatively uniform distribution throughout the alveolated regions.[12,13] More recent studies using scanning electron microscopy have shown that this tendency for deposition at bifurcation points extends to the alveolated regions of the lungs.[14-16] In rats exposed to aerosolized chrysotile asbestos for a brief period of time, fibers in the distal anatomic regions of the lung were localized primarily at alveolar duct bifurcations (Fig. 10-1). The greatest concentration of fibers occurs at bifurcations closest to the terminal bronchiole, and are less numerous at the more distant (e.g., second- and third-order) alveolar duct bifurcations.[6,14,15,17] Very few fibers are observed on the surfaces of adjacent alveoli. A similar pattern is observed for chrysotile and amphibole asbestos fibers.[16]

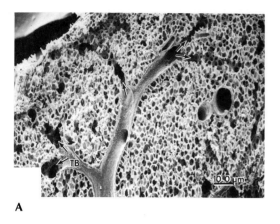

A

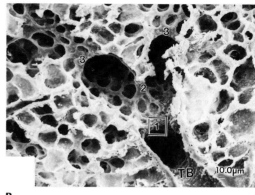

B

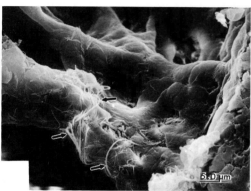

C

FIGURE 10-1. (A) Low-power scanning electron micrograph of rat lung parenchyma showing terminal bronchioles (TB) and alveolar ducts (arrows). (B) Higher magnification of a terminal bronchiole and its alveolar ducts exhibiting three bifurcations. (C) Detailed view of the first alveolar duct bifurcation, outlined in part (B), showing large numbers of chrysotile asbestos fibers (arrows) littering the bifurcation surface. Few fibers are observed on the alveolar surfaces. Reprinted from Ref. 16, with permission.

These observations indicate that the geometry of the tracheobronchial tree is an important determining factor in the deposition of particulates in the lower respiratory tract.[18] Studies in which meticulous dissections of the tracheobronchial tree in asbestos-exposed rats were performed demonstrate that the quantity of asbestos deposited in the lung parenchyma is inversely related to airway path length and the number of airway bifurcations.[19] Variations in airway geometry among different species could result in different patterns of deposition, which in turn could account for some of the variation in species response to asbestos inhalation.[20] In this regard, it should be noted that marked differences in deposition pattern are obtained for dust administered by inhalation versus intratracheal instillation.[21] The distribution of dust resulting from instillation is much less homogeneous than that from inhalation, and penetration to the lung periphery is minimal. The resultant inflammatory responses are also quite different,[22] so that one must use caution in extrapolating results based on intratracheal instillation in experimental animals to human inhalation exposures.[6]

TABLE 10-1. Fractional deposition of chrysotile versus amphibole asbestos fibers in lungs of rats following inhalational exposure*

Authors	Exposure dose	Exposure duration	Fractional deposition	
			Chrysotile	*Amphibole*
Morgan et al.[13]	4, 11, & 32 µg/l	30 min	12–15%	16%
Roggli and Brody[23]	15 µg/l	1 h	23%	—
Roggli et al.[25]	3.5 µg/l	1 h	—	19%
Middleton et al.[24]	1, 5, & 10 µg/l	6 wks	17–36%	65–100%

*The studies by Morgan et al.,[13] Roggli and Brody,[23] and Roggli et al.[25] employed nose-only exposure chambers, whereas the studies by Middleton et al.[24] used open-chamber (i.e., whole animal) exposures.

Opinions differ regarding the fractional deposition of chrysotile versus amphibole asbestos fibers in the lower respiratory tract. Morgan et al.,[13] in a study in which rats were exposed to three concentrations (4, 11, and 32 µg/l) of two different samples of radio-labeled chrysotile asbestos for 30 minutes in nose-only chambers, found that 12% and 15% of the respirable mass was deposited in the lower respiratory tract. Roggli and Brody,[23] in a study in which rats were exposed to 15 µg/l of Jeffrey mine chrysotile asbestos (a standardized preparation) for one hour in nose-only chambers, found that 23% of the respirable mass was deposited in the lower respiratory tract. In studies in which rats were exposed to U.I.C.C. (Union Internationale Contre le Cancer) asbestos samples by inhalation for six weeks, Middleton et al.[24] found that the relative retention of chrysotile in the lungs decreases with increasing aerosolized concentrations. For the highest concentration employed in their study (7.8 µg/l), the fractional deposition of chrysotile in the lungs was 17%.[24] Short-term inhalation studies result in a similar fractional deposition for crocidolite as compared to chrysotile asbestos: 16% of the respirable mass in the study by Morgan et al.,[13] and 19% in the study by Roggli et al.[25] In contrast, Middleton et al.[24] determined that, for rats exposed to amphibole fibers for six weeks, the fractional deposition for amosite was 65% and for crocidolite approached 100%. These comparisons are summarized in Table 10-1. Although the reason for these discrepancies is unclear, it is apparent that, with durations of exposure of six weeks or longer, the relative retention of amphibole fibers in the lungs is considerably greater than that of chrysotile.[5,24]

FIBER CLEARANCE

The fate of a fiber that has been deposited in the respiratory tract is dependent to some degree on the site of deposition. Fibers deposited on the surface of the large or small airways may become trapped in the mucous layer, where they will be transported upward by ciliary motion at a rate as high as several millimeters per minute.[10] Fibers deposited on the alveolar epithelium may be transported across the epithelium into the underlying interstitium via a mechanism that

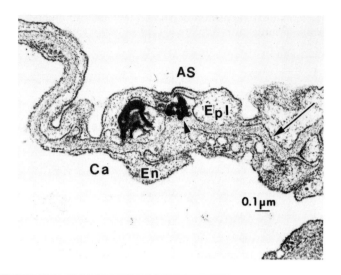

FIGURE 10-2. Transmission electron micrograph showing fibrils of chrysotile asbestos (arrowhead) adjacent to the alveolar capillary basement membrane (arrow). Five hours post-exposure: capillary, Ca; capillary endothelium, En; Type I epithelium, EpI; alveolar spaces, AS. Reprinted from Ref. 14, with permission.

probably involves an actin-containing microfilament system.[6,26,27] Thus, within hours of a brief inhalational exposure, asbestos fibers are observed within the cytoplasm of Type I epithelial cells (Fig. 10-2); within 24 hours, fibers have been translocated into the interstitial compartment, including basement membrane, connective tissue, and cytoplasm of interstitial cells.[6] In addition, there is evidence that transepithelial transport occurs to some extent in the airways as well.[28,29] Once within the interstitium, fibers may then penetrate the cytoplasm of endothelial cells[14,15] and gain access to the vascular and lymphatic systems.[10] Fibers within lymphatic channels may then be carried to the visceral pleura[30] and hence gain access to the pleural space,[31] or be transported to hilar or mediastinal lymph nodes.[32,33] Also, within 24 hours of a brief inhalational exposure to asbestos, there is an influx of alveolar macrophages that proceed to phagocytize any free asbestos fibers on the alveolar surfaces. These macrophages accumulate at the site of initial fiber deposition, and are found on more than 90% of alveolar duct bifurcations by 48 hours post-exposure.[34] Fibers that have been transported to the pulmonary interstitium may similarly be phagocytized by interstitial macrophages. Once ingested within the macrophage, fibers may remain for prolonged periods within alveoli or the interstitium. Alternatively, phagocytized fibers may be removed from the lung when macrophages enter onto the mucociliary escalator of the small airways or into the pulmonary lymphatics.[10]

A number of studies have demonstrated that the average length of fibers retained within the lung increases with time post-exposure, and that this effect is observed for both chrysotile and amphibole asbestos.[23,25,35–39] The presumed mechanism of this effect is the more efficient clearance of short fibers, with preferential retention of longer fibers. This phenomenon can be particularly well demonstrated by measuring the half-times for clearance of fibers in various size categories after a single exposure (Fig. 10-3). In these studies, it can be seen that the residence time within the lung for fibers 10 μ or more in length is particularly prolonged.[39] More direct evidence for the more efficient clearance of shorter fibers comes from the studies of Kauffer et al.,[38] which showed a progressive decrease in mean length of fibers recovered by bronchoalveolar lavage following a brief inhalational exposure, with a concomitant increase in mean length of fibers remaining in the lungs.

With regard to fiber type, short-term inhalational studies have shown similar clearance rates for chrysotile versus amphibole asbestos fibers. Following a one-hour exposure period, the percentage of the original deposited mass remaining one month post-exposure was 25% for crocidolite[25] and 19% for chrysotile asbestos.[23] Middleton et al.[24] also reported that the rate of clearance is similar for chrysotile and amphibole types of asbestos, and that the clearance could be expressed in terms of a three-compartment model with half-lives $(t_\frac{1}{2})$ of 0.38, 8, and 118 days for each respective compartment. These observations are difficult to reconcile with the results of long-term inhalational studies, in which amphibole asbestos fibers accumulate within the lungs to a much greater extent than chrysotile fibers.[5,40] In fact, the lung content of chrysotile appears to level off and remain constant after two or three months of exposure, whereas amphibole fibers continue to accumulate progressively with continued exposure.[5] Middleton et al.[24,41] also noted substantially greater accumulation of amphiboles as compared to chrysotile following a six-week exposure, and attributed the difference to a greater fractional deposition of amphibole fibers (see earlier discussion and Table 10-1). We have similarly observed substantial differences in the pulmonary content of crocidolite versus chrysotile asbestos in rats exposed to similar doses of the two fiber types for a three-month period (Table 10-2). Recent observations using intratracheal instillation of asbestos have demonstrated more rapid clearance of chrysotile fibers as compared to amphiboles beginning almost immediately after exposure.[42,43]

Although the reasons for the preferential retention of amphibole fibers are not entirely clear, one very important factor is undoubtedly the tendency for chrysotile to divide longitudinally into individual fibrils. Roggli and Brody[23] reported a progressive decrease in mean fiber diameter following a one-hour inhalational exposure to chrysotile asbestos, and this observation has been confirmed by a number of investigators.[37,38,42,44] In comparison, no significant alteration in mean fiber diameter is observed for amphibole fibers.[25,37,42,44] The

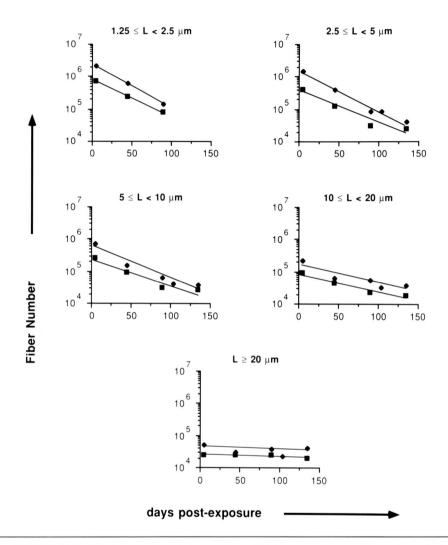

FIGURE 10-3. Washout curves (phase-contrast light microscopy). The points plotted are geometric means of fiber number in each length class. The lines shown are linear regressions of log (fiber number) for each animal vs. time, i.e., a one-compartment model. The slopes of all regression lines for fiber length $< 20\ \mu m$ are significantly different from zero ($p < 0.00001$ in each case). Correlation coefficients range from 0.87–0.96. For length $\geq 20\ \mu m$, the slopes are not significantly different from zero ($p = 0.38$ for washout I, and $p = 0.25$ for washout II). Reprinted from Ref. 39, with permission.

TABLE 10-2. Accumulation of chrysotile versus crocidolite asbestos in rat lungs following inhalational exposure[a]

Fiber type	Fibers/gm[b]	Asbestos/rat (µg)[c]
Crocidolite	1.85×10^8 ($\pm 1.12 \times 10^8$)	814(± 435)
Chrysotile	2.50×10^7 ($\pm 8.4 \times 10^6$)	71.6 (± 28.9)
Sham[d]	3.5×10^4 ($\pm 4.9 \times 10^4$)	0.045 (± 0.025)

[a]Rats sacrificed following 3 months' exposure in inhalation chambers to 10.7 mg/m^3 chrysotile or 11.2 mg/m^3 crocidolite asbestos
[b]Fibers per gram of wet lung ± 1 SE (4 animals in each group)
[c]Calculated mass of asbestos in both lungs ± 1 SE
[d]Animals exposed to room air only

longitudinal splitting of chrysotile fiber bundles creates fibrils with a very fine diameter; short fibrils created by this splitting process are readily cleared from the lung, whereas long, thin chrysotile fibrils are retained.[23,44] Kimizuka et al.[44] reported a further fragmentation of long, thin chrysotile fibers two years post-exposure in hamsters, with a concomitant increase in the percentage of fibers less than 5 µ in length from 13% one year post-exposure to 56% at two years. The decrease in mean fiber diameter of chrysotile has been associated with leaching of magnesium by some investigators[37,44] but not by others.[42] No significant change in elemental composition is observed for amphibole fibers with increasing time post-exposure.[37,44] Progressive leaching of magnesium from chrysotile fibers occurring in an acid environment could result in fiber dissolution, and some investigators believe that this may be an important mechanism of chrysotile clearance from the lung, especially for very small fibrils.[45,46] In this regard, in vitro studies with alveolar macrophages have shown a rate of magnesium leaching from chrysotile asbestos that is comparable to the leaching rate in an acid solution with a pH of 4.[47] Although the in vivo significance of magnesium leaching from chrysotile asbestos fibers is controversial, it is of potential importance, since the cytotoxicity and carcinogenicity of chrysotile asbestos is significantly reduced by in vitro depletion of magnesium.[48]

Additional factors may significantly influence the clearance of asbestos fibers from the lower respiratory tract. Bolton et al.[49] have shown that, once a critical pulmonary burden of asbestos has been reached, there is an overload of the clearance mechanism. This phenomenon occurs at relatively high lung burdens, and may be related to inhibition of clearance by alveolar macrophages. Other studies have shown that administration of a toxic dust such as asbestos or quartz can interfere with the subsequent clearance of a nontoxic dust such as titanium dioxide.[50,51] Furthermore, there is evidence that cigarette smoke interferes with the clearance of asbestos fibers from the lower respiratory tract, largely by increasing the retention of short fibers.[52,53] Exposure to low levels of ozone also enhances pulmonary retention of inhaled asbestos fibers, apparently by interfering with fiber clearance.[54]

Fiber clearance may play an important role in the development and severity of asbestosis following inhalation of asbestos fibers. Experimental studies have shown that high alveolar dust retention precedes the development of asbestosis and that individual variability in alveolar dust clearance capacity may be a major determinant in the development of asbestos-induced pulmonary fibrosis.[55]

FIBROGENESIS

IN VIVO INHALATIONAL STUDIES

Inhalational studies in experimental animals have shown that asbestos produces interstitial pulmonary fibrosis. Three specific lesions have been identified:[3,5,40] (1) peribronchiolar accumulation of dust-containing macrophages, giant cells, and fibrous tissue in association with respiratory bronchioles and alveolar ducts; (2) extension of bronchiolar epithelium into adjacent alveolar ducts and alveoli producing a pattern sometimes referred to as adenomatosis; and (3) diffuse stromal thickening of the alveolar septa associated with proliferation of Type II pneumocytes. Initially, the sites of dust deposition are rich in reticulin fibers, which become more coarse over time and eventually stain strongly for collagen. The earliest lesion is in the vicinity of respiratory bronchioles, and with continuing exposure, appears to extend to involve alveolar ducts and adjacent alveoli.[3,5] All types of asbestos, including chrysotile,[3,5,40] amosite,[5,40] crocidolite,[5,40] anthophyllite,[5,40] and tremolite,[56] produce asbestosis in experimental animal models, and there appears to be a dose–response relationship for each of the fiber types tested.[5,40] Although there is variation in species response to either intratracheal instillation or inhalation of asbestos,[3,6,20] asbestosis has been produced in a wide range of experimental animals, including sheep,[57] mice,[58–60] guinea pigs,[3,52,61,62] hamsters,[44] and the white rat.[3,5,40]

The classic observations regarding experimental asbestos-induced lung injury[3,5,40] have been extended to the cellular level by means of ultrastructural morphometry of animals exposed to asbestos fibers by chronic inhalation.[6] Examination of the lungs of animals exposed to chrysotile asbestos for one week, three months, or one year has demonstrated that the most significant changes occur in the epithelial and interstitial compartments.[63–65] Within the epithelial compartment, an increase in cell number and average cell volume can be largely attributed to alveolar Type II pneumocyte hyperplasia. Similarly, the interstitial compartment shows an increase in cell number and average cell volume, most of which can be attributed to accumulation of interstitial macrophages.[63]

Asbestos fibers may be identified, via transmission electron microscopy, within pulmonary epithelial cells and interstitial macrophages. A decrease in the ratio of magnesium to silicon in some of these fibers, as determined by energy-dispersive x-ray analysis, is indicative of some leaching of magnesium.[64] Microcalcifications also are identified within some interstitial cells. The endothelial and capillary compartments of the lung are for the most part unaffected. Fibers are gradually cleared from epithelial cells and macrophages following cessation of exposure, and these compartments then resolve toward unexposed-control levels. However, significant clearance of fibers from the pulmonary interstitium does not occur even one year following cessation of exposure (Fig. 10-4). This persistence of fibers in the interstitial compartment is associated with continuing fibrogenesis.[65] Long-term studies following intratracheal instillation of chrysotile asbestos in rats have shown, by means of biochemical analysis, significantly increased collagen and elastin content per unit lung weight.[66]

Electron microscopic studies following brief (one-hour) inhalation exposures allow more detailed evaluation of the earliest events in asbestos-induced tissue injury.[6] Within 24 hours of a brief exposure to aerosolized asbestos fibers, the lung responds with an influx of alveolar macrophages at the site of initial fiber deposition.[34] This accumulation of macrophages persists for at least 30 days, and is associated with a significantly increased bifurcation tissue volume as assessed by morphometric studies (Fig. 10-5).[34,67] In the interstitium adjacent to these alveolar duct bifurcations, asbestos fibers can readily be identified one month post-exposure, both intracellularly and extracellularly, and are often associated with microcalcifications.[68] These microcalcifications consist of calcium and phosphate (Fig. 10-6), and may be the consequence of fiber-induced membrane injury of interstitial cells.[68]

Transmission electron microscopy correlated with autoradiography shows that epithelial proliferation is associated with bronchiolar Clara cells and alveolar Type II cells, whereas interstitial proliferation is related to division of interstitial macrophages and fibroblasts.[69,70] Furthermore, blood vessels adjacent to alveolar duct bifurcations show increased labeling of both endothelial and smooth muscle cell nuclei by H^3-TdR 19–72 hours following a brief inhalation exposure to chrysotile asbestos.[71] This mitogenic response may be due to the release of diffusible growth factors presumably deriving from asbestos-stimulated alveolar macrophages (see later discussion). Ultrastructural examination of alveolar duct bifurcations of rats exposed to asbestos for one day has shown persistence of fibers at these sites as long as one year post-exposure.[72]

ROLE OF FIBER DIMENSIONS

The importance of fiber length in asbestos-induced fibrogenesis has been addressed in a number of studies. The classic studies reported by Vorwald et al.[3] suggested that fibers greater than 20 μ in length

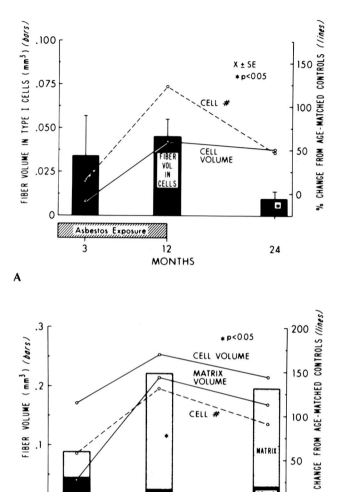

FIGURE 10-4. (A) Morphometrically determined total asbestos fiber volume within Type I alveolar epithelial cells for both lungs (bars), and the corresponding increase in cell number and cell volume (lines), in rats after prolonged inhalation of chrysotile asbestos. Changes in total cell number and tissue volume are expressed as percentage change from age-matched controls. (B) Total asbestos fiber volume present in interstitial cells (solid portion of bars) and extracellular matrix (open portion of bars), and corresponding increase in cell number, cell volume, and matrix volume (lines), in rats after chronic inhalation of chrysotile. Reprinted from Ref. 65, with permission.

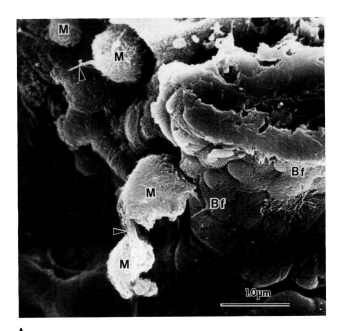

A

B

FIGURE 10-5. (A) Scanning electron micrograph of an alveolar duct bifurcation (Bf) 48 hours after a 1-hour exposure to chrysotile asbestos. Alveolar macrophages (M) are accumulating at sites of fiber deposition and phagocytizing some fibers (arrowheads). (B) Transmission electron micrograph of asbestos-containing macrophages (M) at an alveolar duct bifurcation. The macrophages are tightly adherent to the underlying Type I epithelial cells (arrows): alveolar spaces, AS; interstitial connective tissue, IC; interstitial macrophages, IM. Reprinted from Ref. 34, with permission.

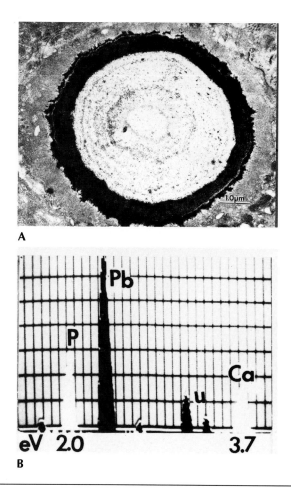

FIGURE 10-6. (A) Transmission electron micrograph of an intracellular microcalcification within the pulmonary interstitium showing a laminated central portion and a dark outer rim. (B) Energy dispersive spectrum from the microcalcification showing peaks for calcium (Ca) and phosphorus (P). Peaks for uranium (U) and lead (Pb) are due to staining with lead citrate and uranyl acetate. Reprinted from Ref. 68, with permission.

are the most fibrogenic, an opinion supported by the studies of Davis et al.[40] Other investigators have also concluded that long-fiber asbestos results in considerably more lung injury than short-fiber asbestos,[59–61,64,73–75] and that there is progression of injury after cessation of exposure only with the long-fiber inhalation.[64] It is difficult to determine a fiber length below which no significant fibrosis will occur regardless of intensity or duration of exposure, in part because of the problem of contamination of "short fiber" samples with a small percentage of "long fibers."[74] However, LeMaire et al.[76] studied rats injected intratracheally with 5 mg of a preparation of very short chrysotile fibers (100% < 8 μ) and found an alveolitis 60 days post-exposure but no apparent fibrosis.

Platek et al.[77] exposed rats by inhalation of short chrysotile asbestos with a mean concentration of fibers in the chamber of 1.0 mg/m^3 and only 0.79 fibers/ml with length exceeding five microns. These investigators showed that a concentration of 23×10^6 chrysotile fibers >5 μ in length per gram of dry lung or 272×10^6 chrysotile fibers <5 μ in length per gram of dry lung or a combination of the two is insufficient to produce pulmonary fibrosis in the rat 18–24 months after initiation of exposure.[77] Adamson and Bowden found no appreciable fibrosis in the lungs of mice following intratracheal instillation of 0.1 mg of short crocidolite asbestos fibers (mean length 0.6 μ, with 98.8% of fibers less than 2.5 μ in length),[59] whereas peribronchiolar fibrosis and significantly increased collagen levels were observed following instillation of 0.1 mg of long crocidolite asbestos fibers (mean length 24.4 μ, with 88% of fibers greater than 2.5 μ in length).[60] Contrary to the findings of most other investigators, Fasske[78] reported the production of interstitial fibrosis following intratracheal instillation of ultrashort-fiber chrysotile asbestos (fiber length between 0.05 μ and 0.2 μ). However, the one published light micrograph shows dense fibrosis at too high a magnification to determine whether the pattern is typical for that observed with asbestosis.[6]

In contrast to fiber length, relatively few studies have examined the role of fiber diameter in the pathogenesis of asbestos-induced tissue injury. The major importance of fiber diameter appears to be its role as a limiting factor for fiber deposition. For fibers with an aspect ratio between 10 and 100, the aerodynamic equivalent diameter is approximately three to four times the actual fiber diameter.[10] Hence, for fibers with an aspect ratio of 10 or more, 2 μ is about the maximum diameter of a fiber that may be deposited in the lower respiratory tract of the rat.[10] Other physical parameters of fibers are also potentially important. Some studies have indicated that fiber surface area is the most important determinant of the severity of pulmonary fibrosis[79] (see also Chap. 11). In this regard, the progressive decrease in mean fiber diameter of chrysotile may be an important feature in its pathogenicity. This decrease in fiber diameter is believed to be due to longitudinal splitting of chrysotile fibers in vivo, which would result in both increased fiber number and increased surface area.[80] Each of these factors has been shown to correlate positively with the severity of fibrosis. Finally, another physical feature of importance is fiber charge, with highly charged fibers being more likely to be deposited in lung tissue.[81] This effect is probably greatest for long fibers, and electrostatically charged chrysotile asbestos produces more fibrosis than a similar level of asbestos that has been charge neutralized.[81]

IN VITRO STUDIES OF MECHANISMS OF ASBESTOS CYTOTOXICITY

There is abundant evidence that asbestos is directly cytotoxic to a variety of cells and tissues in vitro.[82] The mechanisms of asbestos-induced cytotoxicity were first explored in red blood cells[83–85] and later in cell and tissue cultures.[28,29,86,87] Photoelectron spectrometry analysis demonstrated that phospholipid membranes are adsorbed as a bilayer onto the surface of chrysotile asbestos fibers.[84] Scanning electron microscopic examination of red blood cells treated with chrysotile asbestos showed distortion of the cells, and this effect was almost totally ablated by pretreatment of the cells with neuraminidase.[85] Similar observations have been reported for the binding of chrysotile fibers to alveolar macrophages in vitro.[88] These studies suggest that chrysotile binds to sialic acid residues on membrane surfaces. In contrast, neuraminidase treatment had no demonstrable effect on crocidolite binding. Other investigators using cell cultures of rat tracheal epithelium concluded that membrane damage was only a minor component of fiber-induced toxicity, and that a sequence of fiber binding, phagocytosis, nuclear damage, disruption of mitosis, and inhibition of proliferation or cell death is an important alternative pathway of fiber toxicity.[89]

One mechanism whereby asbestos could injure cells is by means of generating active oxygen species, which can produce alterations in membrane fluidity, lipid peroxidation, and breakage of DNA. Asbestos fibers have been shown to catalyze the production of hydroxyl radicals and superoxide anions from hydrogen peroxide in cell-free systems, which may occur by a modified Haber-Weiss (Fenton-like) reaction.[90-92] The potential importance of this pathogenetic mechanism has been illustrated by the prevention of asbestos-induced cell death in rat lung fibroblasts and alveolar macrophages by catalase, superoxide dismutase, and dimethylthiourea—all scavengers of active oxygen species.[93] These observations have been extended in vivo in a model of crocidolite-induced pulmonary interstitial fibrosis, in which continuous administration of polyethylene glycol–conjugated catalase significantly reduced the inflammatory response and severity of fibrosis secondary to inhalation of aerosolized asbestos fibers.[94] The possible role of iron within the asbestos fiber as a driver of the Fenton-type reaction has been shown by the effectiveness of deferoxamine—an iron chelator—as an inhibitor of asbestos toxicity in vitro.[93,95]

Although all forms of asbestos have been shown to be cytotoxic in vitro, results have varied as to which fiber type is the most cytotoxic. Early studies indicated that the order of cytotoxicity is chrysotile > crocidolite > amosite.[86] Other studies indicated that the order of cytotoxicity depends on the target cell type.[87] Most of these studies compared fiber toxicity on an equal-mass basis. However, when cytotoxicity on a fibroblast cell line in vitro is compared on an equal-number basis (i.e., equal numbers of fibers per dish), it is found that crocidolite is more potent in causing cell death than chrysotile.[96] Of particular interest is the observation that erionite, a fibrous zeolite that is a potent cause of mesothelioma in humans (see Chap. 5), is several orders of magnitude more potent on an equal-number basis in causing cell death than either crocidolite or chrysotile.[96] Fiber size is

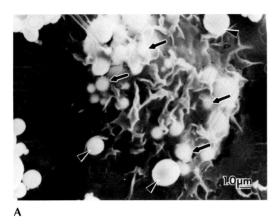 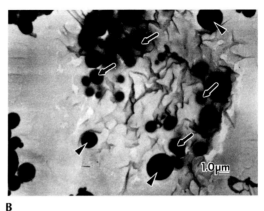

A   B

FIGURE 10-7. (A) Scanning electron micrograph of an alveolar macrophage showing carbonyl iron beads with sharp margins on the cell surface (arrowheads). (B) Back-scattered electron image of the same macrophage showing internalized beads (arrows). These same beads visualized in part (A) have fuzzy borders. Reprinted from Ref. 34, with permission.

also an important factor, with longer and thinner fibers having the greatest cytotoxic effect.[87] Fibers with lengths greater than 8–10 μ and diameters less than 0.25 μ result in greater induction of ornithine decarboxylase activity in tracheal epithelial cells[97] and greater generation of active oxygen species in alveolar macrophages[98] than is observed with shorter, blunter fibers.

In addition to direct cytotoxicity of asbestos fibers, the inflammatory response to asbestos exposure is an extremely important mechanism of asbestos-induced tissue injury. Aerosolized chrysotile asbestos exposure produces a dose-related bronchiolitis and fibrosis associated with significantly elevated numbers of alveolar macrophages, neutrophils, and lymphocytes in bronchoalveolar lavage fluid.[99] Much of the in vitro work in this area has focused on the role of the alveolar macrophage as a mediator of asbestos-induced injury. Asbestos activates complement through the alternative pathway, resulting in the production of C_{5a} from C_5 and the subsequent accumulation of macrophages at first alveolar duct bifurcations.[100–103] This chemoattraction of macrophages is reduced or abolished by depletion of circulating complement, as shown by decreased numbers of macrophages at alveolar duct bifurcations in asbestos-exposed, complement-depleted rats.[102,103] Alterations in macrophage cytoplasmic and surface morphology are observed in animals exposed either briefly or chronically to aerosolized asbestos fibers.[34,104–107] These cells demonstrate diminished phagocytic capacity as assessed by carbonyl iron bead uptake[34,101] (Fig. 10-7).

Alveolar macrophages can produce a wide variety of substances that are potential mediators of asbestos-induced tissue injury and

TABLE 10-3. Potential mediators of asbestos-induced tissue injury and repair produced by alveolar macrophages

Mediator	References
Active oxygen species	
Superoxide anion	98,108,109
Hydroxyl radical	109,110
Hydrolytic enzymes	
Aminopeptidase	111
Acid phosphatase	111,112,118
Esterase	111
Lysozyme	112
Cathepsin	112,118
Ribonuclease	112
Lipase	112
Phospholipase A_1 and A_2	113
Elastase	114
Hyaluronidase	115
Beta-glucuronidase	112
Catalase	116,117
Arachidonic acid metabolites	
Leukotriene B_4	119,121
Prostaglandin E_2	120
Prostaglandin $F_{2\alpha}$	120
Growth factors	
Platelet-derived growth factor	123
Interleukin-1	120,123
Fibroblast growth factor	123
Tumor necrosis factor	121–123

repair (Table 10-3). It has been shown that phagocytosis of asbestos fibers by macrophages can result in the generation of active oxygen species,[98,108–110] which can in turn produce alterations in membrane fluidity, lipid peroxidation, and breakage of DNA. Alveolar macrophages also secrete a number of hydrolytic enzymes, including aminopeptidase, acid phosphatase, esterase, lysozyme, cathepsin, RNase, lipase, phospholipase A_1 and A_2, elastase, hyaluronidase, beta-glucuronidase, and catalase,[111–118] which could enhance tissue breakdown and destruction. In addition, alveolar macrophages may be stimulated to produce a broad spectrum of regulatory molecules that could in turn modulate the acitivty of other cells within the lung. These include the arachidonic acid metabolites, leukotriene B_4, prostaglandin E_2 and prostaglandin $F_{2\alpha}$,[119,120] as well as certain growth factors, such as platelet-derived growth factor, interleukin-1, fibroblast growth factor, and tumor necrosis factor.[121–123] Asbestos exposure in vitro[121] and in vivo[119] stimulates the release by alveolar macrophages of leukotriene B_4, a potent chemotaxin for neutrophils and eosinophils. Furthermore, both in vitro [121] and in vivo [122] exposure of alveolar macrophages to asbestos results in release of tumor necrosis factor, which can augment neutrophil and eosinophil functional activity as well as stimulate fibroblast growth. Fibroblast growth may also be stimulated by prostaglandin $F_{2\alpha}$, interleukin-1, and fibronectin secretion by macrophages.[120,124]

Granulocytes (including neutrophils and eosinophils) have been shown to be present in increased numbers in bronchoalveolar lavage fluid obtained from patients with asbestosis.[119] Granulocytes are also increased in lavage fluid from experimental animals exposed to an asbestos aerosol.[99] Alveolar macrophages may play a key role in this influx of granulocytes[125] through the production and release of leukotriene B_4 (see earlier).[119,121] Neutrophils could then amplify asbestos-induced tissue injury by release of potent hydrolytic enzymes as well as active oxygen species. In vitro studies have shown that asbestos fibers have both a cytotoxic and an activating effect on neutrophils.[126,127] In the presence of extracellular calcium, asbestos-fibers stimulate the release of granule-associated enzymes by exocytosis.[126] Incubation of asbestos fibers with normal human neutrophils also results in generation of active oxygen species as measured by chemiluminescence.[127] Furthermore, asbestos fibers and neutrophils interact to injure cultured human pulmonary epithelial cells in vitro through a mechanism that probably involves hydrogen peroxide production.[128] Fiber dimensions are once again an important factor, with long fibers producing greater neutrophil recruitment than short fibers.[129]

It is also possible that asbestos fibers may exert a direct effect on fibroblasts through the transport of fibers to the interstitium, where they may persist for prolonged periods.[65] In vitro studies in which a normal fibroblast cell line derived from rat lung was exposed to various concentrations of crocidolite asbestos, showed enhanced synthesis of total cellular collagen per ng of DNA associated with asbestos exposure.[130] In vivo studies have also shown increased replication of interstitial fibroblasts in asbestos-exposed animals, as determined by autoradiography.[69,130] This latter effect is probably modulated by the release of fibroblast growth factor,[131,132] tumor necrosis factor,[121,122] interleukin-1,[120] prostaglandin $F_{2\alpha}$,[120] and/or fibronectin[124] by asbestos-activated alveolar macrophages.

Immunologic mechanisms may also contribute to the pathogenesis of asbestos-induced tissue injury.[133] A number of immune derangements have been described in individuals with asbestosis, including impaired cell-mediated immunity and hyperactive B-cell function.[133,134] Impaired cell-mediated immunity may manifest as cutaneous anergy, defective mitogen-induced lymphocyte blastogenesis and cytotoxic effector function, defective production of migration inhibitory factor, defective natural killer cell function, lymphopenia, and elevated T-helper:suppressor ratio in blood and lavage fluid.[133] Hyperactive B-cell function is indicated by polyclonal hypergammaglobulinemia, elevated levels of secretory IgA, high frequency of autoantibodies and circulating immune complexes, enhanced spontaneous immunoglobulin production, and lymphoid neoplasms of

B-cell lineage.[133] These immunologic abnormalities correlate poorly with clinical and radiographic parameters of asbestosis, and may thus represent epiphenomena unrelated to the pathogenesis of asbestos-induced lung disease.[134]

Nevertheless, a number of interesting observations have been reported regarding asbestos effects on lymphocyte function. In vitro studies have shown that asbestos has a direct depressive effect on human lymphocyte mitogen response to phytohemagglutinin (PHA).[135] Asbestos inhalation is also associated with enhanced attachment of lymphocytes to alveolar macrophages,[136] which is followed by a vigorous lymphoproliferative response.[137] As just noted, asbestos exposure stimulates alveolar macrophages to release interleukin-1,[120] which can modulate T-cell function and lymphocyte proliferation.[133] In addition, IgG specifically enhances the production of superoxide anion by alveolar macrophages stimulated by chrysotile (but not crocidolite) asbestos.[138] The effects of asbestos on the immune system are quite complex, and perturbation of the system could lead to unpredictable results. For example, low-dose cyclophosphamide treatment in a sheep model of experimental asbestosis accelerated, rather than suppressed, the fibrotic process.[139]

ASBESTOS-INDUCED FIBROGENESIS

Based on the foregoing discussion, a hypothetical scheme can be proposed for the mechanism of asbestos-induced fibrogenesis (Fig. 10-8).[140-142] According to this scheme, asbestos is deposited on the alveolar surfaces, especially on first alveolar duct bifurcations, where transport across the epithelium begins almost immediately. Asbestos initiates the conversion of C_5 to C_{5a} through the alternative pathway, which results in chemoattraction of alveolar macrophages to the site of asbestos deposition. These alveolar macrophages proceed to phagocytize the asbestos fibers, stimulating the release of active oxygen species and various hydrolytic enzymes. Also released are factors that amplify the inflammatory response through the attraction of granulocytes. In addition, activated macrophages release growth factors that stimulate the replication of interstitial macrophages and fibroblasts. Asbestos fibers translocated to the interstitium produce tissue injury by a combination of generating active oxygen species and direct interaction with cellular membranes of interstitial macrophages and fibroblasts. As a result of some combination of soluble growth factor release from alveolar (and perhaps interstitial) macrophages and direct tissue injury by translocated asbestos fibers, fibroblasts are stimulated to replicate and to synthesize collagen and other extracellular matrix components in increased amounts. Ongoing release of growth factors by activated macrophages and persistence of asbestos fibers within the interstitium would result in continuing fibrogenesis long after the cessation of exposure.

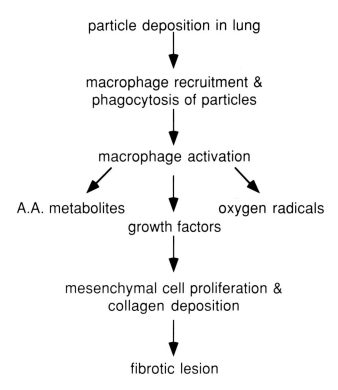

**Macrophage-Mediated
Particle-Induced Fibrogenesis**

particle deposition in lung

macrophage recruitment &
phagocytosis of particles

macrophage activation

A.A. metabolites   oxygen radicals

growth factors

mesenchymal cell proliferation &
collagen deposition

fibrotic lesion

FIGURE 10-8. Hypothetical schema illustrating the pathogenesis of asbestos-induced pulmonary interstitial fibrosis. Fibers deposited on the surfaces of alveolar duct bifurcation stimulate the release of chemoattractants for alveolar macrophages. These cells phagocytize the fibers and become activated, releasing active oxygen species, arachidonic acid (A. A.) metabolites, and various growth factors. These various mediators then stimulate fibroblast replication and collagen synthesis, which eventuate in pulmonary interstitial fibrosis (i.e., asbestosis). Courtesy Dr. Jamie Bonner, NIEHS, Research Triangle Park, NC.

CARCINOGENESIS

IN VIVO INHALATIONAL STUDIES

Inhalational studies in experimental animals have shown that asbestos produces neoplasms of the lung and pleura. These include pulmonary adenoma, adenocarcinoma, and squamous cell carcinoma,[5,40,74,80] and malignant mesothelioma of the pleura and peritoneum.[5,40,74] These tumors have a prolonged latency period (300 days or more in the rat) and there is some evidence of a dose–response relationship, with a greater incidence of tumors in rats exposed for 12 months as compared to six months, but no further

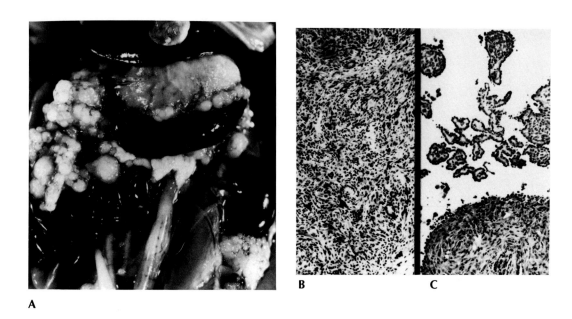

B   C

A

FIGURE 10-9. (A) Diffuse malignant mesothelioma developing in the abdomen of an asbestos-inoculated rat. These lesions exhibit a mixture of epithelial and fibrosarcomatous patterns [parts (B) and (C)]. Reprinted from Ref. 30, with permission.

increase in incidence from 12–24 months of exposure.[5] All types of asbestos, including chrysotile,[5,40,74,80] amosite,[5,73,75] crocidolite,[5] anthophyllite,[5] and tremolite[56] produce pulmonary and pleural neoplasms in experimental animals. In the classic studies of Wagner et al.,[5] chrysotile was as potent as crocidolite in the production of mesothelioma by dust inhalation, with four mesotheliomas developing in 137 animals at risk with chrysotile exposure and four in 141 animals at risk due to crocidolite. Two animals developed mesothelioma after only one day of exposure, one following exposure to crocidolite and the other, to amosite asbestos.[5] The mesotheliomas occurring in experimental animals exposed to asbestos are histologically, histochemically, and ultrastructurally similar to those occurring in humans (Fig. 10-9).[143,144] In addition, experimental pulmonary adenocarcinomas and squamous cell carcinomas are similar histologically to those occurring in humans.[5,40,73]

The studies reported by Wagner et al.[5] and by Davis et al.[40] both showed a close association between the severity of interstitial fibrosis (i.e., asbestosis) and the development of pulmonary neoplasms. This finding suggests that pulmonary parenchymal tumors in asbestos-exposed animals derive from a metaplastic and hyperplastic epithelial response in areas of interstitial fibrosis that in some instances progresses to neoplasia. More recently, Davis and Cowie[145] have addressed this question in greater detail. These authors note that

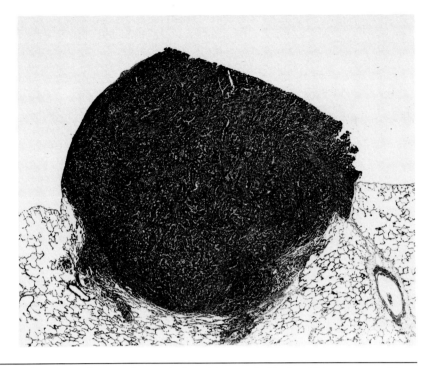

FIGURE 10-10. Pulmonary adenocarcinoma induced in a male Fischer 344 rat exposed to chrysotile asbestos. H&E, ×22. Courtesy Dr. Gene McConnell, Raleigh, NC.

when adenomas or very early carcinomas are found, they are frequently in the center of areas of advanced asbestosis with exuberant epithelial metaplasia/hyperplasia. In studies comparing the pathologic effects of various mineral fibers, there has also been a close association between the severity of pulmonary fibrosis and tumor development.[146–148] In an analysis of data from several different studies,[40,74,75] a strong correlation was observed between the percentage of lung occupied by fibrosis and the occurrence of pulmonary tumors ($p < 0.001$).[145] In animals in which tumors developed in association with low recorded levels of fibrosis (involving less than 4% of the lung area), these were either advanced tumors occupying a single lung lobe or early tumors originating from the center of areas of interstitial fibrosis (Fig. 10-10). These studies do not definitively answer the question as to whether fibrosis is an absolute prerequisite for the development of pulmonary tumors in experimental animals, which would require examination of a relatively large population of rats during the period of early tumor development.[145] Furthermore, the results may not be relevant to the great majority of lung cancers occurring in asbestos workers, in which cigarette smoking is an important cofactor (see Chap. 7 and upcoming subsection on "Asbestos as Promoter vs. Initiator").

ROLE OF FIBER DIMENSIONS

Inhalation studies have indicated that in an analogous fashion to fibrogenic potential, long fibers have the greatest carcinogenic potential in experimental animal models.[5] Davis et al.,[75] using an amosite preparation with extremely few fibers greater than 5 μ in length, reported no tumors in rats following long-term inhalation, whereas a clear excess of lung carcinomas and pleural mesotheliomas developed in rats breathing an amosite cloud containing considerable numbers of fibers 5 μ or greater in length. Similar but less clear-cut results were obtained in a study of long and short preparations of chrysotile asbestos.[74] In this latter study, some longer fibers were still present in the "short-fiber" chrysotile preparation, although the "long-fiber" preparation (on an equal-mass basis) had five times as many fibers 5 μ or greater in length and 80 times as many fibers 30 μ or greater in length. Both long and short chrysotile preparations produced mesotheliomas in more than 90% of rats following intraperitoneal injection of 25 mg, whereas at a dose level of 2.5 mg, the short-fiber preparation produced only one-third as many mesotheliomas as the long-fiber preparation, which still produced mesotheliomas in more than 90% of the animals injected. At a dose of 0.25 mg, the short-fiber preparation produced no mesotheliomas, whereas the long-fiber preparation still produced these tumors in 66% of rats.[74] The dose of short-fiber chrysotile that resulted in no mesothelial tumors in 24 rats (injected intraperitoneally) was calculated to contain 57 million fibers greater than 8 μ in length.[74] Studies using mineral fibers other than asbestos have also shown a strong association between fiber length and carcinogenicity.[73,149–153] Fasske[154] reported the development of pulmonary carcinomas or malignant pleural mesotheliomas in 24% of 70 rats treated by intratracheal instillation of 1 mg of chrysotile asbestos fibers 0.05–0.2 μ in length. However, the author did not specify details regarding how it was ascertained that there were no long fibers in the samples injected.

The classic studies of Stanton et al.[155,156] showed that, in addition to fiber length, fiber diameter is also an important determinant of carcinogenic potential. The "Stanton hypothesis" has emphasized the dimension and durability of fibers with regard to carcinogenicity, and states that, irrespective of chemical composition, the probability of developing mesothelioma following implantation of mineral fibers into the pleural cavity correlates best with the numbers of fibers 8 μ or greater in length and 0.25 μ or less in diameter.[156] Hesterberg and Barrett[157] reported that in vitro studies with cultured Syrian hamster embryo cells showed the transforming potency to be greatest for long, thin fibers. Furthermore, in organ cultures of rodent tracheobronchial epithelial cells, long fibers (≥8 μ) cause enhanced incorporation of tritiated thymidine, increased biosynthesis of polyamines, and increased amounts of squamous metaplasia and keratinization.[158] These effects are only observed with short fibers (≤2 μ) at several-fold-higher concentrations. In a recent review of asbestos exposure indices, Lippman proposed, on the basis of the available data, that fibers 5 μ or greater in length and 0.1 μ or less in diameter are the most important in the production of mesotheliomas, whereas fibers 10 μ or greater in length and 0.15 μ or greater in diameter are the most important in the production of pulmonary carcinomas.[79] In addition, it has been suggested that surface properties of mineral fibers may be an additional contributing factor to carcinogenic potency.[159] For example, fibrous erionite, which appears to have many times greater potential for mesothelioma induction than asbestos, has an internal surface area (due to "pores" in the crystal lattice) of 200 m²/gm, as compared to a total surface area of 8–10 m²/gm for crocidolite asbestos.[160] The mechanism by which this increased surface area enhances the carcinogenic potential of a fiber is unknown.

IN VITRO MODELS OF ASBESTOS CARCINOGENICITY

A complete understanding of the mechanisms by which fibers induce neoplastic transformation will not be forthcoming until more of the mystery enshrouding the carcinogenic process itself has been unraveled. Nonetheless, a great deal has been learned regarding the mechanisms by which fibers could interact with cells and produce heritable alterations in cellular genetic material. Asbestos differs from most chemical carcinogens in that it tests negatively in bacterial mutation assays[161–163] and is not mutagenic in liver epithelial cells[164] or Syrian hamster embryo fibroblasts.[165] A potential breakthrough in our understanding of asbestos-induced carcinogenicity is the development of methods for growing mesothelial cells in culture.[166–169] Cultured mesothelial cells have been shown to phagocytize chrysotile asbestos fibers in vitro,[170] which results in a slow leaching of magnesium from the chrysotile at a rate comparable to that which occurs in solution at pH 7.[47] Chrysotile asbestos produces intense vacuolization of cultured mesothelial cells[171] and also induces morphologically transformed colonies.[172] Incubation of mesothelial cells with either chrysotile or crocidolite asbestos fibers prolonged the doubling time in culture, although this effect occurred at lower doses of chrysotile as compared to crocidolite. With either fiber type, asbestos fibers were often observed within dividing cells.[171] Wang et al.[173] used scanning electron microscopy to demonstrate the interaction between asbestos fibers and metaphase chromosomes of rat pleural mesothelial cells. Chromosomes were frequently entangled with, adherent to, or severed or pierced by long curvilinear fibers, and this effect was more pronounced for chrysotile than for crocidolite asbestos.[173]

These observations are intriguing, considering that nonrandom chromosomal abnormalities, including translocations, rearrangements, and marker chromosomes, have been identified in both experimental (asbestos-induced)[174] and human malignant pleural mesotheliomas.[175–177] Furthermore, studies with nonneoplastic human pleural mesothelial cells in culture have shown aneuploidy with consistent specific chromosomal losses in mesothelial cells surviving two cytotoxic exposures with amosite fibers.[178] These aneuploid cells exhibited altered growth control properties as well as a population-doubling potential beyond the culture lifespan of control cells. Other studies using crocidolite, chrysotile, or amosite asbestos reported significant increases in numerical and/or structural chromosomal abnormalities in short-term cultured normal human mesothelial cells.[179] Also, crocidolite asbestos has been shown to induce sister chromatid exchanges in rat pleural mesothelial cells in vitro.[180]

Other in vitro approaches have also provided interesting information with respect to asbestos-induced carcinogenicity. Asbestos fibers have been shown to mediate the transfection of exogenous DNA into a variety of mammalian cells in vitro.[181,182] Exposure of Chinese hamster ovary cells to crocidolite asbestos fibers in cell culture resulted in an increased frequency of multinucleate cells, and various mitotic abnormalities were observed in cells containing fibers 20 μ or greater in length.[183] However, crocidolite fibers did not significantly increase the frequency of thioguanine-resistant mutants. Some studies have shown a strong correlation between fiber-induced cytotoxicity in a macrophage-like cell line and the probability of fiber-induced mesothelioma in rats,[184] whereas others have reported no direct relationship between cytotoxicity and carcinogenic potency.[185] Oncogenes and growth factors might also play a role, as suggested by the enhanced expression of the c-sis (PDGF B) oncogene and the platelet-derived growth factor (PDGF) A-chain gene in 10 human malignant mesothelioma cell lines.[186] Growth factors might also be implicated in the individual susceptibility for mesothelioma that has been observed, since a significant interindividual variation in growth rates and response to various growth factors has been reported for normal cultured human mesothelial cells derived from different donors.[187]

In vivo models have also provided useful information regarding the early events of asbestos interaction with the mesothelium. Studies by Moalli et al.[188] using stereomicroscopy and scanning electron microscopy demonstrated the rapid clearance of short asbestos fibers through the opening of diaphragmatic stomata, whereas long fibers (60% ≥ 2 μ in length) were trapped on the peritoneal surface, invoking an intense inflammatory reaction. This was associated with mesothelial cytotoxicity and regeneration at the periphery of asbestos fiber clusters. Maximal incorporation of tritiated-thymidine by mesothelial cells occurred seven days after exposure, and it was hypothesized that repeated episodes of injury and regeneration may promote the development of mesotheliomas.[188] Furthermore, asbestos fiber clusters on the peritoneal surface induce angiogenesis in the form of a capillary network radiating toward the center of the lesion, first notable 14 days after injection.[189] Additional studies are needed to define further the early changes in the mesothelium following in vivo exposures to mineral fibers. Also, the capability of growing mesotheliomas as xenografts in athymic rodents[190–192] should enhance the opportunity for investigators to study the properties of malignant mesothelial cells.

Much of the foregoing discussion has focused on the carcinogenic effects of asbestos fibers on mesothelial cells. However, asbestos is also carcinogenic for the respiratory epithelium (see earlier subsection on "In Vivo Inhalational Studies" and Chap. 7), and much knowledge has been gained by the study of the effects of asbestos on tracheal explants and organ cultures.[28,29] Crocidolite asbestos causes necrosis and desquamation of surface epithelial cells, with subsequent basal cell hyperplasia and squamous metaplasia.[28,193] Furthermore, asbestos-induced squamous metaplasia is inhibited by retinoids (retinyl methyl ether)[194] and vitamin C (ascorbic acid).[195] These studies may have important implications regarding the prevention and prophylaxis of respiratory tract malignancies in workers who have been heavily exposed to asbestos in the past (see Chap. 9).

ASBESTOS AS PROMOTER VS. INITIATOR

In the previous discussion, mechanisms by which asbestos fibers might interact directly with DNA and chromosomes, and thus as an initiator of carcinogenesis, were emphasized. However, there is considerable epidemiologic data indicating that, with respect to carcinoma of the lung, asbestos interacts in a multiplicative fashion with cigarette smoke to enhance greatly the rate of neoplastic transformation. In this sense, asbestos behaves as a classic promoter of carcinogenesis. Numerous studies have explored various mechanisms by which asbestos could interact with cigarette smoke components in the process of carcinogenesis.[196]

One mechanism of interaction might be the adsorption of polycyclic aromatic hydrocarbons or other carcinogenic compounds within cigarette smoke onto the surface of the asbestos fiber, which then could act as a carrier particle, providing prolonged and intimate contact of the adsorbed carcinogens with respiratory epithelial cells. In vitro studies have demonstrated the adsorption of benzo[a]pyrene, nitrosonornicotine, and N-acetyl-2-aminofluorene onto the surface of all types of asbestos as well as other mineral fibers, with chrysotile binding significantly more carcinogen than the other mineral fibers tested.[197] Carcinogen binding is greatly enhanced by the prior adsorption of phospholipids (such as occur in surfactant) onto the asbestos fibers.[198] Studies using cell and organ cultures of tracheobronchial epithelium exposed to asbestos with and without adsorbed 3-methyl-cholanthrene (3-MC) show increased aryl hydrocarbon hydroxylase activity in cells treated with both asbestos and 3-MC as compared to 3-MC alone.[199] Furthermore, asbestos fibers and adsorbed carcinogens display a synergistic effect in the production of cell transformation in BALB/3T3 cells in vitro[200] and in the formation of malignant tumors from treated tracheal explants that were subsequently implanted into syngeneic animals.[201] Intratracheal instillation studies using chrysotile administered concomitantly with subcutaneously injected *N*-nitrosoheptamethyleneimine have also demonstrated a synergistic effect between these two agents in the induction of pulmonary neoplasms in rats.[202] Although cigarette smoking is not thought to be a cofactor in the production of malignant mesothelioma in humans (see Chap. 5), the administration of 3-MC along with chrysotile asbestos by intrapleural or intraperitoneal injection greatly enhances the production of mesotheliomas over that observed by chrysotile injection alone.[203]

Additional mechanisms whereby asbestos might interact with cigarette smoke or other environmental agents have also been explored. A novel hypothesis regarding the synergistic effect between asbestos fibers and polycyclic aromatic hydrocarbons suggests that the adsorption of lung surfactant phospholipids onto asbestos fibers[84,198] provides the opportunity for lipophilic carcinogens to diffuse within an all-lipid environment, with the asbestos fiber behaving like a chemical and physical bridge across the 5-μ-thick aqueous regions of the bronchial lining layer.[204] Others have reported results indicating that cigarette smoke and asbestos synergistically increase DNA damage by means of active oxygen species, such as hydroxyl radical formation.[110] Furthermore, cigarette smoke potentiates the uptake of asbestos fibers by the tracheobronchial epithelium.[53] This latter effect is blocked by prior treatment with superoxide dismutase, catalase, and deferoxamine, which are inhibitors of active oxygen species.[205] Studies have also suggested that asbestos might interact with ionizing radiation in the process of oncogenic transformation.[206] In this regard, ionizing radiation has been reported to augment the production of mesotheliomas in rats injected with chrysotile asbestos as compared to animals treated with chrysotile alone.[203]

CONCLUSION

It appears that asbestos is a complete carcinogen, possessing both initiating and promoting properties.[163,207] The carcinogenic process is complex, and there are multiple ways in which asbestos can interact with the individual cell during the process of neoplastic transformation (Fig. 10-11).

In the tracheobronchial tree, asbestos acts primarily as a promoter agent. Important steps in this process include epithelial cell injury, with subsequent basal cell hyperplasia and squamous metaplasia, cocarcinogenic effect of asbestos as a carrier for polycyclic aromatic hydrocarbons, and stimulation of aromatic hydrocarbon hydroxylase activity and DNA synthesis.[199] Squamous metaplasia interferes with mucociliary clearance mechanisms, and thus may encourage the transepithelial uptake of fibers otherwise cleared from the lung. This uptake in turn would bring fibers in contact with basal epithelium, where these cells would then be exposed to any carcinogens adsorbed to the surface of the asbestos fibers.[208] Asbestos exposure

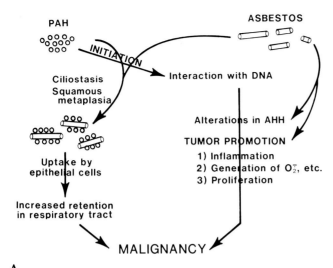

A

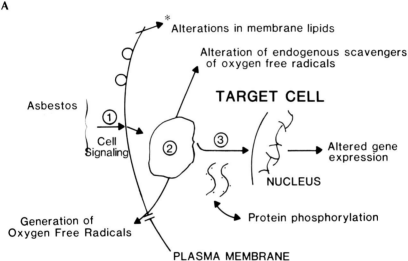

① = Interaction with plasma membrane.

② = Transport in lysosomes or in cytoplasm.

③ = Interaction with macromolecules such as DNA, RNA and proteins.

B

FIGURE 10-11. (A) Hypothetical schema illustrating several mechanisms of synergism between asbestos and polycyclic aromatic hydrocarbons in the induction of bronchogenic carcinoma. (B) Direct interaction of asbestos fibers with target cell nuclear macromolecules (DNA, RNA, and proteins) could lead to altered gene expression and possible malignant transformation. Courtesy of Dr. Brooke Mossman, University of Vermont, Burlington, VT. Part (A) reprinted from Mossman BT and Craighead JE: Mechanisms of asbestos-associated bronchogenic carcinoma. In: *Asbestos-Related Malignancy* (Antman K, Aisner J, eds.), Orlando, FL: Grune & Stratton, 1987, pp. 137–150, with permission.

alone may also produce carcinomas in the lung periphery through the poorly understood mechanism of interstitial fibrosis with bronchiolar and alveolar cell hyperplasia proceeding to neoplastic transformation (scar carcinoma concept).[145,207]

In the pleural and peritoneal cavities, asbestos acts like a complete carcinogen, exhibiting both initiating and promoting activities.[207] A critical step appears to be the transport of durable fibers of appropriate dimensions to the pleura, through either the air spaces or the interstitial lymphatics (or both).[30] Peritoneal transport mechanisms include direct penetration of the intestinal wall by swallowed fibers, diaphragmatic penetration, or lymphatic pathways. Once fibers have come into contact with mesothelial cells, these cells seem to be particularly susceptible to asbestos-mediated cellular injury, as compared, for example, to bronchial epithelial cells or fibroblasts.[178]

Important steps in the neoplastic transformation of mesothelial cells probably include cellular injury with subsequent regeneration and hyperplasia, new blood vessel formation (angiogenesis), and chromosomal alterations as a result of either direct interaction of asbestos fibers with mesothelial cells during cellular division or indirectly through the generation of active oxygen species by asbestos fibers or inflammatory cells. The role of growth factors and oncogenes is an important area requiring further study,[163] and variable response of mesothelial cells to growth factors may be an important determinant of individual susceptibility to the development of fiber-induced mesotheliomas.[187]

REFERENCES

1. Gardner LU: Experimental pneumoconiosis. In: *Silicosis and Asbestosis* (Lanza, AJ, ed.), New York: Oxford University Press, 1938, pp. 282–283.
2. King EJ, Clegg JW, Rae VM: The effect of asbestos and of aluminum on the lungs of rabbits. *Thorax* 1:188–195, 1946.
3. Vorwald AJ, Durkan TM, Pratt PC: Experimental studies of asbestosis. *Arch Ind Hyg Occup Med* 3:1–43, 1951.
4. Timbrell V: The inhalation of fibrous dusts. *Ann NY Acad Sci* 132:255–266, 1965.
5. Wagner JC, Berry G, Skidmore JW, Timbrell V: The effects of inhalation of asbestos in rats. *Br J Cancer* 29:252–269, 1974.
6. Roggli VL, Brody AR: The role of electron microscopy in experimental models of pneumoconiosis. In: *Electron Microscopy of the Lung* (Schraufnagel D, ed.), New York: Marcel Dekker, 1990, pp. 315–343.
7. Green GM, Jakab GJ, Low RB, Davis GS: Defense mechanisms of the respiratory membrane. *Am Rev Respir Dis* 115:479–514, 1977.
8. Raabe OG: Deposition and clearance of inhaled particles. In: *Occupational Lung Disease* (Gee JBL, Morgan WKC, Brooks SM, eds.), New York: Raven Press, 1984, pp. 1–37.
9. Timbrell V: Aerodynamic considerations and other aspects of glass fiber. In: *Occupational Exposure to Fibrous Glass.* Washington, DC: HEW Publ. No. (NIOSH) 76-151, 1976, pp. 33–53.
10. Lee KP: Lung response to particulates with emphasis on asbestos and other fibrous dusts. *CRC Crit Rev Toxicol* 14:33–86, 1985.

11. Turnock AC, Bryks S, Bertalanffy FD: The synthesis of tritium-labelled asbestos for use in biological research. *Environ Res* 4:86–94, 1971.
12. Evans JC, Evans RJ, Holmes A, Hounam RF, Jones DM, Morgan A, Walsh M: Studies on the deposition of inhaled fibrous material in the respiratory tract of the rat and its subsequent clearance using radioactive tracer techniques. I. UICC crocidolite asbestos. *Environ Res* 6:180–201, 1973.
13. Morgan A, Evans JC, Evans RJ, Hounam RF, Holmes A, Doyle SG: Studies on the deposition of inhaled fibrous material in the respiratory tract of the rat and its subsequent clearance using radioactive tracer techniques. II. Deposition of the U.I.C.C. Standard Reference samples of asbestos. *Environ Res* 10:196–207, 1975.
14. Brody AR, Hill LH, Adkins B, O'Connor RW: Chrysotile asbestos inhalation in rats: Deposition pattern and reaction of alveolar epithelium and pulmonary macrophages. *Am Rev Respir Dis* 123:670–679, 1981.
15. Brody AR, Hill LH: Deposition pattern and clearance pathways of inhaled chrysotile asbestos. *Chest* 80:64S–67S, 1981.
16. Brody AR, Roe MW: Deposition pattern of inorganic particles at the alveolar level in the lungs of rats and mice. *Am Rev Respir Dis* 128:724–729, 1983.
17. Roggli VL, Brody AR: Imaging techniques for application to lung toxicology. In: *Toxicology of the Lung* (Gardner DE, Crapo JD, Massaro EJ, eds.), New York: Raven Press, 1988, pp. 117–145.
18. Schlesinger RB: Particle deposition in model systems of human and experimental animal airways. Ch. 28 In: *Generation of Aerosols and Facilities for Exposure Experiments* (Willeke K, ed.), Ann Arbor, MI: Ann Arbor Sci., 1980, pp. 553–575.
19. Pinkerton KE, Plopper CG, Mercer RR, Roggli VL, Patra AL, Brody AR, Crapo JD: Airway branching patterns influence asbestos fiber location and the extent of tissue injury in the pulmonary parenchyma. *Lab Invest* 55:688–695, 1986.
20. Brain JD, Mensah GE: Comparative toxicology of the respiratory tract. *Am Rev Respir Dis* 128:S87–S90, 1983.
21. Pritchard JN, Holmes A, Evans JC, Evans N, Evans RJ, Morgan A: The distribution of dust in the rat lung following administration by inhalation and by single intratracheal instillation. *Environ Res* 36:268–297, 1985.
22. Brain JD, Knudson DE, Sorokin SP, Davis MA: Pulmonary distribution of particles given by intratracheal instillation or by aerosol inhalation. *Environ Res* 11:13–33, 1976.
23. Roggli VL, Brody AR: Changes in numbers and dimensions of chrysotile asbestos fibers in lungs of rats following short-term exposure. *Exp Lung Res* 7:133–147, 1984.
24. Middleton AP, Beckett ST, Davis JMG: Further observations on the short-term retention and clearance of asbestos by rats, using U.I.C.C. reference samples. *Ann Occup Hyg* 22:141–152, 1979.
25. Roggli VL, George MH, Brody AR: Clearance and dimensional changes of crocidolite asbestos fibers isolated from lungs of rats following short-term exposure. *Environ Res* 42:94–105, 1987.
26. Brody AR, Hill LH, Adler KB: Actin-containing microfilaments of pulmonary epithelial cells provide a mechanism for translocating asbestos to the interstitium. *Chest* 83:11–12, 1983.
27. Brody AR, Hill LH, Hesterberg TW, Barrett JC, Adler KB: Intracellular transport of inorganic particles. In: *The Cytoskeleton: A Target for Toxic Agents* (Clarkson TW, Sager PR, Syverson TL, eds.), New York: Plenum Pub., 1986, pp. 221–227.
28. Mossman BT, Kessler JB, Levy BW, Craighead JE: Interaction of crocidolite asbestos with hamster respiratory mucosa in organ culture. *Lab Invest* 36:131–139, 1977.

29. Topping DC, Nettesheim P, Martin DH: Toxic and tumorigenic effects of asbestos on tracheal mucosa. *J Environ Pathol Toxicol* 3:261–275, 1980.
30. Craighead JE: Current pathogenetic concepts of diffuse malignant mesothelioma. *Hum Pathol* 18:544–557, 1987.
31. Viallat JR, Raybuad F, Passarel M, Boutin C: Pleural migration of chrysotile fibers after intratracheal injection in rats. *Arch Environ Health* 41:282–286, 1986.
32. Holt PF: Transport of inhaled dust to extrapulmonary sites. *J Pathol* 133:123–129, 1981.
33. Vincent JH, Jones AD, Johnston AM, McMillan C, Bolton RE, Cowie H: Accumulation of inhaled mineral dust in the lung and associated lymph nodes: Implications for exposure and dose in occupational lung disease. *Ann Occup Hyg* 31:375–393, 1987.
34. Warheit DB, Chang LY, Hill LH, Hook GE, Crapo JD, Brody AR: Pulmonary macrophage accumulation and asbestos-induced lesions at sites of fiber deposition. *Am Rev Respir Dis* 129:301–310, 1984.
35. Morgan A, Talbot RJ, Holmes A: Significance of fibre length in the clearance of asbestos fibres from the lung. *Br J Ind Med* 35:146–153, 1978.
36. Holmes A, Morgan A: Clearance of anthophyllite fibers from the rat lung and the formation of asbestos bodies. *Environ Res* 22:13–21, 1980.
37. Bellman B, Muhle H, Pott F, König H, Klöppel H, Spurny K: Persistence of man-made mineral fibres (MMMF) and asbestos in rat lungs. *Ann Occup Hyg* 31:693–709, 1987.
38. Kauffer E, Vigneron JC, Hesbert A, Lemonnier M: A study of the length and diameter of fibres, in lung and in broncho-alveolar lavage fluid, following exposure of rats to chrysotile asbestos. *Ann Occup Hyg* 31:233–240, 1987.
39. Coin P: Pulmonary clearance of asbestos fibers. Doctoral Thesis, University of Minnesota, Minneapolis, 1989.
40. Davis JMG, Beckett ST, Bolton RE, Collings P, Middleton AP: Mass and number of fibers in the pathogenesis of asbestos-related lung disease in rats. *Br J Cancer* 37:673–688, 1978.
41. Middleton AP, Beckett ST, Davis JMG: A study of the short-term retention and clearance of inhaled asbestos by rats, using U.I.C.C. standard reference samples. In: *Inhaled Particles IV* (Walton WH, ed.), Oxford: Pergamon Press, 1977, pp. 247–257.
42. Churg A, Wright JL, Gilks B, Depaoli L: Rapid short-term clearance of chrysotile compared with amosite asbestos in the guinea pig. *Am Rev Respir Dis* 139:885–890, 1989.
43. Sebastien P, Begin R: Alveolar clearance of chrysotile and amphibole asbestos (abstr.). *Am Rev Respir Dis* 137:315A, 1988.
44. Kimizuka G, Wang N-S, Hayashi Y: Physical and microchemical alterations of chrysotile and amosite asbestos in the hamster lung. *J Toxicol Environ Health* 21:251–264, 1987.
45. Morgan A, Holmes A, Gold C: Studies of the solubility of constituents of chrysotile asbestos in vivo using radioactive tracer techniques. *Environ Res* 4:558–570, 1971.
46. Parry WT: Calculated solubility of chrysotile asbestos in physiological systems. *Environ Res* 37:410–418, 1985.
47. Jaurand MC, Gaudichet A, Halpern S, Bignon J: In vitro biodegradation of chrysotile fibres by alveolar macrophages and mesothelial cells in culture: Comparison with a pH effect. *Br J Ind Med* 41:389–395, 1984.
48. Morgan A, Davies P, Wagner JC, Berry G, Holmes A: The biological effects of magnesium-leached chrysotile asbestos. *Br J Exp Pathol* 58:465–473, 1977.
49. Bolton RE, Vincent JH, Jones AD, Addison J, Beckett ST: An overload hypothesis for pulmonary clearance of UICC amosite fibres inhaled by rats. *Br J Ind Med* 40:264–272, 1983.

50. Ferin J, Leach LJ: The effect of amosite and chrysotile asbestos on the clearance of TiO$_2$ particles from the lung. *Environ Res* 12:250–254, 1976.
51. McMillan CH, Jones AD, Vincent JH, Johnston AM, Douglas AN, Cowie H: Accumulation of mixed mineral dusts in the lungs of rats during chronic inhalation exposure. *Environ Res* 48:218–237, 1989.
52. McFadden D, Wright JL, Wiggs B, Churg A: Smoking inhibits asbestos clearance. *Am Rev Respir Dis* 133:372–374, 1986.
53. McFadden D, Wright J, Wiggs B, Churg A: Cigarette smoke increases the penetration of asbestos fibers into airway walls. *Am J Pathol* 123:95–99, 1986.
54. Pinkerton KE, Brody AR, Miller FJ, Crapo JD: Exposure to low levels of ozone results in enhanced pulmonary retention of inhaled asbestos fibers. *Am Rev Respir Dis* 140:1075–1081, 1989.
55. Bégin R, Sébastien P: Excessive accumulation of asbestos fibre in the bronchoalveolar space may be a marker of individual susceptibility to developing asbestosis: Experimental evidence. *Br J Ind Med* 46:853–855, 1989.
56. Davis JMG, Addison J, Bolton RE, Donaldson K, Jones AD, Miller BG: Inhalation studies on the effects of tremolite and brucite dust. *Carcinogenesis* 6:667–674, 1985.
57. Begin R, Rola-Pleszczynski M, Masse S, Lemaire I, Sirois P, Boctor M, Nadeau D, Drapeau G, Bureau MA: Asbestos induced injury in the sheep model: The initial alveolitis. *Environ Res* 30:195–210, 1983.
58. Bozelka BR, Sestini P, Gaumer HR, Hammad Y, Heather CJ, Salvaggio JE: A murine model of asbestosis. *Am J Pathol* 112:326–337, 1983.
59. Adamson IYR, Bowden DH: Response of mouse lung to crocidolite asbestos. I. Minimal fibrotic reaction to short fibres. *J Pathol* 152:99–107, 1987.
60. Adamson IYR, Bowden DH: Response of mouse lung to crocidolite asbestos. II. Pulmonary fibrosis after long fibres. *J Pathol* 152:109–117, 1987.
61. Wright GW, Kuschner M: The influence of varying lengths of glass and asbestos fibres on tissue response in guinea pigs. In: *Inhaled Particles*, Vol. IV (Walton WH, ed.), Oxford: Pergamon Press, 1977, pp. 455–474.
62. Filipenko D, Wright JL, Churg A: Pathologic changes in the small airways of the guinea pig after amosite asbestos exposure. *Am J Pathol* 119:273–278, 1985.
63. Barry BE, Wong KC, Brody AR, Crapo JD: Reaction of rat lungs to inhaled chrysotile asbestos following acute and subchronic exposures. *Exp Lung Res* 5:1–22, 1983.
64. Crapo JD, Barry BE, Brody AR, O'Neill JJ: Morphological, morphometric, and x-ray microanalytical studies on lung tissue of rats exposed to chrysotile asbestos in inhalation chambers. In: *Biological Effects of Mineral Fibres*, Vol. 1 (Wagner JC, ed.), Lyon: IARC Scientific Pub. No. 30, 1980, pp. 273–283.
65. Pinkerton KE, Pratt PC, Brody AR, Crapo JD: Fiber localization and its relationship to lung reaction in rats after chronic inhalation of chrysotile asbestos. *Am J Pathol* 117:484–498, 1984.
66. Hirano S, Ono M, Aimoto A: Functional and biochemical effects on rat lung following instillation of crocidolite and chrysotile asbestos. *J Toxicol Environ Health* 24:27–39, 1988.
67. Chang LY, Overby LH, Brody AR, Crapo JD: Progressive lung cell reactions and extracellular matrix production after a brief exposure to asbestos. *Am J Pathol* 131:156–170, 1988.
68. Brody AR, Hill LH: Interstitial accumulation of inhaled chrysotile asbestos fibers and consequent formation of microcalcifications. *Am J Pathol* 109:107–114, 1982.

69. Brody AR, Overby LH: Incorporation of tritiated thymidine by epithelial and interstitial cells in bronchiolar-alveolar regions of asbestos-exposed rats. *Am J Pathol* 134:133–140, 1989.

70. McGavran PD, Brody AR: Chrysotile asbestos inhalation induces tritiated thymidine incorporation by epithelial cells of distal bronchioles. *Am J Respir Cell Mol Biol* 1:231–235, 1989.

71. McGavran PD, Moore LB, Brody AR: Inhalation of chrysotile asbestos induces rapid cellular proliferation in small pulmonary vessels of mice and rats. *Am J Pathol* 136:695–705, 1990.

72. Pinkerton KE, Roggli VL: The role of fiber number, size, and mass in asbestos-induced lung disease. In: *Microbeam Analysis—1986* (Romig Jr. AD, Chambers WF, eds.), San Francisco: San Francisco Press, 1986, pp. 553–555.

73. Lee KP, Barras CE, Griffith FD, Waritz RS, Lapin CA: Comparative pulmonary responses to inhaled inorganic fibers with asbestos and fiberglass. *Environ Res* 24:167–191, 1981.

74. Davis JMG, Jones AD: Comparisons of the pathogenicity of long and short fibres of chrysotile asbestos in rats. *Br J Exp Pathol* 69:717–737, 1988.

75. Davis JMG, Addison J, Bolton RE, Donaldson K, Jones AD: The pathogenicity of long versus short fibre samples of amosite asbestos administered to rats by inhalation and intraperitoneal injection. *Br J Exp Pathol* 67:415–430, 1986.

76. LeMaire I, Nadeau D, Dunnigan J, Massé S: An assessment of the fibrogenic potential of very short 4T30 chrysotile by intratracheal instillation in rats. *Environ Res* 36:314–326, 1985.

77. Platek SF, Groth DH, Ulrich CE, Stettler LE, Finnell MS, Stoll M: Chronic inhalation of short asbestos fibers. *Fundament Appl Toxicol* 5:327–340, 1985.

78. Fasske E: Pathogenesis of pulmonary fibrosis induced by chrysotile asbestos: Longitudinal light and electron microscopic studies on the rat model. *Virch Arch* [Pathol Anat] 408:329–346, 1986.

79. Lippman M: Asbestos exposure indices. *Environ Res* 46:86–106, 1988.

80. Davis JMG, Addison J, Bolton RE, Donaldson K, Jones AD: Inhalation and injection studies in rats using dust samples from chrysotile asbestos prepared by a wet dispersion process. *Br J Exp Pathol* 67:113–129, 1986.

81. Davis JMG, Bolton RE, Douglas AN, Jones AD, Smith T: Effects of electrostatic charge on the pathogenicity of chrysotile asbestos. *Br J Ind Med* 45:292–299, 1988.

82. Fisher GL, Gallo MA, eds: *Asbestos Toxicity.* New York: Marcel Dekker, 1987.

83. Harington JS, Miller K, Macnab G: Hemolysis by asbestos. *Environ Res* 4:95–117, 1971.

84. Jaurand MC, Thomassin JH, Baillif P, Magne L, Touray JC, Bignon J: Chemical and photoelectron spectrometry analysis of the adsorption of phospholipid model membranes and red blood cell membranes on to chrysotile fibres. *Br J Ind Med* 37:169–174, 1980.

85. Brody AR, George G, Hill LH: Interactions of chrysotile and crocidolite asbestos with red blood cell membranes: Chrysotile binds to sialic acid. *Lab Invest* 49:468–475, 1983.

86. Chamberlain M, Brown RC: The cytotoxic effects of asbestos and other mineral dusts in tissue culture cell lines. *Br J Exp Pathol* 59:183–189, 1978.

87. Reiss B, Solomon S, Weisburger JH, Williams GM: Comparative toxicities of different forms of asbestos in a cell culture assay. *Environ Res* 22:109–129, 1980.

88. Gallagher JE, George G, Brody AR: Sialic acid mediates the initial binding of positively charged inorganic particles to alveolar macrophage membranes. *Am Rev Respir Dis* 135:1345–1352, 1987.

89. Hesterberg TW, Ririe DG, Barrett JC, Nettesheim P: Mechanisms of cytotoxicity of asbestos fibres in rat tracheal epithelial cells in culture. *Toxic in Vitro* 1:59–65, 1987.
90. Weitzman SA, Graceffa P. Asbestos catalyzes hydroxyl and superoxide radical generation from hydrogen peroxide. *Arch Biochem Biophys* 228:373–376, 1984.
91. Eberhardt MK, Roman-Franco AA, Quiles MR: Asbestos-induced decomposition of hydrogen peroxide. *Environ Res* 37:287–292, 1985.
92. Zalma R, Bonneau L, Jaurand MC, Guignard J, Pezerat H: Formation of oxy-radicals by oxygen reduction arising from the surface activity of asbestos. *Canad J Chem* 65:2338–2341, 1987.
93. Shatos MA, Doherty JM, Marsh JP, Mossman BT: Prevention of asbestos-induced cell death in rat lung fibroblasts and alveolar macrophages by scavengers of active oxygen species. *Environ Res* 44:103–116, 1987.
94. Mossman BT, Marsh JP, Sesko A, Hill S, Shatos MA, Doherty J, Petruska J, Adler KB, Hemenway D, Mickey R, Vacek P, Kagan E: Inhibition of lung injury, inflammation, and interstitial pulmonary fibrosis by polyethylene glycol–conjugated catalase in a rapid inhalation model of asbestosis. *Am Rev Respir Dis* 141:1266–1271, 1990.
95. Weitzman SA, Chester JF, Graceffa P: Binding of deferoxamine to asbestos fibers in vitro and in vivo. *Carcinogenesis* 9:1643–1645, 1988.
96. Palekar LD, Brown BG, Coffin DL: Correlation between *in vitro* tumorigenesis, *in vitro* CHO cytotoxicity and *in vitro* V79 cytotoxicity after exposure to mineral fibers. In: *Short-term Bioassay in the Analysis of the Complex Environmental Mixtures IV* (Waters MD, Sandu SF, Lewtas J, Claxton J, Strauss G, Nesnow S, eds.), New York: Plenum Press 1985, pp. 155–169.
97. Marsh JP, Mossman BT: Mechanisms of induction of ornithine decarboxylase activity in tracheal epithelial cells by asbestiform minerals. *Cancer Res* 48:709–714, 1988.
98. Hansen K, Mossman BT: Generation of superoxide (O_2^-) from alveolar macrophages exposed to asbestos and non-asbestos fibers. *Cancer Res* 47:1681–1686, 1987.
99. Smith CM, Batcher S, Catanzaro A, Abraham JL, Phalen R: Sequence of bronchoalveolar lavage and histopathologic findings in rat lungs early in inhalation asbestos exposure. *J Toxicol Environ Health* 20:147–161, 1987.
100. Wilson MR, Gaumer HR, Salvaggio JE: Activation of the alternative complement pathway and generation of chemotactic factors by asbestos. *J Allergy Clin Immunol* 60:218–222, 1977.
101. Warheit DB, Hill LH, Brody AR: In vitro effects of crocidolite asbestos and wollastonite on pulmonary macrophages and serum complement. *Scanning Electron Microsc* II:919–926, 918, 1984.
102. Warheit DB, George G, Hill LH, Snyderman R, Brody AR: Inhaled asbestos activates a complement-dependent chemoattractant for macrophages. *Lab Invest* 52:505–514, 1985.
103. Warheit DB, Hill LH, George G, Brody AR: Time course of chemotactic factor generation and the corresponding macrophage response to asbestos inhalation. *Am Rev Respir Dis* 134:128–133, 1986.
104. Warheit DB, Hill LH, Brody AR: Surface morphology and correlated phagocytic capacity of pulmonary macrophages lavaged from the lungs of rats. *Expl Lung Res* 6:71–82, 1984.
105. Warheit DB, Hartsky MA: Assessments of pulmonary macrophage clearance responses to inhaled particulates. *Scanning Microsc* 2:1069–1078, 1988.
106. Miller K: Alterations in the surface-related phenomena of alveolar macrophages following inhalation of crocidolite asbestos and quartz dusts: An overview. *Environ Res* 20:162–182, 1979.

107. Kagan E, Oghiso Y, Hartmann D-P: The effects of chrysotile and crocidolite asbestos on the lower respiratory tract: Analysis of bronchoalveolar lavage constituents. *Environ Res* 32:382–397, 1983.

108. Case BW, Ip MPC, Padilla M, Kleinerman J: Asbestos effects on superoxide production: An in vitro study of hamster alveolar macrophages. *Environ Res* 39:299–306, 1986.

109. Goodglick LA, Kane AB: Role of active oxygen metabolites in crocidolite asbestos toxicity to mouse macrophages. *Cancer Res* 46:5558–5566, 1986.

110. Jackson JH, Schraufstatter IU, Hyslop PA, Vosbeck K, Sauerheber R, Weitzman SA, Cochrane CG: Role of oxidants in DNA damage: Hydroxyl radical mediates the synergistic DNA damaging effects of asbestos and cigarette smoke. *J Clin Invest* 80:1090–1095, 1987.

111. Dannenberg AM, Burstone MS, Walter PC, Kinsley JW: A histochemical study of phagocytic and enzymatic functions of rabbit mononuclear and polymorphonuclear exudate cells and alveolar macrophages. I. Survey and quantitation of enzymes, and states of cellular activation. *J Cell Biol* 17:465–486, 1963.

112. Cohn ZA, Wiener E: The particulate hydrolases of macrophages. I. Comparative enzymology, isolation, and properties. *J Exp Med* 118:991–1008, 1963.

113. Fanson RC, Waite M: Lysosomal phospholipases A_1 and A_2 of normal and bacillus Calmette-Guerin-induced alveolar macrophages. *J Cell Biol* 56:621–627, 1973.

114. Janoff A: Elastase-like protease of human granulocytes and alveolar macrophages. In: *Pulmonary Emphysema and Proteolysis* (Mittman C, ed.), New York: Academic Press, 1972, pp. 205–224.

115. Goggins JF, Lazarus GS, Fullmer HM: Hyaluronidase activity of alveolar macrophages. *J Histochem Cytochem* 16:688–692, 1968.

116. Gee JBL, Vassallo CL, Bell P, Kaskin J, Basford RE, Field JB: Catalase-dependent peroxidative metabolism in the alveolar macrophage during phagocytosis. *J Clin Invest* 49:1280–1287, 1970.

117. Paul BB, Strauss RR, Selvaraj RJ, Sbarra AJ: Peroxidase-mediated antimicrobial activities of alveolar macrophage granules. *Science* 181:849–850, 1973.

118. Sjöstrand M, Rylander R, Bergström R: Lung cell reactions in guinea pigs after inhalation of asbestos (amosite). *Toxicology* 57:1–14, 1989.

119. Garcia JGN, Griffith DE, Cohen AB, Callahan KS: Alveolar macrophages from patients with asbestos exposure release increased levels of leukotriene B_4. *Am Rev Respir Dis* 139:1494–1501, 1989.

120. Sestini P, Tagliabue A, Bartalini M, Boraschi D: Asbestos-induced modulation of release of regulatory molecules from alveolar and peritoneal macrophages. *Chest* 89:161S–162S, 1986.

121. Dubois CM, Bissonnette E, Rola-Pleszczynski M: Asbestos fibers and silica particles stimulate rat alveolar macrophages to release tumor necrosis factor: Autoregulatory role of leukotriene B_4. *Am Rev Respir Dis* 139:1257–1264, 1989.

122. Bissonnette E, Rola-Pleszczynski M: Pulmonary inflammation and fibrosis in a murine model of asbestosis and silicosis: Possible role of tumor necrosis factor. *Inflammation* 13:329–339, 1989.

123. Kumar RK, Bennett RA, Brody AR: A homologue of platelet-derived growth factor produced by rat alveolar macrophages. *FASEB J* 2:2272–2277, 1988.

124. Davies R, Erdogdu G: Secretion of fibronectin by mineral dust-derived alveolar macrophages and activated peritoneal macrophages. *Expl Lung Res* 15:285–297, 1989.

125. Schoenberger CI, Hunninghake GW, Kawanami O, Ferrans VJ, Crystal RG: Role of alveolar macrophages in asbestosis: Modulation of neutro-

phil migration to the lung after acute asbestos exposure. *Thorax* 37:803–809, 1982.

126. Elferink JGR, Deierkauf M, Kramps JA, Koerten HK: An activating and cytotoxic effect of asbestos on polymorphonuclear leukocytes. *Agents Actions* 26:213–215, 1989.

127. Doll NJ, Stankus RP, Goldbach S, Salvaggio JE: In vitro effect of asbestos fibers on polymorphonuclear leukocyte function. *Int Archs Allergy Appl Immunol* 68:17–21, 1982.

128. Kamp DW, Dunne M, Weitzman SA, Dunn MM: The interaction of asbestos and neutrophils injures cultured human pulmonary epithelial cells: Role of hydrogen peroxide. *J Lab Clin Med* 114:604–612, 1989.

129. Donaldson K, Brown GM, Brown DM, Bolton RE, Davis JMG: Inflammation generating potential of long and short fibre amosite asbestos samples. *Br J Ind Med* 46:271–276, 1989.

130. Mossman BT, Gilbert R, Doherty J, Shatos MA, Marsh J, Cutroneo K: Cellular and molecular mechanisms of asbestosis. *Chest* 89:160S–161S, 1986.

131. LeMaire I, Beaudoin H, Massé S, Grondin C: Alveolar macrophage stimulation of lung fibroblast growth in asbestos-induced pulmonary fibrosis. *Am J Pathol* 122:205–211, 1986.

132. Lemaire I, Beaudoin H, Dubois C: Cytokine regulation of lung fibroblast proliferation. Pulmonary and systemic changes in asbestos-induced pulmonary fibrosis. *Am Rev Respir Dis* 134:653–658, 1986.

133. Kagan E: Current perspectives in asbestosis. *Ann Allerg* 54:464–474, 1985.

134. DeShazo RD, Daul CB, Morgan JE, Diem JE, Hendrick DJ, Bozelka BE, Stankus RP, Jones R, Salvaggio JE, Weill H: Immunologic investigations in asbestos-exposed workers. *Chest* 89:162S–165S, 1986.

135. Barbers RG, Shih WWH, Saxon A: In vitro depression of human lymphocyte mitogen response (phytohemagglutinin) by asbestos fibres. *Clin Exp Immunol* 48:602–610, 1982.

136. Miller K, Weintraub Z, Kagan E: Manifestations of cellular immunity in the rat after prolonged asbestos inhalation. I. Physical interaction between alveolar macrophages and splenic lymphocytes. *J Immunol* 123:1029–1038, 1979.

137. Miller K, Kagan E: Manifestations of cellular immunity in the rat after prolonged asbestos inhalation. II. Alveolar macrophage–induced splenic lymphocyte proliferation. *Environ Res* 26:182–194, 1981.

138. Scheule RK, Holian A: IgG specifically enhances chrysotile asbestos-stimulated superoxide anion production by the alveolar macrophage. *Am J Respir Cell Mol Biol* 1:313–318, 1989.

139. Bégin R, Cantin A, Massé S, Côté Y, Fabi D: Effects of cyclophosphamide treatment in experimental asbestosis. *Expl Lung Res* 14:823–836, 1988.

140. Brody AR: Pulmonary cell interactions with asbestos fibers in vivo and in vitro. *Chest* 89:155S–159S, 1986.

141. Brody AR, Hill LH, Warheit DB: Induction of early alveolar injury by inhaled asbestos and silica. *Fed Proc* 44:2596–2601, 1985.

142. Brody AR, Hill LH: Initial epithelial and interstitial events following asbestos inhalation. Ch. 9 In: *Health Issues Related to Metal and Nonmetallic Mining* (Wagner WL, Rom WN, Merchant JA, eds.). Boston: Butterworth, 1983, pp. 161–172.

143. Davis JMG: Histogenesis and fine structure of peritoneal tumors produced in animals by injections of asbestos. *J Natl Cancer Inst* 52:1823–1837, 1974.

144. Kannerstein M, Churg J: Mesothelioma in man and experimental animals. *Environ Hlth Persp* 34:31–36, 1980.

145. Davis JMG, Cowie HA: The relationship between fibrosis and cancer in experimental animals exposed to asbestos and other fibers. *Environ Hlth Persp* 88:305–309, 1990.

146. Wagner JC, Berry GB, Hill RJ, Munday DE, Skidmore JW: Animal experiments with man-made mineral (vitreous) fibers: Effects of inhalation and intrapleural inoculation in rats. In: *Biological Effects of Man-Made Mineral Fibers* (Wagner JC, ed.), Copenhagen: World Health Organization, 1985, pp. 209–233.

147. McConnell EE, Wagner JC, Skidmore JW, Moore JA: A comparative study of the fibrogenic and carcinogenic effects of UICC Canadian chrysotile B asbestos and glass microfibre (JM100). In: *Biological Effects of Man-Made Mineral Fibers* (Wagner JC, ed.), Copenhagen: World Health Organization, 1985, pp. 234–252.

148. Smith DM, Ortiz LW, Archuleta RF, Johnson NF: Long-term health effects in hamsters and rats exposed chronically to man-made vitreous fibres. *Ann Occup Hyg* 31:731–754, 1987.

149. Maltoni C, Minardi F, Morisi L: Pleural mesotheliomas in Sprague-Dawley rats by erionite: First experimental evidence. *Environ Res* 29:238–244, 1982.

150. Suzuki Y: Carcinogenic and fibrogenic effects of zeolites: Preliminary observations. *Environ Res* 27:433–445, 1982.

151. Suzuki Y, Kohyama N: Malignant mesothelioma induced by asbestos and zeolite in the mouse peritoneal cavity. *Environ Res* 35:277–292, 1984.

152. Özesmi M, Patiroglu TE, Hillerdal G, Özesmi C: Peritoneal mesothelioma and malignant lymphoma in mice caused by fibrous zeolite. *Br J Ind Med* 42:746–749, 1985.

153. Wagner JC, Skidmore JW, Hill RJ, Griffiths DM: Erionite exposure and mesotheliomas in rats. *Br J Cancer* 51:727–730, 1985.

154. Fasske E: Experimental lung tumors following specific intrabronchial application of chrysotile asbestos: Longitudinal light and electron microscopic investigations in rats. *Respiration* 53:111–127, 1988.

155. Stanton MF, Layard M, Tegeris A, Miller E, May M, Kent E: Carcinogenicity of fibrous glass: Pleural response in the rat in relation to fiber dimension. *J Natl Cancer Inst* 58:587–603, 1977.

156. Stanton MF, Layard M, Tegeris A, Miller A, May M, Morgan E, Smith A: Relation of particle dimension to carcinogenicity in amphibole asbestoses and other fibrous minerals. *J Natl Cancer Inst* 67:965–975, 1981.

157. Hesterberg TW, Barrett JC: Dependence of asbestos- and mineral-dust-induced transformation of mammalian cells in culture on fiber dimension. *Cancer Res* 44:2170–2180, 1984.

158. Mossman BT: *In vitro* studies on the biologic effects of fibers: Correlation with *in vivo* bioassays. *Environ Hlth Persp* 88:319–322, 1990.

159. Bonneau L, Malard C, Pezerat H: Studies on surface properties of asbestos: II. Role of dimensional characteristics and surface properties of mineral fibers in the induction of pleural tumors. *Environ Res* 41:268–275, 1986.

160. Coffin DL, Peters SE, Palekar LD, Stahel EP: A study of the biological activity of erionite in relation to its chemical and structural characteristics. In: *Biological Interactions of Inhaled Mineral Fibers and Cigarette Smoke* (Wehner AP, ed.), Columbus, OH: Battelle Memorial Inst., 1989, pp. 313–323.

161. Chamberlain M, Tarmy EM: Asbestos and glass fibers in bacterial mutation tests. *Mutat Res* 43:159–164, 1977.

162. Light WG, Wei ET: Surface charge and a molecular basis for asbestos toxicity, In: *In Vitro Effects of Mineral Dusts* (Brown RC, Gormley JP, Chamberlain M, Davies R, eds.), Berlin: Springer-Verlag, 1980, pp. 139–146.

163. Barrett JC, Lamb PW, Wiseman RW: Multiple mechanisms for the carcinogenic effects of asbestos and other mineral fibers. *Environ Hlth Persp* 81:81–89, 1989.

164. Reiss B, Solomon S, Tong C, Levenstein M, Rosenberg SH, Williams GM: Absence of mutagenic activity of three forms of asbestos in liver epithelial cells. *Environ Res* 27:389–397, 1982.

165. Oshimura M, Hesterberg TW, Tsutsui T, Barrett JC: Correlation of asbestos-induced cytogenetic effects with cell transformation of Syrian hamster embryo cells in culture. *Cancer Res* 44:5017–5022, 1984.

166. Thiollet J, Jaurand MC, Kaplan H, Bignon J, Hollande E: Culture procedure of mesothelial cells from the rat parietal pleura. *Biomedicine* 29:69–73, 1978.

167. Jaurand MC, Bernaudin JF, Renier A, Kaplan H, Bignon J: Rat pleural mesothelial cells in culture. *In Vitro* 17:98–106, 1981.

168. Rennard SI, Jaurand M-C, Bignon J, Kawanami O, Ferrans VJ, Davidson J, Crystal RG: Role of pleural mesothelial cells in the production of the submesothelial connective tissue matrix of lung. *Am Rev Respir Dis* 130:267–274, 1984.

169. Brown DG, Johnson NF, Wagner MMF: Multipotential behavior of cloned rat mesothelioma cells with epithelial phenotype. *Br J Cancer* 51:245–252, 1985.

170. Jaurand M-C, Kaplan H, Thiollet J, Pinchon M-C, Bernaudin J-F, Bignon J: Phagocytosis of chrysotile fibers by pleural mesothelial cells in culture. *Am J Pathol* 94:529–538, 1979.

171. Jaurand MC, Bastie-Sigeac I, Bignon J, Stoebner P: Effect of chrysotile and crocidolite on the morphology and growth of rat pleural mesothelial cells. *Environ Res* 30:255–269, 1983.

172. Paterour MJ, Bignon J, Jaurand MC: In vitro transformation of rat pleural mesothelial cells by chrysotile fibres and/or benzo[a]pyrene. *Carcinogenesis* 6:523–529, 1985.

173. Wang NS, Jaurand MC, Magne L, Kheuang L, Pinchon MC, Bignon J: The interactions between asbestos fibers and metaphase chromosomes of rat pleural mesothelial cells in culture: A scanning and transmission electron microscopic study. *Am J Pathol* 126:343–349, 1987.

174. Libbus BL, Craighead JE: Chromosomal translocations with specific breakpoints in asbestos-induced rat mesotheliomas. *Cancer Res* 48:6455–6461, 1988.

175. Popescu NC, Chahinian AP, DiPaolo JA: Nonrandom chromosome alterations in human malignant mesothelioma. *Cancer Res* 48:142–147, 1988.

176. Tiainen M, Tammilehto L, Mattson K, Knuutila S: Nonrandom chromosomal abnormalities in malignant pleural mesothelioma. *Cancer Genet Cytogenet* 33:251–274, 1988.

177. Tiainen M, Tammilehto L, Rautonen J, Tuomi T, Mattson K, Knuutila S: Chromosomal abnormalities and their correlations with asbestos exposure and survival in patients with mesothelioma. *Br J Cancer* 60:618–626, 1989.

178. Lechner JF, Tokiwa T, LaVeck M, Benedict WF, Banks-Schlegel S, Yeager H, Jr., Banerjee A, Harris CC: Asbestos-associated chromosomal changes in human mesothelial cells. *Proc Natl Acad Sci USA* 82:3884–3888, 1985.

179. Olofsson K, Mark J: Specificity of asbestos-induced chromosomal aberrations in short-term cultured human mesothelial cells. *Cancer Genet Cytogenet* 41:33–39, 1989.

180. Achard S, Perderiset M, Jaurand M-C: Sister chromatid exchanges in rat pleural mesothelial cells treated with crocidolite, attapulgite, or benzo 3-4 pyrene. *Br J Ind Med* 44:281–283, 1987.

181. Dubes GR, Mack LR: Asbestos-mediated transfection of mammalian cell cultures. *In Vitro Cell Develop Biol* 24:175–182, 1988.

182. Appel JD, Fasy TM, Kohtz DS, Kohtz JD, Johnson EM: Asbestos fibers mediate transformation of monkey cells by exogenous plasmid DNA. *Proc Natl Acad Sci USA* 85:7670–7674, 1988.

183. Kenne K, Ljungquist S, Ringertz NR: Effects of asbestos fibers on cell division, cell survival, and formation of thioguanine-resistant mutants in Chinese hamster ovary cells. *Environ Res* 39:448–464, 1986.

184. Lipkin LE: Cellular effects of asbestos and other fibers: Correlations with in vivo induction of pleural sarcoma. *Environ Hlth Persp* 34:91–102, 1980.

185. Jaurand M-C, Fleury J, Monchaux G, Nebut M, Bignon J: Pleural carcinogenic potency of mineral fibers (asbestos, attapulgite) and their cytotoxicity on cultured cells. *J Natl Cancer Inst* 79:797–804, 1987.

186. Versnel MA, Hagemeijer A, Bouts MJ, van der Kwast TH, Hoogsteden HC: Expression of c-sis (PDGF B-chain) and PDGF A-chain genes in ten human malignant mesothelioma cell lines derived from primary and metastatic tumors. *Oncogene* 2:601–605, 1988.

187. Lechner JF, LaVeck MA, Gerwin BI, Matis EA: Differential responses to growth factors by normal human mesothelial cultures from individual donors. *J Cell Physiol* 139:295–300, 1989.

188. Moalli PA, MacDonald JL, Goodglick LA, Kane AB: Acute injury and regeneration of the mesothelium in response to asbestos fibers. *Am J Pathol* 128:426–445, 1987.

189. Branchaud RM, MacDonald JL, Kane AB: Induction of angiogenesis by intraperitoneal injection of asbestos fibers. *FASEB J* 3:1747–1752, 1989.

190. Suzuki Y, Chahinian AP, Ohnuma T: Comparative studies of human malignant mesothelioma in vivo, in xenografts in nude mice, and in vitro: Cell origin of malignant mesothelioma. *Cancer* 60:334–344, 1987.

191. Lindén C-J, Johansson L: Progressive growth of a human pleural mesothelioma xenografted to athymic rats and mice. *Br J Cancer* 58:614–618, 1988.

192. Lindén C-J, Johansson L: Xenografting of human pleural mesotheliomas to athymic rats and mice. *In Vivo* 2:345–348, 1988.

193. Mossman BT, Craighead JE: Use of hamster tracheal organ cultures for assessing the carcinogenic effects of inorganic particulates on the respiratory epithelium. *Prog Exp Tumor Res* 24:37–47, 1979.

194. Mossman BT, Craighead JE, MacPherson BV: Asbestos-induced epithelial changes in organ cultures of hamster trachea: Inhibition by retinyl methyl ether. *Science* 207:311–313, 1980.

195. Holtz G, Bresnick E: Ascorbic acid inhibits the squamous metaplasia that results from treatment of tracheal explants with asbestos or benzo[a]pyrene-coated asbestos. *Cancer Letts* 42:23–28, 1988.

196. Wehner AP, ed: *Biological Interactions of Inhaled Mineral Fibers and Cigarette Smoke.* Columbus, OH: Battelle Memorial Inst., 1989.

197. Harvey G, Pagé M, Dumas L: Binding of environmental carcinogens to asbestos and mineral fibres. *Br J Ind Med* 41:396–400, 1984.

198. Gerde P, Scholander P: Adsorption of benzo[a]pyrene onto asbestos and man-made mineral fibers in an aqueous solution and in a biological model solution. *Br J Ind Med* 45:682–688, 1988.

199. Mossman BT, Craighead JE: Mechanisms of asbestos carcinogenesis. *Environ Res* 25:269–280, 1981.

200. Lu Y-P, Lasne C, Lowy R, Chouroulinkov I: Use of the orthogonal design method to study the synergistic effects of asbestos fibres and 12-0-tetradecanoylphorbol-13-acetate (TPA) in the BALB/3T3 cell transformation system. *Mutagenesis* 3:355–362, 1988.

201. Mossman BT, Craighead JE: Comparative cocarcinogenic effects of cro-
     cidolite asbestos, hematite, kaolin and carbon in implanted tracheal or-
     gan cultures. *Ann Occup Hyg* 26:553–567, 1982.
202. Harrison PTC, Heath JC: Apparent synergy between chrysotile asbestos
     and *N*-nitrosoheptamethyleneimine in the induction of pulmonary tu-
     mours in rats. *Carcinogenesis* 9:2165–2171, 1988.
203. Warren S, Brown CE, Chute RN, Federman M: Mesothelioma relative
     to asbestos, radiation, and methylcholanthrene. *Arch Pathol Lab Med*
     105:305–312, 1981.
204. Gerde P, Scholander P: A hypothesis concerning asbestos carcinogenic-
     ity: The migration of lipophilic carcinogens in adsorbed lipid bilayers.
     Ann Occup Hyg 31:395–400, 1987.
205. Churg A, Hobson J, Berean K, Wright J: Scavengers of active oxygen
     species prevent cigarette smoke-induced asbestos fiber penetration in
     rat tracheal explants. *Am J Pathol* 135:599–603, 1989.
206. Hei TK, Hall EJ, Osmak RS: Asbestos, radiation and oncogenic trans-
     formation. *Br J Cancer* 50:717–720, 1984.
207. Mossman BT, Gee JBL: Asbestos-related diseases. *N Engl J Med*
     320:1721–1730, 1989.
208. Mossman B, Light W, Wei E: Asbestos: Mechanisms of toxicity and car-
     cinogenicity in the respiratory tract. *Ann Rev Pharmacol Toxicol* 23:595–
     615, 1983.

11. Analysis of Tissue Mineral Fiber Content

Victor L. Roggli, Philip C. Pratt, and Arnold R. Brody

The development of techniques for assaying the mineral fiber content of tissues has provided the opportunity to correlate the occurrence of various fiber-related diseases with the cumulative fiber burdens in the target organ. Exposure to mineral fibers generally occurs through the inhalation of airborne fibers, and thus the respiratory tract is the site of most asbestos-related diseases. Consequently, most studies of tissue fiber burdens have concentrated on the analysis of lung parenchyma.[1] This chapter reviews the various techniques that have been developed for the analysis of tissue fiber burdens, noting the advantages and limitations of each. (The morphologic, crystallographic, and chemical features of the various types of asbestos are reviewed in Chap. 1, and the structure and nature of asbestos bodies in Chap. 3.) This chapter also explores the relationship between tissue asbestos burden and the various asbestos-associated diseases (see Chaps. 4–7) and the various categories of occupational and environmental exposures (see Chap. 2). Finally, the overall total contribution of the various types of asbestos and nonasbestos mineral fibers to the total mineral fiber burden are discussed in relation to the biological activity and pathogenicity of the various fiber types.

HISTORICAL BACKGROUND

Throughout the twentieth century, there has been considerable interest in the correlation of dusts in the workplace environment with lung diseases resulting from the inhalation of these dusts (i.e., the pneumoconioses). Analysis of lung dust burdens required considerable cooperation between the basic physical sciences and the biological and medical sciences.[2] The distinctive behavior of fibrous materials as compared to other particulates has required many pointed studies as to inhalability, deposition, and subsequent disposal or accumulation of airborne fibers (see Chap. 10). Generally, bulk analytical techniques were employed, such as x-ray diffraction, chemical analysis, and polarizing microscopy, which were adequate in most circumstances because of the well-defined source of the dust in the workplace and the relatively large amounts of dust recoverable from the lungs of patients dying with pneumoconiosis. However, analysis of dust content from individuals exposed to asbestos posed a number of difficulties for the traditional bulk analytical approaches. First, the quantities of dust present within the lung samples were often relatively small. Second, the size of the particles posed some difficulty, since most of the asbestos fibers were less than a micron in diameter. Third, other dusts were often present in similar or even greater amounts than the asbestos component. Fourth, alteration of the chemical or crystalline properties of some types of fibers during prolonged residence in tissues complicated the precise identification of such agents. Furthermore, many of the techniques used for microfiber extraction from tissues tended to alter or destroy some of the mineral phases present.[2]

Clearly, the development of unique approaches for the identification of asbestos fibers in tissues was necessary before progress in this area could become possible. In the 1970s, the use of analytical electron microscopy for the identification and characterization of individual asbestos fibers isolated from human tissues was pioneered, in large part, by the innovative studies of investigators such as Arthur Langer in the United States and Fred Pooley in Great Britain.[3-8] The usefulness of these techniques has since been confirmed by other investigators.[9-14] In the 1980s and since, these techniques have been employed to correlate the tissue asbestos burden with various asbestos-related diseases.[11,15-18]

METHODS FOR ANALYSIS OF TISSUE MINERAL FIBER CONTENT

TISSUE SELECTION

As noted earlier, most studies of tissue mineral fiber content have examined lung parenchyma. There is no inherent reason why the techniques developed for this purpose cannot be applied to other tissues. However, little published information exists on the expected values of mineral fiber content of tissues other than the lung. Therefore, any investigator wishing to study such tissues must establish normal ranges for his or her laboratory and for the analytical technique employed. In addition, the expected levels of fibers in extrapulmonary tissues would be at or below the limits of detection for current techniques, and background contamination can be a considerable problem. In this section, comments regarding selection of tissue for mineral fiber analysis will be confined to lung parenchyma.

In most circumstances, formalin-fixed lung tissue is utilized, although fresh specimens work just as well. In some instances, paraffin-embedded tissue is all that is available. Such samples can be deparaffinized in xylene and rehydrated with 95% ethanol. The dehydration process removes some components of tissue, mainly lipids, so that a correction factor must be applied to equate the values obtained from paraffin blocks to those obtained from formalin-fixed tissue. In the authors' laboratory, the correction factor has been determined to be approximately 0.7 (i.e., the asbestos fiber concentration determined from a paraffin block should be multiplied by 0.7).[17]

In selecting tissue for digestion, areas of consolidation, congestion, or tumor should be avoided as much as possible. Such pathologic alterations would affect the denominator in calculations of the tissue concentration of fibers or asbestos bodies. Since there is some site-to-site variation of mineral fiber content within the lung, the more tissue that is available for analysis the better. Ideal specimens include autopsy, pneumonectomy, and lobectomy specimens, with analysis of multiple sites. In the authors' laboratory, two or three samples are typically analyzed for a lobectomy or pneumonectomy specimen, whereas four sites (upper and lower lobes of each lung) are sampled when both lungs are available at autopsy. Samples usually include lung parenchyma abutting against the visceral pleura, with each sample typically weighing 0.25–0.35 gm (wet weight). However, analyses may be performed on as little as 0.1 gm (sometimes less) of wet tissue. Although some studies have reported analyses of transbronchial biopsy specimens,[19,20] the small size of such samples (usually 2–5 mg of tissue, at best) makes them unlikely to be representative.[21,22]

DIGESTION TECHNIQUES

Techniques for mineral fiber analysis generally involve three basic steps: (1) dissolution and removal of the organic matrix material of the lung in which the fibers are embedded; (2) recovery and concentration of the mineral fibers; and (3) analysis of the fiber content by some form of microscopy.[1] Dissolution steps involve either wet chemical digestion or ashing. Wet chemical digestion can be accomplished with sodium hydroxide, potassium hydroxide, hydrogen peroxide, 5.25% sodium hypochlorite solution (commercial bleach), formamide, or proteolytic enzymes.[12] Most investigators prefer an alkali wet chemical digestion using either sodium hypochlorite, sodium hydroxide, or potassium hydroxide. Tissue ashing is an alternative approach. Ashing in a muffle furnace at 400–500°C is unsuitable, because the drying and shrinkage of the tissue causes fragmentation of the fibers, artefactually increasing fiber numbers and decreasing mean fiber lengths. This problem is largely avoided by ashing the sample in a low-temperature-plasma asher.[23]

Once the digestion of the tissue is complete, the inorganic residue may then be collected on an acetate or polycarbonate filter, or an aliquot can be transferred into a Fuchs-Rosenthal counting chamber for direct counting of fibers by phase-contrast light microscopy.[15] However, a permanent sample cannot be prepared with this latter technique, so most investigators prefer filtration, with a pore size of 0.2–0.45 μm. Use of a pore size too large in relation to the size of fibers to be analyzed can result in significant loss of fibers and underestimation of the mineral fiber content of the sample.[24] (Details of the digestion procedure employed by the authors are provided in the Appendix.)

FIBER IDENTIFICATION AND QUANTIFICATION

A number of analytical techniques have been used for the identification of asbestos fibers in bulk samples, including x-ray diffractometry, infrared spectroscopy, differential thermal analysis, and polarization microscopy with dispersion staining.[2,6,11] For a variety of reasons, as noted earlier in the section on "Historical Background," these techniques have severe limitations in regard to the identification of fibers from human lung tissue samples, and in practice bulk analytical techniques have been ineffective for this purpose.[2,6,11] As a result, investigators have turned to various forms of microscopy for the analysis of pulmonary mineral fiber content. These include conventional bright-field light microscopy, phase-contrast light microscopy, scanning electron microscopy, and transmission electron microscopy.

Conventional bright-field light microscopy is a simple, inexpensive technique that requires no special instrumentation. This technique (detailed in Chap. 3) is ideal for the quantification of asbestos bodies.[1,14,17] A few uncoated asbestos fibers can also be observed, but the vast majority of fibers are beyond the resolution of this technique. Furthermore, conventional light microscopy cannot distinguish among the various fiber types. Asbestos bodies can be counted at a magnification of 200–400×, and the results reported as numbers per gram of wet lung tissue.[12,17] Alternatively, a piece of lung tissue adjacent to the one actually analyzed can be dried to constant weight to obtain a wet-to-dry weight ratio, and the results reported as asbestos bodies per gram of dry weight.[11,14]

Phase-contrast light microscopy (PCLM) has also been used by investigators to quantitate the tissue mineral fiber burden.[15,18] This technique can resolve fibers with a diameter of $0.2\,\mu$ or greater, and it reveals that uncoated fibers greatly outnumber coated ones (i.e., asbestos bodies).[25] However, a substantial proportion of asbestos fibers have diameters less than $0.2\,\mu$ and thus are not detected by PCLM. As is the case for conventional light microscopy, one cannot distinguish among the various types of asbestos fibers or differentiate asbestos from nonasbestos fibers by PCLM. Investigators using this technique have generally reported results as total fibers per gram of dry lung tissue[15] or separately as asbestos bodies and uncoated fibers per gram of dry lung tissue.[26] Some investigators have also reported results as fibers per cm^3 of lung tissue.[27] As a rule of thumb, 1 fiber/gm wet lung $\cong$ 1 fiber/cm^3 $\cong$ 10 fibers/gm dry lung.[22]

Scanning electron microscopy (SEM) has been used by some investigators for the quantification of tissue mineral fiber content.[17,23,28] This technique offers several advantages over PCLM and conventional bright-field light microscopy. At low magnifications (1000×), asbestos bodies and uncoated fibers can be counted, yielding quantitative results similar to those obtained with PCLM (Fig. 11-1).[17] At higher magnifications (10,000–20,000×), the superior resolution of SEM permits the detection of fibers not visible by PCLM, that is, fibers as small as $0.3\,\mu$ long and $0.05\,\mu$ in diameter.[28] Furthermore, SEM can be coupled with energy-dispersive x-ray analysis (EDXA) to determine the chemical composition of individual fibers (Fig. 11-2). This information can in turn be used to classify a fiber as asbestos or

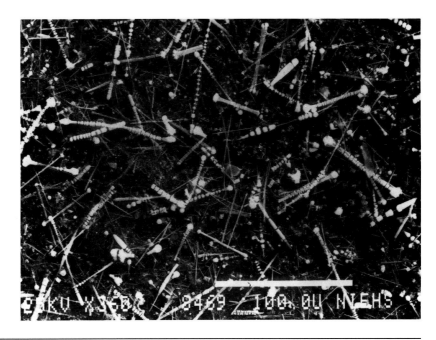

FIGURE 11-1. Scanning electron micrograph of Nuclepore filter preparation of lung tissue from an asbestos insulator with malignant pleural mesothelioma and asbestosis. Numerous asbestos bodies and uncoated asbestos fibers are visible. This patient's lung tissue contained nearly 3 million asbestos bodies and more than 9 million uncoated fibers 5 μm or greater in length per gram of wet lung. Magnified ×360. Reprinted from Ref. 22, with permission.

nonasbestos and to determine the specific asbestos fiber type.[17,28–30] Sample preparation for SEM is relatively simple, requiring only that the filter be mounted on a suitable substrate (such as a carbon disc) with carbon paste, and then coated with a suitable conducting material (such as carbon or gold). Also, SEM analysis of mineral fibers has the potential for automation using commercially available automated image x-ray analyzers[31] and software programs that discriminate between fibers and other particles.[32,33] Disadvantages of SEM include the high cost of the instrumentation and the considerable time required for analysis (several hours per sample).

Transmission electron microscopy (TEM) has been the analytical technique preferred by most investigators for the determination of mineral fiber content in tissue digest preparations.[7,8,11,16,18,20,26] This technique provides the highest resolution for the identification of the smallest fibers and can be coupled with EDXA for determination of the chemical composition of individual fibers. TEM has the further advantage that selected-area electron diffraction (SAED) can also be performed, providing information on the crystalline structure of an individual particle. The diffraction pattern of a fiber (Fig. 11-3) can provide information useful for identification purposes, especially when the chemical compositions of two fibers are similar.[35,35] For

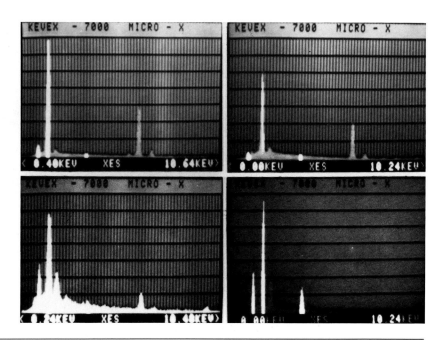

FIGURE 11-2. Energy-dispersive x-ray spectra of four different amphibole asbestos fibers. (A, *upper left*) Amosite has peaks for silicon, iron, magnesium, and sometimes manganese. (B, *upper right*) Crocidolite has peaks for silicon, iron, sodium, and magnesium. (C, *lower left*) Anthophyllite has peaks for silicon, magnesium, and iron. (D, *lower right*) Tremolite has peaks for silicon, magnesium, and calcium. The peak in each spectrum immediately to the right of silicon is due to the gold used to coat the specimen. Reprinted from Ref. 17, with permission.

example, SAED can readily distinguish chrysotile from anthophyllite asbestos, or anthophyllite from talc.[35] Methods for preparation of tissue samples for TEM analysis have been described;[35,36] however, these techniques are more complex than preparative steps for light microscopy or SEM. Therefore, there is increased opportunity for loss of fibers or contamination of the sample. Also, only a small proportion of a filter can be mounted on a TEM grid, so that one must be concerned with whether the portion of the filter sampled is truly representative.[22] As is the case for SEM, analysis of mineral fiber content of tissue by TEM is both time-consuming and expensive. Results are generally reported in terms of fibers per gram of wet or dry lung tissue. The magnifications used are generally too high to accurately assess the tissue asbestos-body content by TEM.

Two other techniques deserve brief mention as potentially useful for tissue mineral fiber analysis. The confocal scanning optical microscope uses a focused light beam to scan across the sample, and the image is detected and processed electronically.[37,38] This light microscopy technique has a resolution of 0.1μ or better, which is superior to that of PCLM and thus would permit detection of considerably more

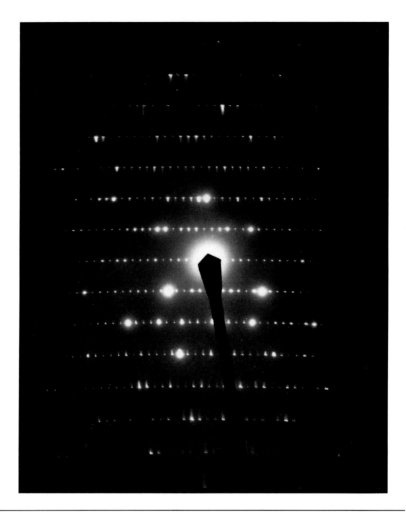

FIGURE 11-3. Selected-area electron diffraction pattern obtained from an asbestos-body core of an insulation worker. The pattern shows discrete dots along each layer line, with a calculated 5.3-Å interlayer–line spacing typical of amphibole asbestos. Reprinted from Roggli VL et al.: New techniques for imaging and analyzing lung tissue. *Environ Hlth Persp.* 56:163–183, 1984 (Fig. 4).

fibers. The image is focused in a discrete plane with a thickness of less than 1 μ. Since asbestos fibers may be present at different depths in a filter preparation, quantitative examination of a filter with this imaging technique could be time-consuming. Another technique with potential value is scanning transmission electron microscopy (STEM). This technique has the high resolution and the capacity for electron diffraction characteristic of TEM.[39,40] Furthermore, the scanning mode of operation produces an image amenable to automated analysis. Hence STEM has many characteristics that would be ideal for a standardized and automated approach to mineral fiber analysis.

TABLE 11-1. Factors affecting fiber burden data

I. Digestion Procedure
   A. Wet chemical digestion (alkali, enzymes)
   B. Low-temperature-plasma ashing
   C. Number of sites sampled
II. Recovery Procedure
   A. Inclusion of centrifugation step
   B. Inclusion of a sonication step
   C. Filtration step (type of filter, pore size)
III. Analytical Procedure
   A. Microscopic technique (LM, PCLM, SEM, TEM)*
   B. Magnification used
   C. Sizes of fibers counted and other "counting rules"
   D. Numbers of fibers or fields actually counted
IV. Reporting of Results
   A. Asbestos bodies or fibers (or both)
   B. Sizes of fibers counted
   C. Concentration of fibers (per gram wet or dry lung or per cm^3)

SOURCE: Reprinted from Ref. 1.
*LM = Light microscopy; PCLM = Phase-contrast light microscopy; SEM = Scanning electron microscopy; TEM = Transmission electron microscopy

VARIABILITY OF RESULTS

The wide variety of preparative techniques and analytical methodologies that have been employed by various investigators makes it difficult to extrapolate results from one laboratory to another. The actual analytical result obtained on any one sample can be profoundly influenced by the steps employed in the analytical procedure (Table 11-1).[1] Interlaboratory comparison trials demonstrate some striking differences among laboratories, even when the same sample is analyzed.[41] Some asbestos bodies and fibers may be lost during preparation,[42,43] and some of the smallest fibers are difficult to recognize and count in a reproducible fashion.[44] On the other hand, including a sonication step or ashing of the specimen can enhance the fragmentation of chrysotile fibers, artefactually increasing fiber numbers.[21,42] Nonetheless, there is evidence for internal consistency within individual laboratories, with similar ranking of samples among different laboratories from the lowest to the highest tissue fiber concentration. Still, one must use caution in comparing results between laboratories, bearing in mind any differences in the analytical procedures employed.[1]

In addition to interlaboratory variation, intralaboratory variation can occur, which may be due either to changes in a laboratory's procedure over time[45] or to variation in fiber content from one site to another within the lung.[25,46] Morgan and Holmes[25,46] have reported a five- to ten-fold site-to-site variation based on analyses of multiple samples from a single lung using phase-contrast light microscopy. In the authors' experience using light microscopy for asbestos-body quantification (Fig. 11-4) or SEM for asbestos-body and uncoated-

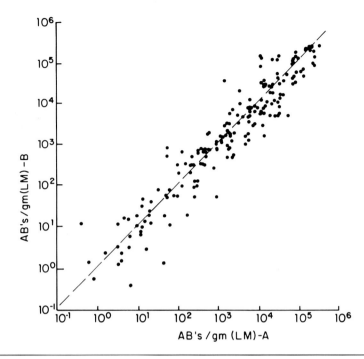

FIGURE 11-4. Correlation of asbestos-body counts by light microscopy in 136 cases where multiple sites were sampled. Graph shows all pairwise comparisons, with the linear regression equation given by log y = 0.96 log x + 0.09 (correlation coefficient r = 0.95, p < 0.00001).

fiber quantification (Fig. 11-5), paired samples have asbestos-body and fiber-concentration values ranging from identical to within a factor of two or three. Rarely, two samples from the same patient may differ by as much as a factor of 10. The coefficient of variation for counting the same sample on multiple occasions is on the order of 10%.[47] When interpreting fiber burden data, one must keep in mind that the analysis is occurring at a single point in time, usually when advanced disease is present. The fiber burden at that time may or may not relate to the tissue fiber content at the time when disease was actively evolving.[1] Nonetheless, there is a growing consensus that the fiber burdens that persist in the lung are the primary determinant of subsequent disease.[48,49]

ASBESTOS CONTENT OF LUNG TISSUE IN ASBESTOS-ASSOCIATED DISEASES

ASBESTOSIS

Relatively few studies have been published in which the asbestos content of lung tissue was examined in a series of patients with asbestosis.[15,16,18,26,50] The data from these studies are summarized in

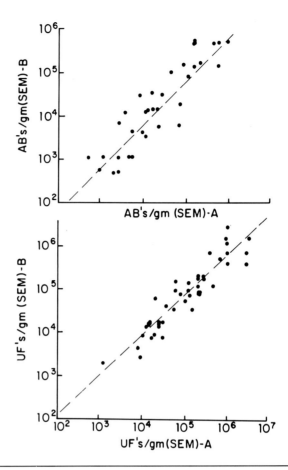

FIGURE 11-5. (*Top*) Correlation of asbestos-body counts by scanning electron microscopy (SEM) in 23 cases where multiple sites were sampled. Graph shows
all pairwise comparisons, with the linear regression equation given by
$\log y = 1.06 \log x - 0.34$ (correlation coefficient $r = 0.90$, $p < 0.0001$). (*Bottom*) Correlation of uncoated-fiber concentrations for fibers 5 µm or greater
in length by SEM in 30 cases where multiple sites were sampled. Graph
shows all pairwise comparisons, with the linear regression equation given
by $\log y = 0.92 \log x + 0.24$ ($r = 0.93$, $p < 0.0001$).

Table 11-2. Except for the unusually high median count for asbestos
bodies in the study by Ashcroft and Heppleston,[26] and the high mean
count for uncoated fibers by electron microscopy in the study by
Wagner et al.,[18] the values are roughly similar among the reported
series. This is rather remarkable when one considers the wide range
of values obtained when different laboratories examine the same
sample[41] and the different techniques employed in the various
studies referred to in the table. For example, Whitwell et al.[15] used
PCLM and counted all fibers greater than or equal to 6 µ in length,
counting asbestos bodies and uncoated fibers together. Ashcroft and
Heppleston[26] used PCLM at a magnification of 400× and counted all

TABLE 11-2. Asbestos content of lung tissue in reported series of patients with asbestosis

Source	Number of cases	Method[a]	Asbestos bodies per gram dried lung[b]	Uncoated fibers per gram dried lung[b]
Whitwell et al.[15]	23	PCLM	—	8 (1.0–70)
Ashcroft and Heppleston[26]	22	PCLM	12.2 (0.49–192)	32 (1.3–493)
Warnock et al.[16]	22	TEM[c]	0.123 (0.001–7.38)	5.68 (1.6–121)
Wagner et al.[18]	100	PCLM	—	1.5 (0.001–31.6)
	170	TEM	—	372 (<1.0–10,000)
Roggli[50]	76	SEM[c]	0.378[d] (0.006–16)	3.3[d] (0.18–125)

SOURCE: Reprinted from Ref. 50, with permission.
[a]PCLM = Phase-contrast light microscopy; TEM = Transmission electron microscopy; SEM = Scanning electron microscopy
[b]Values reported are the median counts for millions (10^6) of asbestos bodies or uncoated fibers per gram of dried lung tissue, with ranges indicated in parentheses, except for the study of Wagner et al.,[18] where only the mean value could be determined from the data presented.
[c]In these two studies, asbestos bodies were counted by conventional light microscopy.
[d]Values multiplied by a factor of 10 (approximate ratio of wet to dry lung weight) for purposes of comparison.

visible fibers, reporting coated and uncoated fibers separately. Warnock et al.[16] used TEM and counted all fibers exceeding 0.25 μ in length and with an aspect ratio (length to width) of three or greater. Wagner et al.[18] used the PCLM method of Ashcroft and Heppleston[26] as well as TEM. Roggli[50] employed SEM at a magnification of 1000×, counting all fibers with a length greater than or equal to 5 μ. The study by Warnock et al.[16] and that of Roggli[50] also counted asbestos bodies by conventional light microscopy. The median uncoated fiber count exceeds 1 million fibers per gram of dried lung tissue in all five studies. For comparison, the median count by SEM in the authors' laboratory for uncoated fibers 5 μ or greater in length from individuals with normal lungs and no known occupational asbestos exposure is approximately 0.031×10^6 fibers/gm.

The asbestos-body content of the lung in 76 patients with histologically confirmed asbestosis is shown in comparison to that of 16 patients with idiopathic pulmonary fibrosis (IPF) and 64 nonexposed "controls" in Fig. 11-6. The median count for the patients with asbestosis is 37,800 asbestos bodies per gram of wet lung tissue, which can be converted approximately to bodies per gram of dry lung tissue by multiplying by a factor of 10.[11] In comparison, the median

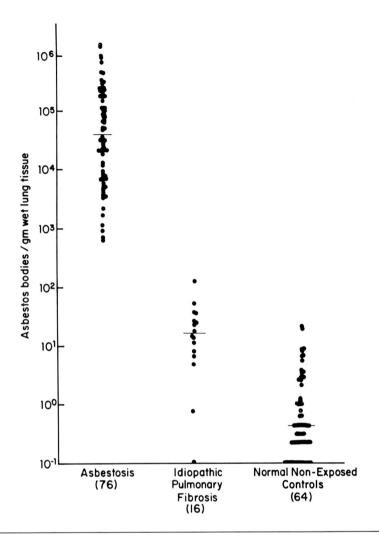

FIGURE 11-6. Histogram of asbestos body counts in 76 patients with asbestosis, 16 patients with idiopathic pulmonary fibrosis, and 64 nonexposed "controls." Horizontal bars indicate median values. Note logarithmic scale. Reprinted from Ref. 50, with permission.

count for the patients with IPF is 16 AB/gm and for the controls is 0.4 AB/gm. Although there is substantial overlap between the IPF and "control" groups, a few IPF patients with low-level asbestos exposure have slightly elevated values. In 95% of the cases of asbestosis, the asbestos-body content is 1700 AB/gm or greater. At this tissue asbestos-body concentration, several asbestos bodies should be observed on most 2×2-cm histologic sections stained for iron and examined systematically (see Chap. 3).[51] Thus the finding of asbestos bodies in histologic sections is a reasonable histopathologic discriminator between asbestosis and IPF (see Chap. 4).[50]

TABLE 11-3. Severity of asbestosis vs. tissue asbestos content as total fibers per gram dried lung*

Study	Asbestosis grade				
	0	½+	1+	2+	3+
Whitwell et al.[15]			8×10^6	14×10^6	37×10^6
Ashcroft and Heppleston[26]	2.4×10^6		20×10^6	200×10^6	144×10^6
Warnock et al.[16]	4.8×10^6	5.7×10^6	48×10^6	11×10^6	3.6×10^6
Wagner et al.[18]	0.005×10^6	0.009×10^6	0.015×10^6	0.12×10^6	1.2×10^6
	1.3×10^6	31.6×10^6	44×10^6	68×10^6	464×10^6

SOURCE: Reprinted from Ref. 50, with permission.
*Values represent the median counts derived from the data presented in the reference cited. Asbestosis grade is as defined in each original source. First two studies employed phase-contrast light microscopy, whereas the study by Warnock et al.[16] used transmission electron microscopy and the study of Wagner et al.[18] used both (phase contrast results from Fig. 2 of the latter study are listed first, and EM results from Fig. 1 are listed below). Wagner et al.[18] grading scheme of 0 to 4 has been modified to 0 to 3 simply for purposes of tabulation.

A few studies have investigated the relationship between tissue asbestos burden and the fibrotic response in human lungs (Table 11-3). Whitwell et al.[15] found a progressive increase in median total coated- and uncoated-fiber count from patients with mild (1+) to severe (3+) fibrosis. Ashcroft and Heppleston[26] also reported a progression in the severity of fibrosis with increasing uncoated-fiber count from no fibrosis to moderate (2+) fibrosis, but no further increase in fiber count from moderate to severe disease. These authors concluded that additional factors other than tissue fiber burden must be involved in progression from moderate to severe fibrosis.[26] Warnock et al.[16] graded the severity of fibrosis on a scale of 0 to 3+ based on visual inspection of the cut surface of inflation-fixed specimens, with ½+ defined as microscopic fibrosis only. These authors found no apparent correlation between the severity of fibrosis and total fiber content for all fibers 0.25 μ or greater in length as assessed by TEM.[16] Wagner et al.[18] graded the severity of fibrosis microscopically on a scale of 0 to 4. For the sake of convenience, their data as summarized in Table 11-3 have been tabulated as 0 to 3, with their grade-1 fibrosis listed under ½+. These authors found a progressive increase in optically visible and electron microscopically enumerated fibers with increasing severity of asbestosis.[18]

Thus there generally appears to be a correlation between the severity of fibrosis in patients with asbestosis and the tissue mineral fiber burden, although there is a wide scatter in the data.[26,50] In this regard, studies by Timbrell et al.[52] (reviewed by Lippmann[53]) have shown that, among individuals exposed to the various types of amphibole asbestos, the severity of pulmonary fibrosis correlates better with the relative fiber surface area per unit weight of tissue than with the relative fiber number or mass, as determined by magnetic alignment and light scattering. On the other hand, Churg et al.[54] in a study of asbestosis among chrysotile miners and millers found no

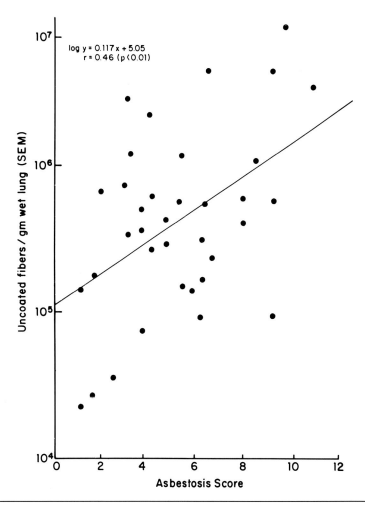

FIGURE 11-7. Correlation between uncoated fiber count by scanning electron microscopy and histologic assessment of the severity of asbestosis for 36 autopsied cases, using grading scheme of College of American Pathologists and National Institute for Occupational Safety and Health.[55] The correlation coefficient (r) for the linear regression line is 0.46 ($p < 0.01$). SEM = Scanning electron microscopy. Reprinted from Ref. 50, with permission.

correlation of fibrosis with fiber size, surface area, or mass for chrysotile and an *inverse* correlation with fiber length, aspect ratio, and surface area for contaminating tremolite asbestos. The authors did show a direct correlation between fiber concentration and severity of fibrosis for both chrysotile and tremolite fibers.[54] Further studies of the mineralogic correlates of fiber-induced pulmonary fibrosis are needed in order to resolve these discrepancies.[1]

The relationship between the tissue content of uncoated fibers 5 μ or greater in length as assessed by SEM in the authors' laboratory and the histologic asbestosis score as determined by the method proposed by the Pneumoconiosis Committee of the College of American Pathologists[55] is shown in Fig. 11-7. These data are based on 36 cases

TABLE 11-4. Correlation of histologic grade of asbestosis with tissue asbestos content and other parameters*

	Correlation coefficient (r)	p
Uncoated fibers/gm (>5 μ), SEM	0.46	<0.01
Total fibers/gm (coated and uncoated), SEM	0.44	<0.01
Asbestos bodies/gm, LM	0.26	NS
Smoking history, pack-years	0.22	NS
Age	0.12	NS
Duration of exposure, years	0.06	NS

SOURCE: Reprinted from Ref. 50, with permission.
*SEM = Scanning electron microscopy; LM = Light microscopy; Pack-years = Packs smoked daily × number of years smoked; NS = Not significant ($p > 0.05$).

of asbestosis for which tissue was available for analysis of asbestos content.[50] There is a statistically significant relationship ($p < 0.01$) between fiber content and histologic score, although as just noted, there is a wide range of scatter of the data points. It is likely that the correlation would improve with more extensive histologic and mineralogic sampling of the lungs and expression of the data as total lung burden rather than as fiber concentration.[17] This is because accumulation of collagen and other cellular components as a result of the scarring process increases the weight of the lungs and hence dilutes the concentration of fibers in the parenchyma, a point often overlooked in dust analysis studies.[56] The intercept of the regression line in Fig. 11-7 is approximately 100,000 fibers per gram of wet lung (or 1 million fibers per gram of dried lung), which coincides with the lower limit of the range of values shown in Table 11-2. It can be seen from this figure that very few patients with alveolar septal fibrosis (grade 4 or higher) have uncoated-fiber counts below 100,000 per gram, although some patients with fibrosis confined to the walls of small airways (grade 3 or less) have values well below this level.[50] This observation is in agreement with the findings of Churg[57] that relatively low tissue asbestos burdens occur in chrysotile miners and millers with fibrosis confined to the walls of small airways. The present authors' data also show a statistically significant association between histologic score and total (coated plus uncoated) fiber content as assessed by SEM, but not between histologic score and asbestos-body content as measured by light microscopy (Table 11-4). Furthermore, as the table shows there was no significant association between histologic score and patient age, duration of occupational exposure, or pack-years of smoking.[50]

In summary, analyses of tissue mineral fiber burdens in patients with asbestosis indicate a heavy lung asbestos burden in the vast majority of cases. This observation is consistent with epidemiologic evidence that asbestosis occurs primarily in individuals with direct and prolonged occupational exposure to asbestos.[1] Since no uniform method for the analysis of tissue mineral fiber content has been established, it is not presently possible to recommend a specific tissue

TABLE 11-5. Asbestos content of lung tissue in reported series of patients with mesothelioma

Source	Number of cases	Method[a]	Asbestos bodies per gram dried lung[b]	Uncoated fibers per gram dried lung[b]
Whitwell et al.[15]	100	PCLM	—	0.75 (0–70)
Gylseth et al.[64]	15	SEM	—	11 (2–490)
Mowé et al.[65]	14	SEM	—	2.4 (0.4–37)
Roggli[22]	67	SEM[c]	13.9[d] (0.01–16,000)	0.321[d] (0.012–93.1)
Churg and Wiggs[66]	10	TEM	—	3.5 (0.1–85.2)
Churg et al.[67]	6	TEM	—	238 (52–2190)
Gaudichet et al.[68]	20	TEM[c]	3.2 (0.04–450)	18
Warnock[69]	27	TEM[c]	18.5 (1.9–3800)	4.9 (0.57–137)

[a]PCLM = Phase-contrast light microscopy; SEM = Scanning electron microscopy; TEM = Transmission electron microscopy
[b]Values are the median counts for thousands (10^3) of asbestos bodies or millions (10^6) of uncoated fibers per gram of dried lung tissue, with ranges indicated in parentheses, except for the study of Gaudichet et al.,[68] where only the mean value for total fibers per gram dried lung could be obtained from the data presented.
[c]In these three studies, asbestos bodies were counted by conventional light microscopy.
[d]Values multiplied by a factor of 10 (approximate ratio of wet to dry lung weight) for purposes of comparison.

asbestos fiber content to be used as a criterion for the pathologic diagnosis of asbestosis. Nonetheless, based on the data summarized in Table 11-2, it seems unlikely that a patient with clinically significant pulmonary interstitial fibrosis who has fewer than 10^6 fibers 5 μ or greater in length per gram of dried lung (10^5 fibers/gm wet lung) tissue is suffering from asbestosis.[50] Whereas the fibrogenicity of asbestos fibers 5 μ or greater in length is well established,[58-62] the fibrogenicity of fibers less than 5 μ in length remains unproven[63] (see Chap. 10). Therefore, no tissue level of fibers in the latter size range should be proposed at the present time as a criterion for the diagnosis of asbestosis.[50]

MALIGNANT MESOTHELIOMA
Several studies have examined the asbestos content of lung tissue in series of patients with mesothelioma.[15,22,64-69] The data from these studies are summarized in Table 11-5. Whitwell et al.[15] studied 100 patients with malignant mesothelioma by means of PCLM. The median count was 750,000 combined fibers and bodies per gram of dried lung, with a range of 0–70 million fibers per gram. In only seven

cases was the combined count less than 20,000 per gram; in six of these, there was no identifiable occupational exposure to asbestos. In contrast, the count was less than 20,000 per gram in 71% of the normal control series in the same study.[15] Gylseth et al.[64] examined 15 cases of malignant mesothelioma counting fibers by means of SEM at a magnification of 4500×, and compared the results with those of 14 cases of parietal pleural plaques and 12 control cases without cancer or chronic respiratory disease. The median fiber count in the patients with mesothelioma was 11 million per gram of dried lung as compared to 2.2 million per gram in the pleural plaque cases and 0.6 million per gram among the control cases. Mowé et al.[65] used SEM at a magnification of 4500× to analyze the asbestos fiber content of lung tissue from 14 cases of mesothelioma and 28 controls matched for age, sex, year of death, and county of residence. These investigators reported a median fiber count of 2.4 million fibers per gram of dried lung among the mesothelioma patients as compared to 0.25 million fibers per gram among the controls. Roggli examined the mineral fiber content of lung tissue from 67 patients with malignant mesothelioma by SEM[17,22,28] (and unpublished observations). The median uncoated-fiber count was 32,100 fibers per gram of wet lung (approximately 321,000 fibers per gram of dried lung), as compared to a median count of 3130 fibers/gm wet lung in 20 normal lungs. These results are more similar to the findings of Whitwell et al.[15] than to those of Gylseth et al.[64] or Mowé et al.[65] (see Table 11-5) because of the magnification used in the study by Roggli (1000×), which primarily detects fibers 5 μ or greater in length.

Other studies have employed TEM to investigate the asbestos content of lung tissue in patients with malignant mesothelioma (see Table 11-5). Churg and Wiggs[66] examined 10 patients with amphibole asbestos-related mesotheliomas, and reported a median value of 3.5 million fibers per gram of dried lung. In contrast, analysis of lung tissue from six patients with malignant mesothelioma among chrysotile miners and millers resulted in a median fiber count of 238 million fibers per gram of dried lung.[67] These authors concluded that patients with mesothelioma due to exposure to chrysotile from mining and milling have large pulmonary fiber burdens relative to patients with mesothelioma secondary to exposure to amosite or crocidolite asbestos. Gaudichet et al.[68] examined lung tissue in 20 patients with mesothelioma and compared the results with those from 40 lung cancer cases and 20 patients who died from nonmalignant, non-asbestos-related processes. The mean total fiber burden for the patients with mesothelioma was 18 million fibers per gram of dried lung, as compared to 16 million fibers per gram for the lung cancer cases and 11.2 million fibers per gram for the nonmalignant control group. The main difference between the mesothelioma cases and the other comparison groups was in regard to the greater numbers of commercial amphibole fibers (amosite and crocidolite) in the former as compared to the latter. Warnock[69] studied the mineral fiber content

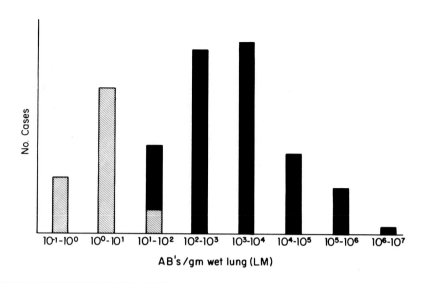

FIGURE 11-8. Distribution of asbestos-body counts in 100 patients with malignant mesothelioma. The normal values are in the range of 0–20 asbestos bodies per gram of wet lung. Note the logarithmic scale, with values ranging from 0.1 (10^{-1}) to 10 million (10^7) asbestos bodies per gram as determined by light microscopy (LM). The data are consistent with a biphasic log normal distribution with 25% of cases having a mean of 0.2 and standard deviation 0.5, while 75% of cases have a mean of 3 and standard deviation 1.5 (chi-square goodness-of-fit test, $\chi^2_6 = 4.57$, $p = 0.6$). The first distribution (hatched area) has values overlapping with those of the general population.

of lung tissue in 27 shipyard and construction workers with mesothelioma. The median total fiber count by TEM was 4.9 million fibers per gram of dried lung. In contrast, the median count in 19 unexposed controls was 0.85 million fibers per gram.

Although valuable information can also be obtained from an analysis of the tissue asbestos-body content in mesothelioma cases, only a few studies have reported such data in a series of patients with malignant mesothelioma. Gaudichet et al.[68] reported a median asbestos-body concentration of 3200 asbestos bodies per gram of dried lung tissue in 20 patients with mesothelioma. The concentration exceeded 1000 asbestos bodies per gram in 70% of mesothelioma patients, but in only 10% of 80 age- and sex-matched control cases. Warnock[69] found a median asbestos-body count of 18,500 bodies per gram of dried lung in 27 patients with mesothelioma, as compared to 300 bodies per gram in 19 nonexposed controls. Kishimoto et al.[70] reported a median asbestos-body concentration of 1360 asbestos bodies per gram of wet lung (approximately 13,600 bodies per gram of dried lung) in eight Japanese workers with mesothelioma. The present authors have had the opportunity to obtain quantitative asbestos-body counts in 100 patients with malignant mesothelioma.[17,22,71] These data are displayed as a histogram in Fig. 11-8. The median asbestos-body count for the entire series is 335 bodies per gram of wet lung (approximately 3350 bodies per gram of dried lung). In comparison, the median count for 70 control cases is less than one asbestos body per gram of wet lung, with a range of 0–20 bodies per gram.[17,71] That 28% of our mesothelioma cases had asbestos-body counts within our normal range correlates well with the findings of Chahinian et al.[72] that 70–80% of patients with mesothelioma have an identifiable exposure to asbestos, whereas 20–30% do not. Although it is possible that patients with asbestos-body counts within the normal range still have asbestos-related mesotheliomas, the distribution in Fig. 11-8 is bimodal, suggesting that these are in fact two distinct populations. It seems more likely that most of those cases with counts within the normal range represent background, or "spontaneous," mesotheliomas, or else cases due to some etiologic factor other than asbestos.[22]

The median asbestos-body count for the 16 mesothelioma cases in the authors' series who also had histologically confirmed asbestosis was 29,200 bodies per gram of wet lung. This value is quite similar to the median count of 38,700 bodies per gram of wet lung in our 76 patients with asbestosis.[50] (see Table 11-2). Excluding patients with asbestosis, the median asbestos-body count in 26 patients with parietal pleural plaques and mesothelioma was 1270 bodies per gram of wet lung, whereas the median count in 44 mesothelioma patients without plaques was 37 bodies per gram. Interestingly, the median asbestos-body count in 11 patients with peritoneal mesothelioma was only 11.3 bodies per gram of wet lung; and in seven cases the count was within our normal range. Furthermore, the median count among the 12 women with mesothelioma was only 14 asbestos bodies per gram of wet lung; and in seven cases the count was within our normal range.[22,71] This finding is consistent with the observations of McDonald and McDonald,[73] who could find a history of occupational exposure to asbestos in only 5% of women in North America with malignant mesothelioma. Asbestos bodies were observed in H&E and/or iron-stained histologic sections in 40 of 69 cases (58%) where this information was available. However, in an additional 12 cases (17%), asbestos-body levels outside our normal range were observed where bodies were not seen in histologic sections. Eight of these cases had tissue asbestos-body counts in the range of 10–100 bodies per gram of wet lung tissue (see Fig. 11-8), and cases with values that fall in this range require careful analysis of multiple samples whenever feasible.[22]

In view of the experimental observations that fibers 8.0 μ or greater in length and 0.25 μ or less in diameter are the most efficient at producing mesotheliomas,[74] it is of interest to examine fiber dimension data in studies of human cases of malignant mesothelioma. In a study of amphibole-asbestos-induced mesotheliomas, Churg and Wiggs[66] reported that 39% of amosite and 23% of crocidolite fibers exceeded 5 μ in length. In contrast, a study of chrysotile-related mesotheliomas showed that only 11% of chrysotile fibers and 13% of tremolite fibers were 5 μ or greater in length.[67] The vast majority of fibers in both studies were less than 0.25 μ in diameter.[66,67] These differences in fiber dimension may explain in part the different potential for amphibole as compared to chrysotile asbestos fibers for the production of malignant mesothelioma in humans.[49] In a recent review of the human and experimental animal data regarding fiber size and mesothelioma induction, Lippmann[53] concluded that it is primarily fibers 5 μ or greater in length and 0.1 μ or less in diameter that are responsible for the development of mesothelioma.

Almost all the studies of fiber burdens in mesothelioma patients have examined lung parenchyma. It is reasonable to assume that fibers actually reaching the pleura are the ones responsible for pleural disease, and the dimensions and types of fibers accumulating in the pleura are not necessarily similar to those accumulating in the lung. Sebastien et al.[27] reported that, in individuals exposed to mixtures of fibers, short chrysotile fibers (<5 μ) tended to accumulate in the pleura whereas longer amphibole fibers accumulated in the lung parenchyma. Churg et al.,[67] on the other hand, found no difference in the length, diameter, or type of fibers isolated from peripheral versus central lung parenchyma in Canadian chrysotile workers. Although there is considerable information available regarding the fiber content of lung parenchyma from the general population, no similar data exist for the visceral and parietal pleura or for the peritoneum. Clearly, the migration and distribution of amphibole versus chrysotile fibers to the pleural and peritoneal cavities is an area needing further investigation.[22]

In summary, patients with mesothelioma who do not also have asbestosis have considerably smaller pulmonary asbestos burdens than patients with asbestosis. This observation is consistent with epidemiologic evidence that mesothelioma can occur in individuals with brief, low-level, or indirect exposures to asbestos.[1] In over half of the patients with mesothelioma in the authors' series, asbestos bodies can be detected in histologic sections with careful scrutiny, and in nearly three-quarters of the cases, tissue digestion studies show an elevated tissue asbestos-body content. The distribution of asbestos-body counts in patients with mesothelioma appears to be bimodal (see Fig. 11-8), suggesting that there are two distinct populations: one with elevated tissue asbestos content in patients with asbestos-induced mesotheliomas, and one with a tissue asbestos content indistinguishable from a reference population in patients with "spontaneous" mesotheliomas.[15,22] Analysis of tissue asbestos content in an individual case can thus provide useful information with regard to an etiologic role for asbestos in the production of a mesothelioma.

BENIGN ASBESTOS-RELATED PLEURAL DISEASES

Relatively few studies have examined the asbestos content of lung tissue in series of patients with benign asbestos-related pleural

TABLE 11-6. Asbestos content of lung tissue in reported series of patients with benign asbestos-related pleural disease

Source	Number of cases	Method[a]	Asbestos bodies per gram dried lung[b]	Uncoated fibers per gram dried lung[b]
Gylseth et al.[64]	14	SEM	—	2.2 (0.1–13)
Roggli et al. (present study)	40	SEM[c]	14.5[d] (0.068–189)	0.26 (0.008–2.43)
Warnock et al.[75]	20	TEM[c]	7.8[d] (0.3–9600)	0.54[d] (0.018–71)
Churg[76]	29	TEM[c]	17.3[d] (0–194)	1.14[d] (ND)
Stephens et al.[77]	7[e]	PCLM	—	0.131 (0.029–0.378)
		TEM	—	28.9 (9.2–83.5)

[a]PCLM = Phase-contrast light microscopy; SEM = Scanning electron microscopy; TEM = Transmission electron microscopy
[b]Values are the median counts for thousands (10^3) of asbestos bodies or millions (10^6) of uncoated fibers per gram of dried lung tissue, with ranges indicated in parentheses, except for the study of Churg,[76] where only the mean value for total fibers per gram was given and a range could not be determined (ND).
[c]In these three studies, asbestos bodies were counted by conventional light microscopy.
[d]Values multiplied by a factor of 10 (approximate ratio of wet to dry lung weight) for purposes of comparison.
[e]Cases in series of Stephens et al.[77] are diffuse pleural fibrosis. All others are parietal pleural plaques.

disease.[64,75–77] Most of these have dealt with parietal pleural plaques, and the studies are summarized in Table 11-6. Gylseth et al.[64] studied 14 cases of parietal pleural plaques by means of SEM, and found a median of 2.2 million fibers per gram of dried lung as compared to 0.6 million fibers per gram in 12 control cases. Warnock et al.[75] reported a median of 0.54 million fibers per gram of dried lung in 20 cases of parietal pleural plaques studied by TEM, whereas Churg[76] found 1.14 million fibers per gram in 29 cases of pleural plaques. Both studies showed a significant increase in the concentrations of commercial amphiboles (amosite or crocidolite) in the lungs of patients with plaques as compared to a reference population, but no significant differences for chrysotile or noncommercial amphiboles. Whitwell et al.[15] included 21 patients with pleural plaques in their normal control series of 100 cases, and found that 55% of the cases with more than 20,000 fibers per gram as determined by PCLM but only 5.5% of cases with fewer than 20,000 fibers per gram had plaques. All of these observations support a role for asbestos fibers in the production of pleural plaques.[1]

The authors have had the opportunity to examine the mineral fiber content of the lung by SEM in 40 patients with parietal pleural plaques but no evidence of parenchymal asbestosis (see Table 11-6).

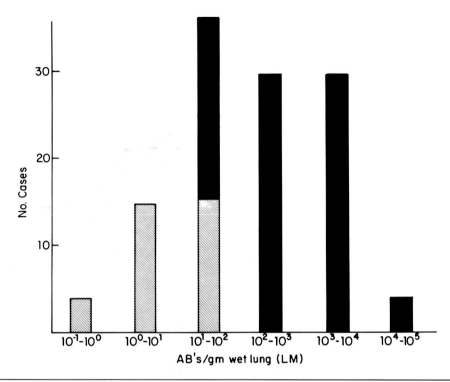

FIGURE 11-9. Distribution of asbestos body counts in 120 patients with parietal pleural plaques. The normal values are in the range of 0–20 asbestos bodies per gram of wet lung. Note the logarithmic scale, with values ranging from 0.1 (10^{-1}) to one hundred thousand (10^5) asbestos bodies per gram as determined by light microscopy (LM). There is no evidence for a biphasic log normal distribution. The hatched area has values overlapping with those of the general population.

The median fiber count for uncoated fibers 5 µ or greater in length was 0.26 million fibers per gram of dried lung, which is less than 10% of the median level in patients with asbestosis[50] (see Table 11-2). The median asbestos-body concentration by light microscopy in these 40 patients was 1450 per gram of wet lung tissue, which is similar to the median value of 780 bodies per gram in the study by Warnock et al.[75] and the value of 1730 per gram wet lung in the series reported by Churg.[76]

Asbestos-body counts made by light microscopy have been performed in the authors' laboratory in 120 cases of parietal pleural plaques, and the distribution of counts is illustrated diagramatically in Fig. 11-9. The median count for all 120 cases (including the 40 cases also studied by SEM) was 145 asbestos bodies per gram of wet lung tissue, with a range of 0–23,000 asbestos bodies per gram. This value is considerably less than the median count of 37,800 bodies per gram in 76 patients with asbestosis (with or without plaques). Among the 120 patients with plaques alone, 28% had asbestos body counts within our normal range of 0–20 asbestos bodies per gram of wet lung (see Fig. 11-9), as compared to 0% of the 76 patients with asbestosis (see

Fig. 11-6). Andrion et al.[78] reported a highly significant association between pleural plaques and the finding of asbestos bodies in 30-μ-thick histologic sections by light microscopy in a study of 191 cases of pleural plaques from a series of 996 consecutive autopsies in Torino, Italy. Whereas the distribution of asbestos-body counts in patients with plaques is unimodal (see Fig. 11-9), that in patients with mesothelioma is bimodal (see Fig. 11-8). The interpretation of this observation is not clear, but it could indicate a lower threshold for pleural plaque formation than for mesothelioma induction. The median asbestos-body count tends to be higher in patients with bilateral plaques when compared to those with unilateral plaques.[17] In addition, the asbestos-body count in histologic sections seems to correlate positively with the severity and extent of plaque formation.[78]

Benign asbestos-related pleural diseases that occur less frequently than pleural plaques include diffuse pleural fibrosis, rounded atelectasis, and benign asbestos effusions (see Chap. 6). Stephens et al.[77] examined the pulmonary mineral fiber content in seven patients with diffuse pleural fibrosis (see Table 11-6). In these seven cases the median uncoated-fiber count by PCLM was 0.131 million fibers per gram dried lung, and by TEM was 28.9 million fibers per gram. These patients on the average have a greater fiber burden than patients with pleural plaques alone, but less than patients with asbestosis (see Tables 11-2 and 11-6). The asbestos content of lung parenchyma in five patients with rounded atelectasis has been examined in the authors' laboratory. All five patients were male, and their ages ranged from 49–72 years. Two patients also had parietal pleural plaques and one had bilateral areas of rounded atelectasis. The asbestos-body counts by light microscopy in these five cases were 14, 1140, 1150, 1680, and 1980 asbestos bodies per gram of wet lung tissue. The uncoated-fiber concentrations (fibers 5 μ or greater in length) as assessed by SEM were 0.087, 0.221, 1.14, 1.58, and 1.89 million fibers per gram of dried lung tissue. These levels are within the range of values we have observed for patients with pleural plaques. We are not aware of any reports in the literature of pulmonary mineral fiber content in series of patients with benign asbestos effusion.

In summary, patients with parietal pleural plaques who do not also have asbestosis have considerably smaller pulmonary asbestos burdens than patients with asbestosis, and levels that are somewhat lower than, but of about the same order of magnitude as, patients with malignant mesothelioma. This observation is consistent with epidemiologic evidence that pleural plaques can occur in individuals with brief, low-level, or indirect exposures to asbestos.[1] Very limited information is available regarding the pulmonary mineral fiber content of patients with other benign asbestos-related pleural diseases. Preliminary observations in this regard seem to indicate that patients with rounded atelectasis have tissue asbestos levels similar to those of patients with plaques, whereas patients with diffuse pleural fibrosis have levels intermediate between those of patients with plaques and patients with asbestosis.

TABLE 11-7. Asbestos content of lung tissue in reported
series of patients with carcinoma of the lung

Source	Number of cases	Selection criteria	Method[a]	Asbestos bodies per gram dried lung[b]	Uncoated fibers per gram dried lung[b]
Whitwell et al.[15]	100	General population	PCLM	—	0.009 (0–0.115)
Gaudichet et al.[68]	40	General population	TEM[c]	0.16 (0–290)	16
Warnock et al.[16]	9	Asbestos workers	TEM[c]	35.6 (0.41–840)	5.83 (3.10–73.3)
Warnock and Isenberg[79]	75	Asbestos workers	TEM[c]	3.75 (0–1000)	2.18 (0.077–97)
Roggli et al. (present study)	48	Asbestosis	SEM[c]	334[d] (6.2–3520)	3.07[d] (0.185–78)
	25	Pleural plaques		18.8[d] (0.23–189)	0.309[d] (0.035–1.6)
	70	Other		1.70[d] (0.01–320)	0.147[d] (0.007–2.62)

[a]PCLM = Phase-contrast light microscopy; SEM = Scanning electron microscopy; TEM = Transmission electron microscopy
[b]Values are the median counts for thousands (10^3) of asbestos bodies or millions (10^6) of uncoated fibers per gram of dried lung tissue, with ranges indicated in parentheses, except for the study of Gaudichet et al.,[68] where only the mean value for total fibers per gram dried lung could be obtained from the data presented.
[c]In these four studies, asbestos bodies were counted by conventional light microscopy.
[d]Values multiplied by a factor of 10 (approximate ratio of wet to dry lung weight) for purposes of comparison.

CARCINOMA OF THE LUNG

The association between asbestos exposure and increased risk for lung cancer has been well established epidemiologically, and cigarette smoking and asbestos appear to act synergistically to increase this risk.[1] (The data supporting these observations and the pathologic features of lung cancers occurring among asbestos-exposed individuals are described in Chap. 7.) Although the association between asbestos exposure and lung cancer among individuals with asbestosis is universally accepted, the causative role for asbestos among cigarette-smoking asbestos workers with lung cancer but without asbestosis is controversial. It is therefore of interest to review what has been learned from fiber burden analysis in this regard.

Studies that have examined the asbestos content of lung tissue in series of patients with lung cancer are summarized in Table 11-7.[15,16,68,79] The values reported are influenced not only by the investigative and analytical techniques employed, but also by the way the cases were selected. Whitwell et al.[15] examined 100 consecutive cases of lung cancer by PCLM and found a similar distribution of fiber content between cancer cases and controls. Gaudichet et al.[68] included 20 patients with squamous carcinoma and 20 with adenocarcinoma of the lung, and found similar asbestos-body counts by light microscopy and fiber counts by TEM in these two groups as compared to 20 patients with pulmonary metastases and 20 with cardiovascular disease. The series of Warnock et al.[16] included seven of nine cases with histologically confirmed asbestosis, and the series of Warnock and Isenberg[79] included 12 of 62 cases with asbestosis. The authors of the latter study concluded that an asbestos-body concentration of 1000 or more per gram of dried lung tissue or a combined amosite and crocidolite fiber concentration of 100,000 or more per gram of dried lung should be used as an indication that a lung cancer may be asbestos-related.[79]

We have had the opportunity to study the asbestos content of lung tissue by SEM in 143 cases of lung cancer, and the results of our analyses are also summarized in Table 11-7. Forty-eight patients also had asbestosis, 25 had parietal pleural plaques without asbestosis, and 70 had neither plaques nor asbestosis. All had some alleged degree of asbestos exposure. The median age was similar for all three groups: 64 years (range, 48–82) for asbestosis, 63 years (range, 44–75) for plaques alone, and 60 years (range, 40–85) for the other lung cancer cases. Smoking histories were available in just over half the cases: All but six were cigarette smokers or exsmokers (see upcoming discussion). Information regarding gender was available in 112 cases, and 107 of these were men. The five women included one with asbestosis, one with pleural plaques, and three other lung cancer cases. The data from Table 11-7 show that patients with asbestosis had a median asbestos-body count that was almost 20 times that of pleural plaque cases, and an uncoated-fiber count that was 10 times greater. Similarly, patients with pleural plaques alone had an asbestos-body count more than 10 times as great and an uncoated-fiber content more than twice as great as lung cancer patients with neither plaques nor asbestosis.

Epidemiologic studies have generally failed to present convincing evidence that patients with pleural plaques alone have a significantly increased risk for developing lung cancer (see Chap. 6). Although our 70 lung cancer patients with neither plaques nor asbestosis are a very heterogeneous group with regard to type, duration, and intensity of exposure to asbestos, comparison of their pulmonary fiber burdens with those of the patients with plaques alone would suggest that *as a group* they would be unlikely to have a significantly increased risk for lung cancer as a result of exposure to asbestos. Others have argued that *in an individual case* it is the fiber burden rather than the fibrogenic response that is likely the important determinant of carcinogenic risk, and therefore patients with a fiber burden within the range of values observed for patients with asbestosis would have a similar lung cancer risk to patients with asbestosis[79] (see also Chap. 7). Among the lung cancer patients we studied, approximately half of those with pleural plaques alone and a fifth of those with neither plaques nor asbestosis had a pulmonary asbestos-body burden as evaluated by light microscopy that exceeded the fifth percentile for lung cancer–asbestosis patients (Fig. 11-10). Similarly, about half of those with plaques and a fourth of those with neither plaques nor

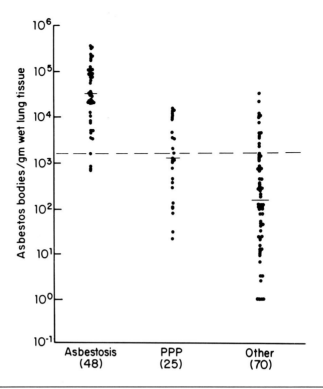

FIGURE 11-10. Histogram of asbestos-body counts in 48 patients with carcinoma of the lung and asbestosis, 25 patients with carcinoma of the lung and parietal pleural plaques (but without asbestosis), and 70 patients with carcinoma of the lung and some history of asbestos exposure but with neither plaques nor asbestosis. Median values are indicated by horizontal bars. Horizontal dashed line indicates the fifth percentile for lung cancer–asbestosis patients. Note logarithmic scale.

asbestosis had an uncoated-fiber content as determined by SEM that exceeded the fifth percentile for lung cancer–asbestosis patients. Multivariate analysis of pulmonary fiber burdens in which other confounding factors (such as pack-years of cigarette smoking, age, and sex) were adequately accounted for in a well-defined population with and without lung cancer would be very important to determine whether fiber burden in the absence of asbestosis is a significant and independent predictor of lung cancer risk. Such an analysis has not yet been reported.

Since lung cancer is quite uncommon in nonsmoking asbestos workers, it is of particular interest to consider separately the six lung cancer cases without plaques or asbestosis who were nonsmokers that we have studied. These included two women and four men, with an age range of 40–75 years (Table 11-8). All had a pulmonary adenocarcinoma, two of which were of the bronchioloalveolar cell type. One of the latter two occurred in the setting of idiopathic pulmonary fibrosis. The tissue asbestos content was outside the normal range for

TABLE 11-8. Asbestos content of lung in six nonsmokers with pulmonary carcinoma*

Case number	Age/sex	Exposure	Diagnosis[a]	Asbestos bodies per gram[b]	Uncoated fibers per gram[b]
1	40/M	Shipyard worker, 20 yr	Poorly differentiated adenocarcinoma	2,700	38,200
2	75/F	Shipyard worker, 1 yr in 1940s	Adenocarcinoma LLL	1,200	32,400
3	73/F	Household exposure, husband insulator	BACA	400	23,700
4	59/M	Merchant marine and boilermaker, 32 yr	BACA, IPF	360	20,400
5	45/M	History of asbestos exposure (details unknown)	Adenocarcinoma, LUL	25	6,340
6	46/M	Worked in building containing asbestos, 20 yr	Adenocarcinoma	14	25,000

[a]BACA = Bronchioloalveolar cell carcinoma; IPF = Idiopathic pulmonary fibrosis; LUL = Left upper lobe; LLL = Left lower lobe
[b]Values reported as asbestos bodies per gram of wet lung as determined by light microscopy and uncoated fibers per gram of wet lung as determined by SEM.

our laboratory in four of the cases (Cases 1–4). Amosite asbestos was identified by EDXA in all four of these cases, chrysotile in two (Cases 1 and 3), and tremolite and anthophyllite in one (Case 2). The tissue asbestos content was not significantly different from normal in the remaining two cases; tremolite was detected in one case by EDXA (Case 5) and amosite in the other (Case 6). Most of the fibers analyzed in these two cases were nonasbestos mineral fibers. A few studies have shown an excess risk of lung cancer among nonsmoking asbestos workers (see Chap. 7), and asbestos has been demonstrated to be a lung carcinogen in experimental animal studies (see Chap. 10). It is the authors' opinion that, in patients with carcinoma of the lung who are nonsmokers and have an elevated pulmonary asbestos burden, asbestos is a substantial contributing cause to these cancers even in the absence of asbestosis.

In summary, tissue asbestos analysis has shown that, in populations with no appreciable occupational exposure to asbestos and with substantial exposure to cigarette smoke, there is no evidence for a contributing role of asbestos in any lung cancers that occur.[15,68] This observation is not surprising when one considers that 85–90% of lung cancers occurring annually in the United States are attributable to cigarette smoking, whereas as few as 2% of cases may be related to asbestos exposure.[80] In populations with some occupational exposure to asbestos but without asbestosis, the tissue asbestos burden is greater than that of the general, unexposed population.[16,17,19] Such results may suggest, but do not *prove*, that asbestos is a substantial contributing factor to the lung cancers in those patients exposed to

asbestos who do not have asbestosis. Fiber dimensions are probably
important with regard to the carcinogenic potential of asbestos;
Lippmann[53] concluded in his review of the human and animal data
that it is primarily fibers greater than 10 μ in length and greater than
0.15 μ in diameter that are responsible for the development of lung
cancer.[1]

OTHER NEOPLASIA
A number of other malignancies have been associated with asbestos
exposure (see Chap. 8). Very little information is available in the literature regarding the pulmonary asbestos content in individuals with
these other malignancies. We have had the opportunity to study the
tissue asbestos content in 32 cases of other neoplasia, most of which
have come to our attention because of the finding of parietal pleural
plaques at autopsy. Others have been referred for analysis of the
pulmonary mineral fiber content because of a history of asbestos exposure. There are six cases of laryngeal carcinoma, six esophageal
carcinomas, eight other gastrointestinal cancers, nine hematopoietic
malignancies, and three renal cell carcinomas. The age, sex, and
asbestos-body content of the lung in these 32 cases are summarized
in Table 11-9. SEM analysis for uncoated fibers was performed in only
10 cases. Since parietal pleural plaques are a fairly common finding in
consecutive autopsy series,[81] the demonstration of an elevated lung
asbestos burden in and of itself does not prove a causal link between
these malignancies and asbestos exposure.

NORMAL LUNGS (NONEXPOSED INDIVIDUALS)
Determination of background levels of fibers to be expected in the
general population is an extraordinarily difficult task, since it is no
simple matter to define what is normal or to exclude unknown exposures. Several investigators have established ranges of fiber burdens
identified in control or reference populations,[15,28,65,68,82,83] and these
are summarized in Table 11-10. The variations in reported values can
be accounted for largely by methodologic differences and patient selection criteria. Our own control cases were selected on the basis of
having macroscopically normal lungs at autopsy and an asbestos-
body count within our previously determined normal range.[17,71] Two
cases with grossly normal lungs but with asbestos-body counts of 620
and 300 per gram of wet lung were excluded. Ten of the 20 cases have
been reported previously.[28] In order to facilitate comparison, the tissue asbestos content in the various asbestos-associated diseases and
reference populations are summarized by analytical technique (i.e.,
conventional light microscopy, PCLM, SEM, or TEM) in Tables 11-11
through 11-13. In any analysis of fiber burden data in a population
with a given disease, it is of paramount importance to compare the
findings with those of an appropriate reference or control population
for which the same analytical technique was employed.[1]

TABLE 11-9. Asbestos content of lung tissue in 32 cases of other neoplasia

Age/sex	Other diagnoses[a]	Asbestos bodies per gram[b]	Uncoated fibers per gram[b]
Laryngeal carcinoma			
64/M	PPP	10,300	51,750
64/M	PPP	7,480	—
65/M	PPP	3,260	—
67/M	PPP	1,700	—
65/M	PPP	210	—
64/M	PPP	21	—
Esophageal carcinoma			
56/M	Asbestosis	2,020,000	6,840,000
60/M	PPP	610	—
63/M	PPP	10	—
61/M		8.9	2,020
39/M		4.5	20,500
58/M	PPP	2.5	—
Other gastrointestinal cancer			
55/M	Colon ca.	28,900	269,000
57/M	Colon ca., PPP	1,190	—
67/M	Colon ca., PPP	1,120	1,600
71/M	Biliary ca.	520	13,500
71/M	Hepatocellular ca., PPP	380	—
84/M	Sq. cell ca., FOM, PPP	130	—
62/M	Sq. cell ca., FOM	19	7,810
43/M	Pancreatic ca.	36	—
Hematopoietic malignancy			
61/M	Primary pulmonary lymphoma	520	—
61/M	Immunoblastic lymphoma, PPP	330	—
61/M	CLL, Richter's syndrome, PPP	250	—
61/M	CML, blast crisis, PPP	215	—
59/M	AMML, PPP	145	—
51/M	Eosinophilic leukemia, PPP	117	—
?/M	Lymphoma	21	8,050
63/M	Nodular PDL, PPP	14	—
71/M	Lymphoma, PPP	9.2	—
Renal cell carcinoma			
59/M	BACA lung, IPF	360	20,400
62/M	Prostate and lung ca., PPP	51	—
76/M	PPP	16	—

[a]AMML = Acute myelomonocytic leukemia; BACA = Bronchioloalveolar cell carcinoma; ca. = carcinoma; CLL = Chronic lymphocytic leukemia; CML = Chronic myelogenous leukemia; FOM = Floor of mouth; IPF = Idiopathic pulmonary fibrosis; PDL = Poorly differentiated lymphocytic lymphoma; PPP = Parietal pleural plaque; Sq. = Squamous
[b]Values are asbestos bodies per gram of wet lung as determined by light microscopy, and uncoated fibers per gram of wet lung as determined by SEM.

TABLE 11-10. Asbestos content of lung tissue in reference or control populations

Source	Number of cases	Method[a]	Asbestos bodies per gram dried lung[b]	Uncoated fibers per gram dried lung[b]
Whitwell et al.[15]	100	PCLM	—	0.007 (0–0.521)
Mowé et al.[65]	28	SEM	—	0.25 (0–4.8)
Roggli et al. (present study)	20	SEM[c]	0.029[d] (0–0.22)	0.031[d] (0.004–0.169)
Gaudichet et al.[68]	20	TEM[c]	0.18 (0–3.2)	11.2
Churg and Warnock[82]	20	TEM[c]	0.28[d] (0.02–0.84)	1.29[d] (0.260–7.55)
Case and Sebastien[83]	23	TEM	—	0.62

[a]PCLM = Phase-contrast light microscopy; SEM = Scanning electron microscopy; TEM = Transmission electron microscopy
[b]Values are the median counts for thousands (10^3) of asbestos bodies or millions (10^6) of uncoated fibers per gram of dried lung tissue, with ranges indicated in parentheses, except for the study of Gaudichet et al.,[68] where only the mean value for total fibers per gram dried lung could be obtained from the data presented.
[c]In these three studies, asbestos bodies were counted by conventional light microscopy.
[d]Values multiplied by a factor of 10 (approximate ratio of wet to dry lung weight) for purposes of comparison.

TABLE 11-11. Asbestos content of lung tissue in asbestos-associated diseases—phase-contrast and conventional light microscopy

	Number of cases	Asbestos bodies per gram ($\times 10^3$)	Uncoated fibers per gram ($\times 10^6$)
Asbestosis			
Whitwell et al.[15]	23	—	8
Ashcroft and Heppleston[26]	22	12,200	32
Wagner et al.[18]	100	—	1.5
Roggli[50]	76	378	—
Warnock et al.[16]	22	123	—
Mesothelioma			
Whitwell et al.[15]	100	—	0.75
Roggli et al. (present study)	100	3.4	—
Gaudichet et al.[68]	20	3.2	—
Warnock[69]	27	18.5	—
Benign Asbestos-Related Pleural Diseases			
Warnock et al.[75]	20	7.8	—
Churg[76]	29	17.3	—
Roggli et al. (present study)	120	1.4	—
Stephens et al.[77]	7	—	0.131
Reference Population			
Whitwell et al.[15]	100	—	0.007
Roggli[50]	64	0.004	—
Churg and Warnock[82]	20	0.28	—
Gaudichet et al.[68]	20	0.18	—

TABLE 11-12. Asbestos content of lung tissue in asbestos-associated diseases—scanning electron microscopy

	Number of cases	Uncoated fibers per gram ($\times 10^6$)
Asbestosis		
Roggli[50]	76	3.3
Mesothelioma		
Gylseth et al.[64]	15	11
Mowé et al.[65]	14	2.4
Roggli[22]	67	0.32
Benign Asbestos-Related Pleural Diseases		
Gylseth et al.[64]	14	2.2
Roggli et al. (present study)	40	0.26
Reference Population		
Roggli et al. (present study)	20	0.031
Mowé et al.[65]	28	0.25

TABLE 11-13. Asbestos content of lung tissue in asbestos-associated diseases—transmission electron microscopy

	Number of cases	Uncoated fibers per gram ($\times 10^6$)
Asbestosis		
Warnock et al.[16]	22	5.68
Wagner et al.[18]	170	372
Mesothelioma		
Churg and Wiggs[66]	10	3.5
Churg et al.[67]	6	238
Gaudichet et al.[68]	20	18
Warnock et al.[69]	27	4.9
Benign Asbestos-Related Pleural Diseases		
Warnock et al.[75]	20	0.54
Churg[76]	29	1.14
Stephens et al.[77]	7	28.9
Reference Population		
Churg and Warnock[82]	20	1.29
Gaudichet et al.[68]	20	11.2
Case et al.[83]	23	0.62

RELATION BETWEEN ASBESTOS CONTENT OF LUNG TISSUE AND EXPOSURE CATEGORY

There have been relatively few studies that attempted to correlate tissue asbestos burdens with occupational exposures. Whitwell et al.[15] reported that the number of asbestos fibers found in the lungs correlated closely with patient occupations but not with their home environment. Patients living near likely sources of atmospheric asbestos pollution had asbestos fiber counts that were similar to the remainder of the patients. Sebastien et al.[27] described the tissue asbestos content in six asbestos workers with heavy exposure, six subjects who handled small amounts of asbestos during their professional life, and six randomly selected cases with no known asbestos exposure history. The mean fiber count by PCLM (400× magnification) for these three groups was 2 million, 2000, and 200 fibers per cubic centimeter of lung parenchyma, respectively. However, the difference between the first two groups was much less striking in terms of fiber counts by TEM: 10 million for the six heavily exposed as compared to 1 million fibers/cm^3 for the casually exposed subjects. Churg and Warnock[84] reported pulmonary asbestos-body counts in 252 urban patients over 40 years of age, and found that 32% of blue-collar men but less than 12% of white-collar men and blue- or white-collar women had more than 100 asbestos bodies per gram of wet lung tissue. In addition, 45% of steelworkers and 65% of construction workers had more than 100 asbestos bodies per gram.

The authors have had the opportunity to examine the pulmonary asbestos content, by LM and SEM, in 188 patients with asbestos-associated diseases and 18 patients with normal lungs whose occupational category was known. The occupational categories for these patients are summarized by disease classification in Table 11-14. The results of tissue asbestos analysis by occupational category are summarized in Table 11-15 and discussed in detail in the following sections.

INSULATORS

The highest levels of pulmonary asbestos content were found in patients categorized as asbestos insulators. These included individuals whose job descriptions involved work as an insulator, pipe fitter, pipe coverer, boilermaker, asbestos sawer, or asbestos plasterer (see Table 11-14). As Table 11-5 shows, the median asbestos-body content among 59 insulators was 20,400 AB/gm, with a range of 16–1,600,000 AB/gm, as determined by LM. The uncoated-fiber content was 224,000 uncoated fibers 5 μ or greater in length per gram of wet lung, with a range of 1660–12,500,000 fibers/gm, as determined by SEM. Thirty of the 59 insulators had histologically confirmed asbestosis (see Table 11-14). Insulators have higher asbestos-body and uncoated-fiber content of the lung than other categories of asbestos-exposed individuals, even when the duration of exposure is similar.[22] These observations correlate well with the reported high prevalence of asbestos-associated diseases among asbestos insulators.[85]

SHIPYARD WORKERS (OTHER THAN INSULATORS)

This category includes individuals whose job descriptions listed their primary occupation as a joiner, welder, rigger, sandblaster, fitter, shipwright, electrician, draftsman, handyman, engineer, or estimator. Shipyard workers whose primary occupation was as an insulator

TABLE 11-14. Occupational category for 188 patients with asbestos-associated diseases and for 18 controls

Disease	Occupational category*								
	Asbestos insulator	Shipyard worker	Railroad worker	Brake line work or repair	Other asbestos	Manual laborer	Household exposure	Building exposure	Other
Asbestosis	30	19	1	0	6	0	1	0	0
Mesothelioma	18	18	3	3	6	9	3	3	3
Parietal pleural plaque	7	11	2	0	4	1	1	0	1
Lung cancer	7	15	4	1	8	1	1	1	0
Normal lungs	0	0	0	0	0	4	0	0	14

*Asbestos insulator: Insulator, pipe fitter, pipe coverer, boilermaker, asbestos sawer, plasterer

Shipyard worker: Joiner, welder, rigger, sandblaster, fitter, shipwright, electrician, draftsman, handyman, engineer, estimator (excluding asbestos insulator)

Other asbestos: Asbestos cement worker, asbestos textile, chemical maintenance worker, welder (nonshipyard), machinist, filter manufacturer, roofing plant worker, refinery worker, sheet metal worker, industrial exposure to asbestos not further specified

Manual laborer: Construction, electrician, maintenance, painter, logger, foundry worker, heavy machinery operator, plumber, mason, carpenter/cabinetmaker, sawmill worker, airplane mechanic

Household exposure: Household contact of an asbestos worker

Building exposure: Worked in building containing asbestos materials as only known exposure. Although no cases with normal lungs are included in this category, such exposure cannot be ruled out among the 18 control cases.

Other: Textile worker, farmer, military, chemical worker, factory worker, dietitian, guard, musician, salesperson, barber, engineer, teacher, tailor, grain mill worker, building contractor, truck driver, office worker

TABLE 11-15. Asbestos content of lung tissue, by exposure category

Exposure category[a]	N	Asbestos bodies per gram (LM)[b]	Uncoated fibers per gram (SEM)[b]
Insulator	59	20,400 (16–1,600,000)	224,000 (1,660–12,500,000)
Shipyard worker (other than insulator)	60	3,600 (1.0–436,000)	37,000 (680–1,890,000)
Railroad workers	10	55 (<5–5,700)	28,800 (3,470–90,000)
Brake line work or repair	8	50 (2.6–7,740)	15,400 (1,220–54,100)
Other asbestos	24	2,360 (<3–322,000)	68,800 (1,750–901,000)
Manual laborer	15	19.6 (0.2–19,500)	8830 (<420–55,400)
Household exposure	6	1,700 (2.0–8,200)	24,300 (17,000–120,000)
Building exposure	4	1.9 (<0.2–14)	9680 (6,120–25,000)
Other	18	2.9 (0–22)	2910 (870–12,700)

[a]Exposure categories are as defined in Table 11-14, with N representing the number of cases in each category.
[b]Data are presented as median values, with range indicated in parentheses underneath, of asbestos bodies per gram of wet lung as determined by light microscopy or uncoated fibers 5 μ or greater in length per gram of wet lung as determined by SEM.

are included in the previous category of asbestos insulators. There were 60 individuals in this group of shipyard workers (see Table 11-15), and most of them did not work directly with asbestos products but rather were exposed as bystanders. The median asbestos-body content among these shipyard workers was 3600 AB/gm, with a range of 1–436,000 AB/gm, as determined by LM. The uncoated-fiber content was 37,000 uncoated fibers 5 μ or greater in length per gram of wet lung, with a range of 680–1,890,000 fibers/gm, as determined by SEM. Nineteen of the 60 shipyard workers had histologically confirmed asbestosis (see Table 11-14). The relatively high pulmonary asbestos burden among individuals with a bystander type of exposure can be related to the fact that these individuals worked side by side with others who directly handled asbestos within the tight confines of the holds of ships. The wide range of values observed in this and other categories of occupational asbestos exposure may be explained by variation in duration and intensity of exposure, cofactors such as cigarette smoking, and individual variability in clearance efficiency.

RAILROAD WORKERS
Railroad workers during the steam engine era often had the opportunity for occupational exposure to asbestos, especially workers in the machine shops or those involved with ripping out old insulation from the steam boilers and replacing it with new insulation. Such exposures virtually disappeared with the replacement of steam locomo-

tives with diesel engines. The authors have had the opportunity to examine the tissue asbestos content of the lungs in 10 individuals whose only known exposure to asbestos was as a railroad worker during the steam engine era (see Table 11-15). The median asbestos-body content among these workers was 55 AB/gm, with a range of less than 5–5700 AB/gm. The median uncoated-fiber content was 28,800 fibers 5 μ or greater in length per gram of wet lung, with a range of 3470–90,000 fibers/gm. Only one of the 10 workers had histologically confirmed asbestosis (see Table 11-14). The median uncoated-fiber content for the railroad workers is similar to that for the shipyard workers (28,000 versus 37,000 fibers/gm), but the asbestos-body counts are strikingly less (55 versus 3600 AB/gm). This may be due to the facts that chrysotile was the primary type of fiber to which the railroad workers were exposed[86] and that chrysotile is less efficient at forming asbestos bodies than are the amphiboles (see Chap. 3). Nonetheless, railroad workers were also exposed to amosite asbestos,[87] and amosite fibers have been identified by the authors in many of these workers' lungs by means of EDXA (unpublished observations).

BRAKE REPAIR WORKERS
Large numbers of workers are involved with the repair and replacement of brake linings and clutch facings in the course of their daily work. Since these friction products contain asbestos, there has been some concern that these workers are at risk for the development of asbestos-associated diseases. The results of tissue asbestos analysis of eight brake line repair workers are summarized in Table 11-15. The median asbestos-body count among these workers was 50 AB/gm, with a range of 2.6–7740 AB/gm. The median uncoated-fiber content was 15,400 fibers 5 μ or greater in length per gram of wet lung, with a range of 1220–54,100 fibers/gm. The patient with the highest asbestos-body count was a brake line grinder in a manufacturing plant for many years, who died at age 85 with advanced pulmonary fibrosis. At autopsy, the uncoated-fiber content was only 13,000 fibers/gm, and most of these were amosite. None of the eight patients had histologically confirmed asbestosis, although four patients (including the 85-year-old man) had pulmonary fibrosis.[88] Three cases of pleural mesothelioma are also included among the eight brake repair workers we have studied, and these have been reported previously.[22] Two additional cases have been described in the literature.[89,90] The low risk of asbestos-related diseases among brake repair workers and their low pulmonary asbestos content are apparently related to the nature of brake dust: It contains a low level of asbestos (about 1%), most of which is short chrysotile fibers (less than 1.0 μ in length), and the crystalline structure of much of the chrysotile in the dust has been altered by the heat generated during the braking process.[91] Experimental animal studies have confirmed the very low fibrogenic and carcinogenic potential of short asbestos fibers (see Chap. 10).

OTHER ASBESTOS WORKERS

This category includes individuals with occupational exposures to asbestos other than those described in the previous four categories. The job descriptions for these individuals listed their primary occupation as asbestos cement worker, asbestos textile worker, chemical maintenance worker, welder (nonshipyard), machinist, asbestos filter manufacturer,[92] roofing plant worker, refinery worker, sheet metal worker, or industrial exposure to asbestos not further specified (see Table 11-14). As Table 11-15 shows, the median asbestos-body content among the 24 workers in this category was 2360 AB/gm, with a range of less than 3–322,000 AB/gm. The median uncoated-fiber content was 68,800 fibers 5 μ or greater in length per gram of wet lung, with a range of 1750–901,000 fibers/gm. As a group, the asbestos-body and uncoated-fiber content of the lung among these 24 asbestos workers was similar to that among the 60 shipyard workers, but considerably less than that observed among the 59 insulators. The asbestos content of these 24 asbestos workers was considerably greater than that of 15 manual laborers with little or no direct exposure to asbestos (see Table 11-15). The manual and skilled laborer category included construction workers, electricians, maintenance workers, painters, loggers, foundry workers, heavy machinery operators, plumbers, masons, carpenters/cabinetmakers, sawmill workers, and airplane mechanics (see Table 11-14). Six of these 24 asbestos workers had histologically confirmed asbestosis, whereas none of the 15 manual laborers did.

HOUSEHOLD EXPOSURES

An increased risk of developing an asbestos-associated disease has been reported among household contacts of asbestos workers,[93,94] apparently secondary to asbestos fibers brought home on the workers' clothing. Whitwell et al.[15] reported a case of mesothelioma in the son of a worker from a gas-mask factory where the workers took crocidolite home to pack into canisters. The worker's son was found to have between 50,000 and 100,000 fibers per gram of dry lung tissue as determined by PCLM. Huncharek et al.[95] reported another case of mesothelioma in the 76-year-old wife of a shipyard machinist who dismantled boilers and other shipyard machinery for 34 years. She was found to have 6.5 million fibers per gram of dry lung as determined by TEM. Gibbs et al.[96] reported 10 cases of malignant pleural mesothelioma among household contacts of asbestos workers. The total fiber count in these individuals ranged from 5.3 million–320 million per gram of dry lung tissue. Amosite and/or crocidolite were found at elevated levels in eight of the 10 cases, whereas two cases had fiber counts within the range of a reference population. The occupations of the asbestos workers included shipyard working, lagging, building, and ordnance. In general, the fiber burdens in the lungs of the household contacts were similar to other groups of workers with light or moderate direct industrial exposure to asbestos.

The authors have had the opportunity to examine the pulmonary asbestos content in six household contacts of asbestos workers, including two housewives and one daughter of asbestos workers with pleural mesothelioma who have been reported previously.[22] The remaining three were cases of lung cancer in housewives of asbestos workers, one of whom also had asbestosis and another of whom had parietal pleural plaques (see Table 11-14). The third patient had neither plaques nor asbestosis, and this patient was also a nonsmoker (see Table 11-8 and Chap. 7). The median asbestos-body count for these six household exposures was 1700 AB/gm, with a range of 2.0–8200 AB/gm. The median uncoated-fiber content was 24,300 fibers 5 μ or greater in length per gram of wet lung, with a range of 17,000–120,000 fibers/gm (see Table 11-15). The tissue asbestos content in these six household contacts is of the same order of magnitude as that of shipyard workers and other asbestos workers (excluding insulators), and is considerably greater than that of 15 manual laborers (see Table 11-15).

ENVIRONMENTAL (BUILDING) EXPOSURES

There has been considerable scientific and public debate concerning possible risks of asbestos-induced disease derived from living or working (or attending school) in buildings containing asbestos. Certainly, the measured fiber levels in buildings are extremely low,[97] and no adverse health effects have been observed in at least one study of workers in buildings with and without asbestos insulation.[98] There is a single case report in the literature of a 54-year-old woman with pleural mesothelioma whose only known exposure to asbestos was as an office worker in a building with ceiling material composed of 70% amosite asbestos.[99] Analysis of lung tissue demonstrated 31 million fibers per gram of dry lung by TEM, the vast majority of which were found by EDXA to be amosite asbestos.

The authors have examined the pulmonary asbestos content in four patients whose alleged exposure was in buildings containing asbestos. Two patients with pleural mesothelioma and one with peritoneal mesothelioma have been reported previously.[22] The remaining patient was a 46-year-old nonsmoking man with pulmonary adenocarcinoma who had worked for 20 years in a building containing asbestos (see Table 11-8). The median asbestos-body count in these four building exposures was 1.9 AB/gm, with a range of less than 0.2–14 AB/gm. The median uncoated-fiber content was 9680 fibers 5 μ or greater in length per gram of wet lung, with a range of 6120–25,000 fibers/gm (see Table 11-15). The asbestos-body counts are indistinguishable from those of 18 individuals with no known occupational exposure to asbestos. The job descriptions for those 18 workers listed their primary occupation as textile worker, farmer, military, chemical worker, factory worker, dietitian, guard, musician, salesperson, barber, engineer, teacher, tailor, grain mill worker, building contractor, truck driver, or officer worker (see Table 11-14). The uncoated-fiber content in the four building exposure cases is slightly greater than that of the 18 individuals without known occupational exposure (see Table 11-15). Of course, the possibility of living or working in a building containing asbestos cannot be excluded in these latter 18 cases.

Although more data is needed in this controversial area, the available information indicates that except under extraordinary circumstances, the asbestos content of the lungs in patients with building exposures is in the range of that found in white-collar workers and manual laborers (see Table 11-15). It is the authors' view that, at these levels of exposure, asbestos-related diseases are extremely unlikely to occur.[100]

IDENTIFICATION OF FIBER TYPES

As noted in the earlier subsection on "Fiber Identification and Quantification," analytical electron microscopy also can be used to identify the types of mineral fibers present in a tissue sample. A number of studies have reported the results of EDXA of mineral fibers from human lung samples.[3–5,16–18,22,28,42,47,49,50,54,57,66,67,69,71,75,76,79,82,83,101–106] These studies have confirmed the observations from animal experimentation, i.e., that amphibole fibers accumulate within the lung parenchyma to a much greater degree than chrysotile fibers, which over long periods of time are more readily cleared from the lungs. The observations regarding types of mineral fibers present in human lung tissue samples from our laboratory as well as results reported in the literature are summarized in the following sections.

ASBESTOS FIBERS
McDonald et al.[107] examined the mineral fiber content of lung tissue in 99 mesothelioma cases and an equal number of age- and sex-matched controls. These investigators noted an excess of amphibole fibers (amosite and crocidolite) in cases as compared to controls, but equal quantities of chrysotile fibers in cases and controls. In a study of 78 additional cases of mesothelioma and matched referents in Canada, McDonald et al.[108] reported that relative risk was related to the concentration of long (≥ 8 μm) amphibole (amosite, crocidolite, or tremolite) fibers with no additional information provided by shorter fibers. The distribution of chrysotile, anthophyllite, and talc fibers and all other inorganic fibers in the two groups were quite similar. In a study of pulmonary mineral fiber content among six cases of malignant mesothelioma among chrysotile miners and millers, Churg et al.[67] reported that the ratio of tremolite (a contaminant of chrysotile ore) to chrysotile is considerably greater in the lungs of workers with mesothelioma as compared to other chrysotile workers. Furthermore, the median total fiber burden in chrysotile workers with mesothelioma is considerably greater than the median fiber concentrations in chrysotile workers with asbestosis.[49] This is the

reverse of the findings in patients with asbestosis versus mesothelioma secondary to amphibole or mixed fiber exposures. These observations and scattered reports of mesothelioma occurring in individuals exposed environmentally to tremolite asbestos (see Chap. 5) have led some investigators to propose that it is the tremolite component of the chrysotile ore that is responsible for the development of mesothelioma in chrysotile mine workers.[49,107,108] Alternatively, chrysotile fibers that have been previously cleared from the lungs may be the primary cause of mesothelioma in these workers, with tremolite serving merely as an indicator of the prior chrysotile dose. More likely, both chrysotile and tremolite fibers contribute to the development of disease in these individuals.

Similar observations have been reported with regard to asbestos fiber types in the lungs of individuals with asbestosis. Warnock et al.[16] found large numbers of commercial amphiboles, noncommercial amphiboles, and chrysotile fibers in patients with asbestosis. Churg[57] reported the presence of both chrysotile and tremolite fibers in the lungs of chrysotile miners and millers with asbestosis, although tremolite fibers were more abundant in the lungs of these miners when compared to the mine dust. Wagner et al.,[18] in a study of naval dockyard workers, found significantly elevated levels of commercial amphiboles in the lungs of workers with asbestosis, whereas chrysotile fibers did not show the same degree of elevation. An elevated pulmonary content of commercial amphibole fibers but not of chrysotile has also been reported for individuals with parietal pleural plaques.[75,76]

The results of the analysis of more than 3400 fibers from more than 250 patients in our laboratory are summarized in Table 11-16. Some of these data have been reported previously.[17,22,28,50,106] Analysis of the types of fibers identified according to disease category indicates that, as the pulmonary asbestos body and fiber burden increases (see Tables 11-11 and 11-12), the proportion of commercial amphiboles (amosite or crocidolite) also increases. These fibers account for only 5% of the fiber burden from individuals with background exposure (i.e., controls), but as much as 92% of the fiber burden among individuals with asbestosis. Commercial amphiboles account for 55% of the fibers identified in the lungs of patients with malignant mesothelioma (the vast majority of whom did *not* have parenchymal asbestosis), 67% of the fibers from patients with parietal pleural plaques (who did not have asbestosis or mesothelioma), and 45% of the fibers from patients with lung cancer and some history of asbestos exposure (but without asbestosis or pleural plaques). Noncommercial amphiboles (tremolite, anthophyllite, and actinolite) accounted for a smaller percentage of the fiber burden, ranging from 1.9% of fibers from patients with asbestosis to 14.5% of fibers from patients with lung cancer. Chrysotile accounted for the lowest percentage of the fiber burden for fibers 5 µm or greater in length, ranging from 0.6% of fibers from patients with asbestosis to 4.5% of fibers from patients with malignant mesothelioma. In general, the percentage of

TABLE 11-16. Energy dispersive x-ray analysis data in patients
with asbestos-associated diseases as compared to controls

Patient group	N		Commercial amphiboles[a]	Noncommercial amphiboles[b]	Chrysotile	Other[c]
Asbestosis	76	C[d]	497	4	0	13
		UC	622	19	8	52
		Total (%)	1119 (92)	23 (1.9)	8 (0.6)	65 (5.5)
Mesothelioma	57	C	183	2	10	1
		UC	289	105	29	239
		Total (%)	472 (55)	107 (12.5)	39 (4.5)	240 (28)
Pleural plaques	39	C	103	2	1	1
		UC	273	43	5	132
		Total (%)	376 (67)	45 (8.0)	6 (1.1)	133 (24)
Lung cancer	66	C	94	11	2	9
		UC	221	91	19	257
		Total (%)	315 (45)	102 (14.5)	21 (3.0)	266 (38)
Controls	20	C	2	0	0	0
		UC	3	14	2	79
		Total (%)	5 (5)	14 (14)	2 (2)	79 (79)

[a]Amosite and crocidolite
[b]Tremolite, anthophyllite, and actinolite
[c]Includes talc, silica, rutile, kaolinite, miscellaneous silicates, fiberglass, aluminum-rich fibers, iron-rich fibers, apatite, copper-zinc, tin, iron-chromium
[d]C = Coated (i.e., asbestos body); UC = Uncoated

noncommercial amphiboles and chrysotile fibers correlated inversely with the total pulmonary fiber burden. Table 11-16 also shows that the vast majority of coated fibers (i.e., ferruginous bodies) have a commercial amphibole core independent of disease category. Chrysotile asbestos bodies do occur but are distinctly uncommon (see Chap. 3).

NONASBESTOS MINERAL FIBERS
If one defines a fiber as an inorganic particle with an aspect (length to diameter) ratio of three or more and with roughly parallel sides, then studies have shown that a number of nonasbestos mineral fibers can be recovered from human lung tissue samples.[109] Among members of the general population, nonasbestos mineral fibers actually outnumber asbestos fibers by a ratio of about 4:1. In a study employing transmission electron microscopy with EDXA and electron diffraction, Churg reported that (in decreasing order of frequency) calcium phosphate (apatite), talc, silica, rutile, kaolinite, micas, feldspar, and other silicates accounted for most nonasbestos mineral fibers recovered from the human lung.[109] These minerals also account for the majority of nonfibrous particulates that can be recovered from human lung samples.[110]

The percentage of nonasbestos mineral fibers from more than 250 patients studied in our laboratory are listed by disease category in Table 11-16. Nonasbestos mineral fibers account for 79% of the fiber burden from individuals with background exposure, but for only 5.5% of the fiber burden among individuals with asbestosis. In general, the percentage of nonasbestos mineral fibers correlated inversely with the total pulmonary fiber burden. In a separate study of 796 nonasbestos mineral fibers from 156 human lung samples,[111] the most commonly encountered fibers, in decreasing order, were talc (31%), silica (18%), rutile (titanium dioxide) (14%), kaolinite (an aluminum silicate) (9%), mica or feldspar (potassium-aluminum silicates) (7%), and iron oxides (4%). The remainder were mostly silicates (10%), with various combinations of silicon with sodium, magnesium, aluminum, potassium, calcium, and iron. Metal oxides other than those of titanium or iron accounted for another 2%, and included aluminum, iron-chromium, iron-aluminum, copper-zinc, and tin fibers. Endogenous calcium fibers (mostly calcium phosphate or apatite) represented 1% of the total. Finally, a small number of fibers (3%) had smooth, parallel sides that consisted mostly of silicon with variable small peaks of aluminum, magnesium, and sodium. These are tentatively classified as fibrous glass based on their morphology and chemical composition. A few ferruginous bodies were identified with nonasbestos fibrous cores (see Table 11-16), and most of these were metal oxides with a few fibrous talc cores identified. Fibrous erionite, a hydrated aluminum silicate belonging to the zeolite family of minerals and known to be associated with malignant mesothelioma and pleural calcification (see Chaps. 3, 5, and 6), has also been identified in human lung tissue samples. Nonetheless, it has thus far not been reported in lung specimens from North America.

Although the biologic significance of nonasbestos mineral fibers is largely unknown, there is no evidence to date (with the exception of erionite) that they are of any significance in the causation of mesothelioma. However, one study has demonstrated a statistically significant increase in the pulmonary content of fibrous and nonfibrous particulates among patients with lung cancer as compared to noncancer controls matched for age, smoking history, and general occupational category.[112] Although it has been suggested that these mineral fibers and particles may play a pathogenic role in the development of lung cancer, these observations may merely imply that smokers who develop lung cancer have genetically determined less efficient clearance mechanisms for fibers, particles, tars, and associated carcinogens that may find their way into the respiratory tract.[1]

REFERENCES

1. Roggli VL: Human disease consequences of fiber exposures—A review of human lung pathology and fiber burden data. *Environ Hlth Persp* 88:295–303, 1990.
2. Berkley C, Langer AM, Baden V: Instrumental analysis of inspired fibrous pulmonary particulates. *NY Acad Sci Trans* 30:331–350, 1967.

3. Langer AM, Selikoff IJ, Sastre A: Chrysotile asbestos in the lungs of persons in New York City. *Arch Environ Health* 22:348–361, 1971.
4. Langer AM, Rubin IB, Selikoff IJ: Chemical characterization of asbestos body cores by electron microprobe analysis. *J Histochem Cytochem* 20:723–734, 1972.
5. Langer AM, Rubin IB, Selikoff IJ, Pooley FD: Chemical characterization of uncoated asbestos fibers from the lungs of asbestos workers by electron microprobe analysis. *J Histochem Cytochem* 20:735–740, 1972.
6. Langer AM, Ashley R, Baden V, Berkley C, Hammond EC, Mackler AD, Maggiore CJ, Nicholson WJ, Rohl AN, Rubin IB, Sastre A, Selikoff IJ: Identification of asbestos in human tissues. *J Occup Med* 15:287–295, 1973.
7. Langer AM, Mackler AD, Pooley FD: Electron microscopical investigation of asbestos fibers. *Environ Hlth Persp* 9:63–80, 1974.
8. Pooley FD: The identification of asbestos dust with an electron microscope analyser. *Ann Occup Hyg* 18:181–186, 1975.
9. Hayashi H: Energy dispersive x-ray analysis of asbestos fibers. *Clay Sci* 5:145–154, 1978.
10. Abraham JL: Recent advances in pneumoconiosis: The pathologists' role in etiologic diagnosis. In: *The Lung*, IAP Monograph 19. Baltimore: Williams & Wilkins, 1978, pp. 96–137.
11. Churg A: Fiber counting and analysis in the diagnosis of asbestos-related disease. *Hum Pathol* 13:381–392, 1982.
12. Roggli VL, Shelburne JD: New concepts in the diagnosis of mineral pneumoconioses. *Sem Respir Med* 4:128–138, 1982.
13. Vallyathan V, Green FHY: The role of analytical techniques in the diagnosis of asbestos-associated disease. *CRC Crit Rev Clin Lab Sci* 22:1–42, 1984.
14. Churg A: Analysis of asbestos fibers from lung tissue: Research and diagnostic uses. *Sem Respir Med* 7:281–288, 1986.
15. Whitwell F, Scott J, Grimshaw M: Relationship between occupations and asbestos fibre content of the lungs in patients with pleural mesothelioma, lung cancer, and other diseases. *Thorax* 32:377–386, 1977.
16. Warnock ML, Kuwahara TJ, Wolery G: The relation of asbestos burden to asbestosis and lung cancer. *Pathol Annu* 18(2):109–145, 1983.
17. Roggli VL, Pratt PC, Brody AR: Asbestos content of lung tissue in asbestos-associated diseases: A study of 110 cases. *Br J Ind Med* 43:18–28, 1986.
18. Wagner JC, Moncrief CB, Coles R, Griffiths DM, Munday DE: Correlation between fibre content of the lungs and disease in naval dockyard workers. *Br J Ind Med* 43:391–395, 1986.
19. Kane PB, Goldman SL, Pillai BH, Bergofsky EH: Diagnosis of asbestosis by transbronchial biopsy: A method to facilitate demonstration of ferruginous bodies. *Am Rev Respir Dis* 115:689–694, 1977.
20. Dodson RF, Hurst GA, Williams MG, Corn C, Greenberg SD: Comparison of light and electron microscopy for defining occupational asbestos exposure in transbronchial lung biopsies. *Chest* 94:366–370, 1988.
21. Roggli VL: Preparatory techniques for the quantitative analysis of asbestos in tissues. *Proceedings of the 46th Annual Meeting of the Electron Microscopy Society of America* (Bailey GW, ed.), San Francisco: San Francisco Press, 1988, pp. 84–85.
22. Roggli VL: Mineral fiber content of lung tissue in patients with malignant mesothelioma. Ch. 6 In: *Malignant Mesothelioma* (Henderson DW, Shilkin KB, Langlois SLP, Whitaker D, eds.), Washington, DC: Hemisphere Pub., 1991, pp. 201–222.
23. Gylseth B, Baunan RH, Bruun R: Analysis of inorganic fiber concentrations in biological samples by scanning electron microscopy. *Scand J Work Environ Health* 7:101–108, 1981.

24. O'Sullivan MF, Corn CJ, Dodson RF: Comparative efficiency of Nuclepore filters of various pore sizes as used in digestion studies of tissue. *Environ Res* 43:97–103, 1987.

25. Morgan A, Holmes A: The distribution and characteristics of asbestos fibers in the lungs of Finnish anthophyllite mine-workers. *Environ Res* 33:62–75, 1984.

26. Ashcroft T, Heppleston AG: The optical and electron microscopic determination of pulmonary asbestos fibre concentration and its relation to the human pathological reaction. *J Clin Pathol* 26:224–234, 1973.

27. Sebastien P, Fondimare A, Bignon J, Monchaux G, Desbordes J, Bonnaud G: Topographic distribution of asbestos fibers in human lung in relation to occupational and nonoccupational exposure. In: *Inhaled Particles* IV (Walton WH, McGovern B, eds.), Oxford: Pergamon Press, 1977, pp. 435–444.

28. Roggli VL: Scanning electron microscopic analysis of mineral fibers in human lungs. Ch. 5 In: *Microprobe Analysis in Medicine* (Ingram P, Shelburne JD, Roggli VL, eds.), New York: Hemisphere Pub., 1989, pp. 97–110.

29. Ferrell RE, Jr., Paulson GG, Walker CW: Evaluation of an SEM-EDS method for identification of chrysotile. *Scanning Electron Microsc* II: 537–546, 1975.

30. Millette JR, McFarren EF: EDS of waterborne asbestos fibers in TEM, SEM and STEM. *Scanning Electron Microsc* III: 451–460, 1976.

31. Johnson GG, White EW, Strickler D, Hoover R: Image analysis techniques. In: *Symposium on Electron Microscopy of Microfibers: Proceedings of the First FDA Office of Science Summer Symposium* (Asher IM, McGrath PP, eds.), Washington, DC: U.S. Government Printing Office, 1976, pp. 76–82.

32. Kenny LC: Asbestos fibre counting by image analysis—The performance of the Manchester Asbestos Program on Magiscan. *Ann Occup Hyg* 28: 401–415, 1984.

33. Kenny LC: Automated analysis of asbestos clearance samples. *Ann Occup Hyg* 32:115–128, 1988.

34. Ruud CO, Barrett CS, Russell PA, Clark RL: Selected area electron diffraction and energy dispersive x-ray analysis for the identification of asbestos fibres, a comparison. *Micron* 7:115–132, 1976.

35. Churg A: Quantitative methods for analysis of disease induced by asbestos and other mineral particles using the transmission electron microscope. Ch. 4 In: *Microprobe Analysis in Medicine* (Ingram P, Shelburne JD, Roggli VL, eds.), New York: Hemisphere Pub., 1989, pp. 79–95.

36. Churg A, Sakoda N, Warnock ML: A simple method for preparing ferruginous bodies for electron microscope examination. *Am J Clin Pathol* 68:513–517, 1977.

37. Schraufnagel D, Ingram P, Roggli VL, Shelburne JD: An introduction to analytical electron microscopy and microprobe analysis: Techniques and tools to study the lung. In: *Electron Microscopy of the Lung* (Schraufnagel D, ed.), New York: Marcel Dekker, 1990, pp. 1–46.

38. Yatchmenoff B: A new confocal scanning optical microscope. *Amer Lab* 20:58, 60–62, 64, 66, 1988.

39. MacDonald JL, Kane AB: Identification of asbestos fibers within single cells. *Lab Invest* 55:177–185, 1986.

40. Geiss RH: Electron diffraction from submicron areas using STEM. *Scanning Electron Microsc* II: 337–344, 1976.

41. Gylseth B, Churg A, Davis JMG, Johnson N, Morgan A, Mowe G, Rogers A, Roggli V: Analysis of asbestos fibers and asbestos bodies in tissue samples from human lung: An international interlaboratory trial. *Scand J Work Environ Health* 11:107–110, 1985.

42. Gylseth B, Baunan RH, Overaae L: Analysis of fibers in human lung tissue. *Br J Ind Med* 39:191–195, 1982.

43. Corn CJ, Williams MG, Jr., Dodson RF: Electron microscopic analysis of residual asbestos remaining in preparative vials following bleach digestion. *J Electron Microsc Tech* 6:1–6, 1987.

44. Steel EB, Small JA: Accuracy of transmission electron microscopy for the analysis of asbestos in ambient environments. *Anal Chem* 57:209–213, 1985.

45. Ogden TL, Shenton-Taylor T, Cherrie JW, Crawford NP, Moorcraft S, Duggan MJ, Jackson PA, Treble RD: Within-laboratory quality control of asbestos counting. *Ann Occup Hyg* 30:411–425, 1986.

46. Morgan A, Holmes A: Distribution and characteristics of amphibole asbestos fibres in the left lung of an insulation worker measured with the light microscope. *Br J Ind Med* 40:45–50, 1983.

47. Roggli VL, Greenberg SD, Seitzman LH, McGavran MH, Hurst GA, Spivey CG, Nelson KG, Hieger LR: Pulmonary fibrosis, carcinoma, and ferruginous body counts in amosite asbestos workers: A study of six cases. *Am J Clin Pathol* 73:496–503, 1980.

48. Wagner JC, Pooley FD: Mineral fibres and mesothelioma. *Thorax* 41:161–166, 1986.

49. Churg A: Chrysotile, tremolite, and malignant mesothelioma in man. *Chest* 93:621–628, 1988.

50. Roggli, VL: Pathology of human asbestosis: A critical review. In: *Advances in Pathology*, vol. 2 (Fenoglio-Preiser CM, ed.), Chicago: Year Book, 1989, pp. 31–60.

51. Roggli VL, Pratt PC: Numbers of asbestos bodies on iron-stained tissue sections in relation to asbestos body counts in lung tissue digests. *Hum Pathol* 14:355–361, 1983.

52. Timbrell V, Ashcroft T, Goldstein B, Heyworth F, Meurman LO, Rendall REG, Reynolds JA, Shilkin KB, Whitaker D: Relationships between retained amphibole fibers and fibrosis in human lung tissue specimens. *Ann Occup Hyg* 32:323–340, 1988.

53. Lippmann M: Asbestos exposure indices. *Environ Res* 46:86–106, 1988.

54. Churg A, Wright JL, De Paoli L, Wiggs B: Mineralogic correlates of fibrosis in chrysotile miners and millers. *Am Rev Respir Dis* 139:891–896, 1989.

55. Craighead JE, Abraham JL, Churg A, et al.: Pathology of asbestos-associated diseases of the lungs and pleural cavities: Diagnostic criteria and proposed grading schema. *Arch Pathol Lab Med* 106:544–596, 1982.

56. Pratt PC: Role of silica in progressive massive fibrosis in coal workers' pneumoconiosis. *Arch Environ Health* 16:734–737, 1968.

57. Churg A: Asbestos fiber content of the lungs in patients with and without asbestos airways disease. *Am Rev Respir Dis* 127:470–473, 1983.

58. Vorwald AJ, Durkan TM, Pratt PC: Experimental studies of asbestosis. *Arch Ind Hyg Occup Med* 3:1–43, 1951.

59. Wright GW, Kuschner M: The influence of varying lengths of glass and asbestos fibers on tissue response in guinea pigs. In: *Inhaled Particles* IV (Walton WH, ed.), Oxford: Pergamon Press, 1977, pp. 455–474.

60. Davis JMG, Beckett ST, Bolton RE, Collings P, Middleton AP: Mass and number of fibres in the pathogenesis of asbestos-related lung disease in rats. *Br J Cancer* 37:673–688, 1978.

61. Crapo JD, Barry BE, Brody AR, O'Neil JJ: Morphological, morphometric, and x-ray microanalytical studies on lung tissue of rats exposed to chrysotile asbestos in inhalation chambers. In: *Biological Effects of Mineral Fibres*, vol. 1 (Wagner JC, ed.), Lyon: IARC Scientific Publications, 1980, pp. 273–283.

62. Lee KP, Barras CE, Griffith FD, Waritz RS, Lapin CA: Comparative pulmonary responses to inhaled inorganic fibers with asbestos and fiberglass. *Environ Res* 24:167–191, 1981.

63. Gross P: Is short-fibered asbestos dust a biological hazard? *Arch Environ Health* 29:115–117, 1974.
64. Gylseth B, Mowé G, Skaug V, Wannag A: Inorganic fibers in lung tissue from patients with pleural plaques or malignant mesothelioma. *Scand J Work Environ Health* 7:109–113, 1981.
65. Mowé G, Gylseth B, Hartveit F, Skaug V: Fiber concentration in lung tissue of patients with malignant mesothelioma: A case-control study. *Cancer* 56:1089–1093, 1985.
66. Churg A, Wiggs B: Fiber size and number in amphibole-asbestos-induced mesothelioma. *Am J Pathol* 115:437–442, 1984.
67. Churg A, Wiggs B, De Paoli L, Kampe B, Stevens B: Lung asbestos content in chrysotile workers with mesothelioma. *Am Rev Respir Dis* 130: 1042–1045, 1984.
68. Gaudichet A, Janson X, Monchaux G, Dufour G, Sebastien P, DeLajartre AY, Bignon J: Assessment by analytical microscopy of the total lung fibre burden in mesothelioma patients matched with four other pathological series. *Ann Occup Hyg* 32[Suppl 1]: 213–223, 1988.
69. Warnock ML: Lung asbestos burden in shipyard and construction workers with mesothelioma: Comparison with burdens in subjects with asbestosis or lung cancer. *Environ Res* 50:68–85, 1989.
70. Kishimoto T, Okada K, Sato T, Ono T, Ito H: Evaluation of the pleural malignant mesothelioma patients with the relation of asbestos exposure. *Environ Res* 48:42–48, 1989.
71. Roggli VL, McGavran MH, Subach JA, Sybers HD, Greenberg SD: Pulmonary asbestos body counts and electron probe analysis of asbestos body cores in patients with mesothelioma: A study of 25 cases. *Cancer* 50:2423–2432, 1982.
72. Chahinian AP, Pajak TF, Holland JF, Norton L, Ambinder RM, Mandel EM: Diffuse malignant mesothelioma: Prospective evaluation of 69 patients. *Ann Int Med* 96:746–755, 1982.
73. McDonald AD, McDonald JC: Malignant mesothelioma in North America. *Cancer* 46:1650–1656, 1980.
74. Stanton MF, Layard M, Tegeris A, Miller E, May M, Morgan E, Smith A: Relation of particle dimension to carcinogenicity in amphibole asbestoses and other fibrous minerals. *J Natl Cancer Inst* 67:965–975, 1981.
75. Warnock ML, Prescott BT, Kuwahara TJ: Numbers and types of asbestos fibers in subjects with pleural plaques. *Am J Pathol* 109:37–46, 1982.
76. Churg A: Asbestos fibers and pleural plaques in a general autopsy population. *Am J Pathol* 109:88–96, 1982.
77. Stephens M, Gibbs AR, Pooley FD, Wagner JC: Asbestos-induced diffuse pleural fibrosis: Pathology and mineralogy. *Thorax* 42:583–588, 1987.
78. Andrion A, Colombo A, Mollo F: Lung asbestos bodies and pleural plaques at autopsy. *La Ricerca Clin Lab* 12:461–468, 1982.
79. Warnock ML, Isenberg W: Asbestos burden and the pathology of lung cancer. *Chest* 89:20–26, 1986.
80. Gaensler EA, McLoud TC, Carrington CB: Thoracic surgical problems in asbestos-related disorders. *Ann Thorac Surg* 40:82–96, 1985.
81. Wain SL, Roggli VL, Foster WL: Parietal pleural plaques, asbestos bodies, and neoplasia: A clinical, pathologic, and roentgenographic correlation of 25 consecutive cases. *Chest* 86:707–713, 1984.
82. Churg A, Warnock ML: Asbestos fibers in the general population. *Am Rev Respir Dis* 122:669–678, 1980.
83. Case BW, Sebastien P: Environmental and occupational exposures to chrysotile asbestos: A comparative microanalytic study. *Arch Environ Health* 42:185–191, 1987.
84. Churg A, Warnock ML: Correlation of quantitative asbestos body counts and occupation in urban patients. *Arch Pathol Lab Med* 101:629–634, 1977.

85. Hammond EC, Selikoff IJ, Seidman H: Asbestos exposure, cigarette smoking, and death rates. In: Health Hazards of Asbestos Exposure (Selikoff IJ, Hammond EC, eds.), *Ann NY Acad Sci* 330:473–490, 1979.

86. Mancuso TF: Relative risk of mesothelioma among railroad machinists exposed to chrysotile. *Am J Ind Med* 13:639–657, 1988.

87. Mancuso TF: Mesothelioma among machinists in railroad and other industries. *Am J Ind Med* 4:501–513, 1983.

88. Roggli VL: Scanning electron microscopic analysis of mineral fiber content of lung tissue in the evaluation of diffuse pulmonary fibrosis. *Scanning Microsc* 5:71–83, 1991.

89. Langer AM, McCaughey WTE: Mesothelioma in a brake repair worker. *Lancet* 2:1101–1103, 1982.

90. Huncharek M, Muscat J, Capotorto JV: Pleural mesothelioma in a brake mechanic. *Br J Ind Med* 46:69–71, 1989.

91. Williams RL, Muhlbaier JL: Asbestos brake emissions. *Environ Res* 29:70–82, 1982.

92. Talcott JA, Thurber WA, Kantor AF, Gaensler EA, Danahy JF, Antman KH, Li FP: Asbestos-associated diseases in a cohort of cigarette-filter workers. *N Engl J Med* 321:1220–1223, 1989.

93. Anderson HA, Lilis R, Daum SM, Selikoff IJ: Asbestosis among household contacts of asbestos factory workers. *Ann NY Acad Sci* 330:387–399, 1979.

94. Newhouse ML, Thompson H: Mesothelioma of pleura and peritoneum following exposure to asbestos in the London area. *Br J Ind Med* 22:261–269, 1965.

95. Huncharek M, Capotorto JV, Muscat J: Domestic asbestos exposure, lung fibre burden, and pleural mesothelioma in a housewife. *Br J Ind Med* 46:354–355, 1989.

96. Gibbs AR, Griffiths DM, Pooley FD, Jones JSP: Comparison of fibre types and size distributions in lung tissues of paraoccupational and occupational cases of malignant mesothelioma. *Br J Ind Med* 47:621–626, 1990.

97. Crump KS, Farrar DB: Statistical analysis of data on airborne asbestos levels collected in an EPA survey of public buildings. *Reg Toxicol Pharmacol* 10:51–62, 1989.

98. Cordier S, Lazar P, Brochard P, Bignon J, Ameille J, Proteau J: Epidemiologic investigation of respiratory effects related to environmental exposure to asbestos inside insulated buildings. *Arch Environ Health* 42:303–309, 1987.

99. Stein RC, Kitajewska JY, Kirkham JB, Tait N, Sinha G, Rudd RM: Pleural mesothelioma resulting from exposure to amosite asbestos in a building. *Respir Med* 83:237–239, 1989.

100. Mossman BT, Bignon J, Corn M, Seaton A, Gee JBL: Asbestos: scientific developments and implications for public policy. *Science* 247:294–301, 1990.

101. Pooley FD: An examination of the fibrous mineral content of asbestos lung tissue from the Canadian chrysotile mining industry. *Environ Res* 12:281–298, 1976.

102. Chen W-j, Mottet NK: Malignant mesothelioma with minimal asbestos exposure. *Hum Pathol* 9:253–258, 1978.

103. Churg A, Warnock ML: Analysis of the cores of asbestos bodies from members of the general population: Patients with probable low-degree exposure to asbestos. *Am Rev Respir Dis* 120:781–786, 1979.

104. Gylseth B, Norseth T, Skaug V: Amphibole fibers in a taconite mine and in the lungs of the miners. *Am J Ind Med* 2:175–184, 1981.

105. Rowlands N, Gibbs GW, McDonald AD: Asbestos fibres in the lungs of chrysotile miners and millers—A preliminary report. *Ann Occup Hyg* 26:411–415, 1982.

106. Roggli VL: Analytical electron microscopy of mineral fibers from human lungs. In: *Proceedings of the 45th Annual Meeting of the Electron Microscopy Society of America* (Bailey GW, ed.), San Francisco: San Francisco Press, 1987, pp. 666–669.
107. McDonald AD, McDonald JC, Pooley FD: Mineral fibre content of lung in mesothelial tumours in North America. *Ann Occup Hyg* 26:417–422, 1982.
108. McDonald JC, Armstrong B, Case B, Doell D, McCaughey WTE, McDonald AD, Sébastien P: Mesothelioma and asbestos fiber type: Evidence from lung tissue analyses. *Cancer* 63:1544–1547, 1989.
109. Churg A: Nonasbestos pulmonary mineral fibers in the general population. *Environ Res* 31:189–200, 1983.
110. Stettler LE, Groth DH, Platek SF, Burg JR: Particulate concentrations in urban lungs. Ch. 7 In: *Microprobe Analysis in Medicine* (Ingram P, Shelburne JD, Roggli VL, eds.), New York: Hemisphere Pub., 1989, pp. 133–146.
111. Roggli VL: Nonasbestos mineral fibers in human lungs. In: *Microbeam Analysis—1989* (Russell PE, ed.), San Francisco: San Francisco Press, 1989, pp. 57–59.
112. Churg A, Wiggs B: Mineral particles, mineral fibers, and lung cancer. *Environ Res* 37:364–372, 1985.

12. Medicolegal Aspects of Asbestos-Related Diseases: Plaintiff's Attorney's Perspective

RONALD L. MOTLEY AND CHARLES W. PATRICK, JR.

When Judge John Minor Wisdom issued the opinion of the United States Court of Appeals for the Fifth Circuit in *Borel* v. *Fibreboard Paper Products Corporation*[1] on September 10, 1973, little did anyone expect that this decision—extending the doctrine of strict product liability to asbestos-related diseases caused by the use of insulation materials—would engender a wave of personal injury litigation never before seen in American jurisprudence. Less than 10 years later, over 16,000 asbestos-related personal injury cases had been filed in the United States, and, in the words of a subsequent opinion by the Fifth Circuit, asbestos litigation "had become the largest area of product liability litigation, far surpassing the number of cases generated by the controversies over Agent Orange, the drug DES, the Dalkon Shield intrauterine device, or even automobile defects."[2] Even after the chapter 11 bankruptcy filings by a number of former manufacturers of asbestos-containing products and efforts by asbestos companies to shield their assets and jettison their liabilities through intricate corporate reorganizations, the asbestos case avalanche continues unabated. It is estimated that there are 90,000 cases pending in state and federal courts,[3] and in the year ending June 30, 1990, an average of 1140 asbestos cases per month were filed in the federal district courts alone.[4]

In the 1990s, the epidemic of asbestos litigation mirrors the pandemic of asbestos disease that has been caused by the extensive use of this mineral in insulation and other products. There have been various estimates of the projected number of asbestos-related diseases that will occur in the next 20–30 years; one projection maintains that 131,200 deaths from asbestos-related cancer alone will occur in the United States between 1985 and 2009.[5] No one knows with any precision the actual number of court cases that will arise from this epidemic of asbestos disease,[6] but it is certain that there will be an enormous number of claims that will serve to further tax an already overburdened judicial system. It is only fitting, therefore, that the federal judicial district that gave birth to asbestos litigation is at the center of the effort to fashion an equitable and lasting solution to the mammoth litigation. On August 20, 1990, Judge Robert Parker of the Eastern District of Texas, the district in which Clarence Borel's case was tried,[7] issued an order allowing a national asbestos personal injury class action to proceed.[8] In order to maximize limited resources, national coordination of asbestos litigation utilizing the class action device and multidistrict discovery is necessary,[9] and certain common issues of law and fact may be decided in a central forum before a determination of other issues unique to the individual cases, such as causation, is made in a local forum.

In all probability, the focus of future asbestos disease trials will shift from liability issues—which may be decided in a national class trial—to medical and causation issues. The role of pathology will, therefore, become more important as the medical issues become more dominant. The task of the plaintiff's lawyer in future asbestos litigation will be to maximize recovery in a trial that may be devoid of evidence of corporate misconduct, which has great emotional impact, and will concentrate on the more technical, but less exciting, issues of causation.

PROVING THE ASBESTOS DISEASE CASE

Unless global resolution of asbestos cases can be accomplished or until a national class action trial is ordered, an asbestos trial consists of plaintiff proving that the manufacturers knew or should have known of the hazards of asbestos, that plaintiff was exposed to the manufacturers' products, that plaintiff's exposure to asbestos caused the disease process, and that plaintiff has suffered damages, such as loss of income or medical expenses, because of the defendant's failure to warn. Additionally, the plaintiff may be able to prove that the defendants acted with reckless disregard, which may justify punitive damages. Absent consolidation, the necessary elements of an asbestos case must be proved anew in each trial. To try the issues of negligence, recklessness, and the hazards of asbestos in each and every asbestos case is, at best, unnecessarily repetitious and, at worst, a colossal waste of time and resources. Nevertheless, until a better solution is found, plaintiff's counsel must prove corporate liability and product defect in each trial.

Under the product liability laws of most states, the plaintiff must prove that the manufacturers either knew or should have known that their asbestos-containing products were hazardous, and that the manufacturers failed to give adequate warnings of those dangers. Establishing this burden can be accomplished in two ways. The plaintiff may prove through oral testimony or documentary evidence that a manufacturer was actually aware that its products containing asbestos could cause harm to the users of those products.[10] Alternatively, a plaintiff may prove that, if a manufacturer were to have reviewed the scientific and medical literature at the time its products were sold, such an analysis would have revealed that asbestos was known to be dangerous. Under the law of product liability, a manufacturer is presumed to know the hazards of its products, and *Borel* established that a manufacturer is considered to be an expert with regard to the dangers of its products.

At trial, a plaintiff may establish the manufacturers' actual knowledge by introducing as exhibits the internal correspondence and memoranda of the companies. For instance, a plaintiff may seek introduction of the correspondence between Johns-Manville and Raybestos Manhattan in 1935 that discussed whether the medical evidence of the hazards of asbestos should be published in a trade magazine known as *Asbestos*. As the publisher of the journal stated in a letter to Sumner Simpson, the president of Raybestos Manhattan, in 1935: "Always you have requested that for certain obvious reasons we publish nothing, and, naturally your wishes have been respected."[11] On October 1, 1935, Simpson forwarded the letter from the magazine's publisher to Vandiver Brown, secretary and general counsel of Johns-Manville. In reference to the study financed by the companies and performed by Dr. Anthony Lanza, Simpson stated:

As I see it personally, we would be just as well off to say nothing about it until our survey is complete. I think the less said about asbestos, the better off we are, but at the same time, we cannot lose track of the fact that there have been a number of articles on asbestos dust control and asbestosis in the British trade magazines.[12]

On October 3, 1935, Brown responded by saying, "I quite agree with you that our interests are best served by having asbestosis receive the minimum of publicity."[13]

The attitude of these corporate executives regarding whether to reveal the hazards of asbestos to the public is representative of that found in many other documents. In face of the mounting evidence concerning the relationship between asbestos and lung cancer, there was a proposal that the Asbestos Textile Institute, a trade organization, sponsor a study on the incidence of lung cancer among American asbestos workers. In minutes of the meeting of March 7, 1957, the member companies rejected their proposal and stated: "There is a feeling among certain members that such an investigation would stir up a hornets' nest and put the whole industry under suspicion."[14] The history of Johns-Manville's conduct with regard to the hazards of asbestos was reviewed in 1979 by an executive of that company, and his memorandum to the chief executive officer of Johns-Manville, John McKinney, sums up that company's attitude regarding the health and safety of the workers who would be exposed to their products. As the asbestos trials began to increase in number, C. G. Linke wrote, on January 12, 1979, "We must now face reality and ask ourselves whether or not we are playing semantic games in constructing our defense which may be appropriate for a court of law, but fade into incredulity under the stare of public opinion."[15] He continues by contrasting the position of Johns-Manville in trials against historical facts: "From an 'average man' point of view, here are a few examples: 1. *J. M. position:* Prior to 1964, we lacked scientific knowledge about cancer hazards of asbestos. *Fact:* In mid-'50s, J. M. officials knew of scientific studies showing a relationship between cancer and asbestos." Further along, he states, "*J. M. position:* We have communicated openly with employees about illnesses. *Fact:* A current J. M. employee tells me it was company practice until the early '70s not to tell a person about his illness." Mr. Linke concludes: "John, looking at this company and its statements from a general public point of view, I can easily see why we have members of Congress calling us liars."

Documentary evidence concerning Manville's conduct with regard to the health and safety of its workers shows it was sordid; and, unfortunately, the conduct of the other principal manufacturers of asbestos products was not much better. Before Owens-Corning Fiberglas purchased the manufacturing facilities for Kaylo from Owens-Illinois, it knew that asbestos insulation workers were becoming ill from asbestosis.[16] In 1963, one of its executives wrote that asbestos in Kaylo "when breathed in the lungs causes asbestosis which often leads to lung cancer."[17] In 1969, the medical director of Owens-Corning Fiberglas was asked his opinions as to when the hazards of asbestos were first known. In a memorandum, he stated that the dangers have been "well known and well documented" since at least the early 1940s.[18]

When the companies were finally forced to place caution labels on their products in order to limit liability, a Pittsburgh Corning executive wrote to one of its lawyers in Texas, who, in 1969, was defending one of the first asbestos-related-disease lawsuits. The executive informed the lawyer that a decision had been made to place a caution label on Unibestos, a Pittsburgh Corning product, but that the company would delay placement of the caution label if the lawyer believed the decision to do so would prejudice the company's defense.[19]

Against this background of documents that will be introduced at trial, evidence concerning the medical and scientific literature seems to pale in comparison. In fact, the industrial physicians knew as much, if not more, about the hazards of asbestos-containing products than the rest of the scientific community. However, a plaintiff may present evidence—through a medical historian or a scientist who lived and worked through that period of time—that asbestos-related diseases have been recognized throughout the century. As stated by Dr. David Ozonoff, a professor of public health at Boston University and a medical historian:

The knowledge that exposure to asbestos could cause a serious chronic pulmonary disease called asbestosis was irrefutable and generally accepted by 1930. The suspicion that asbestos could cause cancer of the lung was first voiced in the 1930s, was considered a probable relationship by 1942, and was generally accepted by 1949. Epidemiological studies in the mid-1950s left little room for doubt. The index of suspicion relating asbestos exposure to the rare tumors called mesothelioma was high by 1953, and by 1960, the full extent of the relationship was being revealed. Exposure to asbestos in the course of work with asbestos-containing products posed the same hazards as exposures in the factory setting; The simple fact that "asbestos was asbestos" was evident from the medical record and confirmed by numerous case reports and studies showing harm to those who worked with asbestos products.[20]

Ironically, the asbestos companies usually present a medical historian to offer their defense that it was not until the publication of the Selikoff studies in 1964 that they either knew or should have known of the hazards of asbestos to insulation workers. The asbestos companies present evidence that the threshold limit value (TLV) for asbestos was established in 1946 as 5 million particles of asbestos per cubic foot of air, and this standard was not changed until 1969. Additionally, they contend that, prior to 1964, it was thought that exposures to asbestos below this TLV were safe and that insulation work usually produced concentrations of atmospheric asbestos less than 5 million particles per cubic foot of air.

The weakness in this defense is that several of the companies had actual knowledge that the TLV was not reliable.[21] In fact, the medical director of Johns-Manville, Dr. Kenneth Smith, testified that he was aware in the late 1940s and early 1950s that insulation workers were developing asbestosis.[22] Indeed, insulation workers were filing workers' compensation claims against the companies throughout the 1950s and 1960s, and these companies included Fibreboard, Owens-Corning, and Armstrong Contracting and Supply.[23] One corporate executive, in reviewing the number of workers' compensation claims filed by insulators, wrote in 1962 that the list of claims was "rather imposing."[24] Although the state-of-the-art expert for the manufacturers may be able to construct a defense solely with reference to the medical literature, a review of the corporate documents reveals not only that the companies should have known of the hazards, but that they did know that asbestos was causing disease in the workers who were using their products.

Not only must the plaintiff prove that the manufacturers knew or should have known about the hazards of asbestos, the plaintiff must demonstrate that he or she breathed asbestos fibers liberated from the use of one or more of the manufacturers' products. Since exposures to asbestos may have occurred decades earlier, recollection of the use of a specific product by name is extremely difficult. Plaintiffs have developed evidence concerning the market share of particular manufacturers over time, but, unlike the DES litigation, market share liability usually is unavailable in asbestos cases. However, evidence that a particular manufacturer sold its products to a specific shipyard or were placed on a specific job site is admissible in the form of sales records. A plaintiff may testify that she or he used a specific product over time, and this testimony may be buttressed by the testimony of co-workers that particular products were used. Court decisions concerning product identification evidence have usually required that, before a co-worker may testify as to the use of specific products, that co-worker must testify that the products were in the general vicinity of the plaintiff.[25]

Finally, the plaintiff must prove that he or she has developed an asbestos-related disease and has suffered damages. In order to prove medical causation, plaintiff's counsel will usually retain an expert medical witness such as a pulmonary specialist, occupational physician, or lung pathologist. The role of the family physician should not be minimized, and even though the treating physician may not be expert in the diagnosis of asbestosis, it is critical that the local doctor support the diagnosis.

Whether or not the diagnosis of an asbestos-related disease can be made is usually the most controversial issue in an asbestos trial. Unless there is no room for a debate, the defendants will attempt to shift the focus of the trial from the evidence of corporate misconduct to creation of doubt in the jurors' minds about the propriety of the diagnosis.

In an asbestosis case, where tissue is not available, the defendants argue that numerous criteria must be met before a diagnosis can be established. In 1986, the American Thoracic Society (ATS) issued a statement concerning the diagnosis of asbestosis, and the manufacturers have seized on a misreading of that document in order to confuse juries about medical causation. The ATS statement reads as follows:

In the absence of pathologic examination of lung tissue, the diagnosis of asbestosis is a judgement based on a careful consideration of all relevant clinical findings. In our opinion, it is necessary that there be:

1. A reliable history of exposure.
2. An appropriate time interval between exposure and detection.

Furthermore, we regard the following clinical criteria to be of recognized value:

1. Chest roentgenographic evidence of type "s," "t," "u," small irregular opacifications of a profusion of 1/1 or greater.
2. A restrictive pattern of lung impairment with a forced vital capacity below the lower limit of normal.
3. A diffusing capacity below the lower limit of normal.
4. Bilateral late or pan-inspiratory crackles at the posterior lung bases not cleared by cough.[26]

As can be seen from the statement itself, there are only two mandatory criteria that must be met before the diagnosis of asbestosis can be made. Obviously, there must be a history of exposure to asbestos, and a sufficient time must have passed between first exposure to asbestos and the development of the disease process. The defendants, however, argue that the other criteria that the ATS regards as "of recognized value" must all be met as well, and this reading, if accepted by the jury, would exclude many legitimate diagnoses.

One of the most controversial criteria in the ATS statement is the requirement for a chest x-ray reading of 1/1 according to the International Labor Organization's (ILO) profusion rating for interstitial fibrosis. From a pathologic standpoint, asbestosis can exist in the absence of chest x-ray findings; and even from a clinical standpoint, other criteria can establish the diagnosis in the absence of a positive chest x-ray reading. Indeed, a 1/0 reading is considered by the ILO to be indicative of an abnormal chest x-ray.[27]

Also hotly contested is the significance of pleural disease. In fact, pleural disease is notably absent from the ATS statement. Although there can be reasonable debate on the issue on the extent to which pleural disease can cause pulmonary dysfunction,[28] no one can argue that pleural plaques and thickening are almost always caused by asbestos in those persons who are occupationally exposed, and the existence of pleural disease in those people is strong evidence that fibrosis on the chest x-ray, however slight, is also due to asbestos exposure.

The remaining criteria, although "of recognized value" in establishing the diagnosis, are certainly not mandatory and are more helpful in assessing impairment. For instance, a reduction in the forced vital capacity (FVC) to below 80% of predicted certainly is indicative of an abnormal FVC, but the ATS document fails to take into consideration the extent to which the lung volumes may have declined over time. A worker with asbestosis, whose FVC has declined from 110% to 82% of predicted still has a "normal" FVC in the absolute sense, but the drop in values is anything but normal. Although more difficult to reproduce, the diffusing capacity shares the same problem.

The issue of restriction versus obstruction is also hotly debated in asbestos disease cases. The defendants argue that obstruction is not caused by asbestos exposure, but is most likely attributable to cigarette smoking if such history is present. Although cigarettes are a frequent cause of obstructive disease, recent data indicate that asbestos can also cause an obstructive disease process.[29]

The cigarette smoking defense is probably the most powerful argument offered by the asbestos manufacturers, and it is raised by them in cases ranging from pleural disease to mesothelioma. In asbestosis cases, the defendants argue that cigarette smoke may increase presence of pleural plaques,[30] cause or contribute to interstitial fibrosis,[31] reduce lung volumes,[32] and impair diffusing capacity.[33] In lung cancer cases, the defendants argue that cigarettes are a powerful carcinogen, and they try to establish that smoking is the sole cause of the cancer. Although the defendants cannot dispute that smoking is not a cause of mesothelioma, they argue that cigarette smoke paralyzes the defense mechanisms of the lungs and allows for increased penetration and retention of asbestos fibers that cause mesothelioma.[34]

In sum, establishing medical causation not only requires that the plaintiff present evidence of an asbestos-related disease, but forces the plaintiff to defuse defense arguments that the diagnosis is incorrect and should not be made on the evidence. Plaintiff's counsel must persuade the jury that the defendants have created an unreasonable diagnostic criteria so that few, if any, claimants, will be able to prove the existence of the disease. The defendants' contentions require that the plaintiff offer a skilled pulmonary or occupational expert to testify and that plaintiff's counsel become well-versed in the medical criteria necessary to establish a diagnosis.

THE SHIFT FROM LIABILITY TO MEDICINE— THE PATHOLOGIST'S ROLE

With the increasing proliferation of mass trials in which liability issues are decided separately, and by different juries, from causation issues, plaintiff's counsel must be prepared to present strong medical testimony[35] and cannot expect to rely on evidence of corporate misconduct to sway a jury in a difficult case.

One of the best ways to demonstrate that a worker has developed an asbestos-related disease is to obtain a lung tissue specimen, have it analyzed, and demonstrate to the jury the presence of asbestos bodies or fibers. The results of chest x-rays, CT scans, and pulmonary function tests are all useful in demonstrating to the jury that an asbestos-related disease is present, but there is nothing more persuasive than evidence, preferably visual, that asbestos is in the plaintiff's lung tissue in elevated concentrations. Also considerably useful to the plaintiff is the detection of a particular type of asbestos fiber that may be in the defendants' products. As is often stated at trial, the pathologist has the "final word" on the diagnosis of asbestosis. And when there is enough lung tissue available for examination, this observation is certainly true. If a plaintiff's lawyer has tissue available, it is certainly advantageous to have the tissue examined by a pulmonary pathologist, and, if possible, to have it analyzed for the presence and type of asbestos fiber. If asbestosis is present, this establishes without question the existence of that disease process; and if lung cancer is coexistent, it is strong, if not conclusive, evidence that the lung cancer was caused by asbestos exposure.

In the absence of a fiber burden analysis, the diagnosis of asbestosis by light microscopy is usually debated only in borderline cases. If asbestosis is severe, multiple asbestos bodies can usually be found in the presence of diffuse interstitial fibrosis. In questionable cases, however, fibrosis may be present but asbestos bodies may be difficult to identify. In the asbestos trial setting, the debate usually centers around the number of asbestos bodies necessary to support the diagnosis. A publication by the College of American Pathologists suggests that a minimum of two asbestos bodies must be present in the areas of fibrosis before the diagnosis can be established.[36] One of the members of the committee that issued this statement has remarked that "the requirement for two asbestos bodies is probably overcautious" and that "the chance of overdiagnosing asbestosis from the observation of only one asbestos body seems very small indeed."[37] Although he continues that "the problem is more theoretic than real,"[38] it unfortunately becomes a matter of frequent dispute in the courtroom. Sometimes only one asbestos body can be identified; in some cases, there are none. In the case of fibrosis alone, one may argue that it is *occult* asbestosis, but the frequency of such cases is probably rare.[39] In the courtroom, however, the frequency of the claim is not.

The type of fibrosis necessary to support the diagnosis of asbestosis is also a disputed subject. Although some lung pathologists require a pattern of peribronchiolar fibrosis,[40] it is not always present in cases that are taken to court. Once again, juries are asked to decide issues that are controversial even among the experts, and they are forced to decide whether peribronchiolar fibrosis is necessary to make the diagnosis or whether "its absence in no way mitigates against the diagnosis."[41] In cases that are not so clear-cut, the trial can indeed become a battle of the experts.

The pathologic diagnosis of asbestosis is not only central to the nonmalignant case, but it is significant in relating a lung cancer to asbestos exposure. The problem lies not in those cases where asbestosis is readily diagnosed—because most commentators are willing to relate a bronchogenic carcinoma to asbestos if coexisting asbestosis can be found.[42] If asbestosis cannot be found but there are numerous asbestos bodies, a strong case can also be made that the underlying lung burden is sufficient to have triggered the cancerous process. However, many defense experts are unwilling to relate a cancer to asbestos exposure unless all of the diagnostic features of asbestosis are present. This idea has been criticized in a report to the British government, which argued that, because the mechanisms of fibrogenesis and carcinogenesis are separate, there is no good reason why asbestosis must necessarily be present.[43] A better indicator of whether lung cancer can be related to asbestos is an elevated fiber burden, and it has been suggested that a fiber burden in excess of 100,000 fibers per gram of dry lung tissue should be used as a minimum for relating a lung cancer to asbestos.[44]

The use of electron microscopy to assess the lung burden of asbestos can be of enormous benefit to the plaintiff in relating a lung cancer or mesothelioma to asbestos exposure. Additionally, an energy-dispersive x-ray analysis that specifically identifies the asbestos fiber type can be used to determine which products may have caused the disease process. For instance, in a mesothelioma case where the plaintiff's lung tissue reveals an elevated asbestos fiber count and the majority of asbestos fibers are amosite, the plaintiff can point as the cause to a defendant whose product contains mostly amosite. By the same token, if the plaintiff worked primarily with chrysotile—and tremolite fibers are identified—the plaintiff may be able to implicate as the culprit a defendant who utilized chrysotile in its products.

On the other hand, a defendant may use a fiber analysis to excul-
pate itself from the case by demonstrating that the fiber type in its
products is not present in the plaintiff's lung tissue, or that other fiber types, such as crocidolite, are present in excessive quantities.
Ninety-five percent of all asbestos used in the United States in insulation products historically was of the chrysotile variety, and the remaining 5% was mostly amosite. Crocidolite was rarely, if ever, used
in insulating materials in the United States,[45] and this fiber type was
primarily imported into the United States for use in asbestos-cement
pipes and certain specialty gaskets.[46] Nevertheless, lung burden
analyses often reveal relatively little chrysotile, greater amounts of
amosite, and, not infrequently, the presence of crocidolite. Tremolite,
a contaminant of chrysotile, is often detected in lung tissue, and it is
a marker of previous chrysotile exposure.[47] Chrysotile tends to dissolve in lung tissue and may be removed from the lung, whereas
amphiboles, specifically crocidolite, are more durable and are retained. A brief crocidolite exposure may still be evident in lung tissue
after decades have passed, whereas heavier chrysotile exposure may
be undetected.

Differences in the methods of analysis by various laboratories may
also result in different findings. Some investigators count all fibers,
whereas some do not count those below five microns in length. In
one case, lung tissue was evaluated by three investigators. One found
an elevated amount of only chrysotile using transmission electron
microscopy.[48] Another, also using transmission electron microscopy,
identified crocidolite, amosite, tremolite, and chrysotile.[49] Finally,
another, using scanning electron microscopy, identified tremolite.[50]
The overall lung burden of asbestos also varied from laboratory to
laboratory.[51] The variability between laboratories for fiber burden assessments often results in the parties having different investigators
perform studies on the same lung tissue. Under the Rules of Civil
Procedure, a party may use a favorable lung burden assessment as
evidence while suppressing as undiscoverable work product an unfavorable report.[52] The extent to which unfavorable lung burden assessments are not revealed by the parties demonstrates the potency
of such reports at trial.

In no case is the pathologist's role greater than in the mesothelioma
case. A pathologist is necessary in rendering the diagnosis, identifying asbestos in the lung tissue, and determining whether the type
of asbestos found was responsible for the development of mesothelioma.

Although the diagnosis of mesothelioma is difficult, recent
immunohistochemical-staining techniques are allowing more certainty in the diagnosis. The defense in most mesothelioma cases is
centered on the difficulty in making a conclusive diagnosis. Even if
the full battery of histochemical and immunohistochemical stains is
performed, the defendants are usually able to find an "expert" to

contest the diagnosis.[53] If the asbestos manufacturers are unable to present testimony that the tumor is not a mesothelioma, they may argue that a mesothelioma diagnosis cannot be made to a reasonable degree of medical certainty. From a plaintiff's perspective, it is certainly necessary in the mesothelioma case to have all possible diagnostic tests performed on the tumor tissue in order to ensure diagnostic certainty. Additionally, an autopsy of the patient is certainly advisable in order to defeat a potential defense claim that the mesothelioma was a metastasis from some other site.[54]

Once the diagnosis of mesothelioma is established, it is necessary to prove that asbestos was the cause. From a practical standpoint, asbestos is the only known cause of mesothelioma that exists in the American workplace.[55] The defendants, however, will engage in tactics of confusion by arguing that there are cases of mesothelioma caused by erionite, therapeutic radiation, certain drugs, and agents that are unknown.[56] These claims will be made even in cases where there is a significant occupational exposure to asbestos and where asbestos can be identified in the lung.

Finally, one of the most hotly contested issues in asbestos litigation is whether chrysotile asbestos can cause mesothelioma.[57] Since insulators are developing mesothelioma at an alarming rate and 95% of all asbestos used in insulating material was chrysotile, it would seem that chrysotile is certainly capable of causing mesothelioma. Nevertheless, certain studies of workers exposed only to chrysotile indicate that chrysotile may be a weaker cause of mesothelioma,[58] and the defendants maintain that these studies demonstrate that chrysotile—in and of itself—does not cause mesothelioma at all. Most authorities now accept that the amphibole, tremolite, is a cause of mesothelioma, and tremolite contaminates most of the chrysotile that has been used in this country.[59] If tremolite can be identified in the lung tissue, it is reasonable to assume that the source of the contamination was the chrysotile asbestos used by the plaintiff.

A few defense experts even contend that amosite is not a cause of mesothelioma and that all mesotheliomas are caused by crocidolite.[60] This position is untenable, and good evidence exists that the likelihood for exposure to crocidolite by most construction or insulation workers is nonexistent. In England, crocidolite was used for insulation purposes, and there is evidence that some British ships have been overhauled in United States shipyards. Consequently, in a mesothelioma case arising from an American shipyard exposure, the defendants argue that the potential for crocidolite exposure existed and this exposure is responsible. The defendants will strongly and consistently argue the potency of crocidolite in mesothelioma causation. And if the defendants can convince the jury that crocidolite was the likely cause, the manufacturers can usually succeed because few, if any, manufacturers utilized crocidolite in their asbestos-containing insulation materials.[61]

PATHOLOGY AT TRIAL

To ensure success in a case where pathologic material is available, plaintiff's counsel should consult with a pulmonary pathologist who has knowledge of asbestos-related diseases, to establish the diagnosis, to identify asbestos in a lung tissue, and to testify that asbestos was responsible for the disease process. When lung tissue is available, it is not enough to rely on clinical evidence alone. Plaintiff's counsel can be sure that, if pathologic evidence is available, the defendants will have it reviewed by a pathologist and will, in all probability, have a pathologist testify at trial. In many cases, the only tissue available is from a transbronchial biopsy, and the manufacturers will present evidence that the pathologic examination did not reveal the presence of either any disease process or asbestos bodies. It should be emphasized on cross-examination that, as explained by one prominent pulmonary pathologist, "transbronchial biopsy is totally unsuited for diagnosing asbestosis; diagnoses of asbestosis made on the basis of transbronchial biopsy are statistically equivalent to guessing, no matter how perfect the histologic pattern may be. . . . [T]issue submitted for mineral analysis should be at least the size of a large open biopsy; analysis of transbronchial biopsies is to be avoided."[62]

When sufficient tissue is available, plaintiff's counsel should utilize the information to be gained from a pathologic examination to the greatest extent possible. The materials should be submitted for microscopic examination, and pictures should be taken that can then be presented in evidence. Visual evidence of asbestos in lung tissue is extremely persuasive to a jury, and pictures of asbestos bodies coupled with the pathologist's opinion that asbestos was responsible for the disease process may sway an otherwise indecisive jury. Additionally, a fiber burden analysis is extremely helpful in convincing a jury that asbestos caused or contributed to the disease process.

CONCLUSION

With the likelihood that future asbestos trials will consist of large numbers of cases and will have separate medical and causation phases, plaintiff's counsel may not have the benefit of evidence of corporate misconduct when compensatory damages are decided by the jury. The plaintiff's lawyer must, therefore, emphasize the hazards of asbestos exposure and the numbers of preventable diseases that have been caused by asbestos exposure. The following points should be emphasized to the jury that will decide the medical phase of the asbestos trial:

1. The extensive industrial use of asbestos throughout this century has caused an epidemic of asbestos-related diseases.

2. Asbestos-related diseases are man-made; i.e., these are diseases that could have been prevented by the elimination of asbestos or through the use of proper respiratory protection.

3. Asbestos—and only asbestos—can cause an incurable, untreatable, irreversible, progressive, and often fatal disease known as asbestosis. It has been demonstrated beyond reasonable doubt that asbestos is a cause of human lung cancer, and asbestos alone is carcinogenic.[63] The combination of cigarette smoking and asbestos exposure is an explosive interaction, and an asbestos worker who smokes has a 50–90 times greater chance of developing lung cancer than the person who neither smokes nor is exposed to asbestos.[64]

4. Asbestos causes malignant mesothelioma, an incurable and invariably fatal tumor of the lining of the lung or abdomen. Mesothelioma is rare in the general population, but it is rampant among asbestos workers.[65]

5. After extensive hearings on the hazards of asbestos, the Occupational Safety and Health Administration of the U.S. government concluded that it was "aware of no instance in which exposure to a toxic substance has more clearly demonstrated detrimental health effects on humans than has asbestos exposure. The diseases caused by asbestos exposure are life-threatening or disabling. Among these diseases are lung cancer, cancer of the mesothelial lining of the pleura and peritoneum, asbestosis, and gastrointestinal cancer."[66]

6. After considering "45,000 pages of analyses, comments, testimony, correspondence and other materials," the U.S. Environmental Protection Agency banned the use of most asbestos-containing products.[67]

7. There is no known safe level for exposure to asbestos.[68]

8. Brief exposures to asbestos have caused mesothelioma in persons decades later, and persons have developed mesothelioma whose only exposure was living near an asbestos mine or plant or residing in the home of an asbestos worker.[69]

The jury must be informed that asbestos is by no means a benign substance, as the defendants would have them believe, and that dangerous concentrations of asbestos can be invisible and undetectable. Furthermore, the jury needs to understand that asbestos fibers are inhaled into the lung, act like tiny spears or splinters, and cause scarring of the lung tissue microscopically. This information must be presented visually, graphically, and, most importantly, simply.

Asbestos litigation has created a major challenge for the American judicial system. During the last 20 years, the growth of asbestos litigation has resulted in landmark court decisions and judicial innovations. However, to ensure that the tens of thousands of asbestos victims or their families receive compensation within the next half-century will require even more creative efforts by both lawyers and the courts. The solution to the asbestos litigation crisis will not be easy. But through national coordination and mass consolidation, the cases can be resolved. Hopefully, the system that is created to solve the asbestos litigation crisis will remain as a blueprint for managing future complex litigation.

END NOTES

1. *Borel* v. *Fibreboard Paper Products Corp.*, 493 F.2d 1076 (5th Cir. 1973), *cert. denied*, 419 U.S. 869 (1974).
2. *Jackson* v. *Johns-Manville Sales Corp.*, 750 F.2d 1314, 1335–36 (5th Cir. 1985) (*en banc*).
3. *In re* Asbestos Products Liability Litigation (No. VI), No. 875 at 1 n.3 and 2 n.6 (J.P.M.D.L. Jan. 17, 1991).
4. Committee Report on Asbestos Litigation Pending in Federal Courts, reported in *New York Times*, March 6, 1991, p. C2, col. 1.
5. Lilienfeld DE: Projection of asbestos-related diseases in the United States, 1985–2009 I. Cancer, *Brit J Ind Med* 45:283–91, 1988. A recent report indicated that 265,000 total asbestos-related deaths will occur by the year 2015. *New York Times*, supra note 4, p. 1.
6. One study for Johns-Manville, which was conducted in 1982, severely underestimated the number of asbestos lawsuits that would arise from asbestos exposure. The authors concluded that "[a] reasonable central projection of the number of lawsuits stemming from all diseases seen from 1982 on is likely to be about 45,000, with a reasonably firm lower bound of 30,000, and a very indefinite upper bound on the order of 120,000." Walker AM: Projections of asbestos-related disease 1980–2009, *J Occ Med* 25:409, 424, 1983. Eighteen years before the end of the projection, the number of cases already approaches the "very indefinite upper bound on the order of 120,000." Ibid.
7. The *Borel* case was the first asbestos lawsuit tried to a plaintiff's verdict. But the first case to be filed in the Eastern District of Texas was that of Claude Tomplait in December 1966. The mere filing of this case by an asbestos worker against multiple defendants was a seminal event. The case was tried, but ended in a defense verdict on the issue of exposure. Brodeur P: *Outrageous Misconduct.* New York: Pantheon, 1985, p. 36.
8. *In re* National Asbestos Litigation, No. 1:90 CV 11,000 (E.D. Tex., Beaumont Div., Aug. 20, 1990). The order stated that the class action shall proceed as *Linscomb* v. *Pittsburgh-Corning Corp.*, No. 1:86-MC-456.
9. *In re* Asbestos Products Liability Litigation (No. VI), supra note 3, p. 2. In its order, issued on January 17, 1991, the Judicial Panel on Multidistrict Litigation stated:

Our goals here are to utilize Section 1407 in order to streamline the common questions in this litigation to the greatest extent possible; to eliminate duplication and overlap; to encourage a uniform case management plan; to allow for division of responsibility among the assigned judges; to provide a mechanism for the transferee judges to fully explore the uniform use of the dispositive techniques (such as [a] classes and subclasses under Fed. R. Civ. P. Rule 23, [b] pleural registries, [c] separately consolidated pretrial or trial on any common issues or claims, and [d] separated reverse trials on various issues); to avoid inconsistent rulings; to facilitate settlement; to focus the circuit appellate process regarding centralized rulings; to provide a method whereby repetition in newly filed actions is eliminated; to provide a focal point to facilitate coordination with the mammoth number of asbestos actions pending in state court; and, most importantly, to better implement Fed. R. Civ. P. Rule 1's edict to secure the just, speedy and inexpensive determination of federal litigation. Matters unique to any actions or subgroups of actions could proceed concurrently with any centralized efforts.

On July 29, 1991, the Judicial Panel on Multidistrict Litigation transferred all asbestos-related disease cases pending in the U.S. District Courts, which were not in trial, to the Eastern District of Pennsylvania. Judge Charles Weiner of Philadelphia, Pa., has been assigned to supervise management of these federal court cases. On August 28, 1991, Judge Weiner met with numerous plaintiffs' and defense counsel regarding resolution of these cases, and he indicated that asbestos-related malignancies should be considered for trial or settlement first. Cases pending in state courts remain unaffected by the transfer.

10. Testimony has been repeatedly taken from such industry consultants as Dr. Gerrit W. H. Schepers, former director of the Saranac laboratory, and Dr. Thomas F. Mancuso, the consultant to the Philip Carey Corp., the predecessor of Celotex.
11. Letter from A. S. Rossiter to S. Simpson, Sept. 25, 1935.
12. Letter from S. Simpson to V. Brown, Oct. 1, 1935.
13. Letter from V. Brown to S. Simpson, Oct. 3, 1935.
14. Minutes of the Air Hygiene and Manufacturing Committee of the Asbestos Textile Institute, Mar. 7, 1957.
15. Memorandum from C. G. Linke to J. A. McKinney, Jan. 12, 1979.
16. Memorandum from K. S. Johnson to M. D. Burch, May 23, 1957.
17. Memorandum from W. A. Lots to A. J. Pearson, Sept. 17, 1963.
18. Memorandum from J. L. Konzen to H. L. Logan, Feb. 9, 1968.
19. Letter from R. Packard to G. Duncan, June 24, 1968.
20. D. Ozonoff, Report concerning *Medical Literature Review* (1981).
21. W. C. L. Hemeon, Report of Preliminary Dust Investigation for Asbestos Textile Institute (Industrial Hygiene Foundation, 1947 unpublished).
22. Deposition of K. Smith in *Louisville Trust Co.* v. *Johns-Manville Corp.*, No. 174–922 (Jefferson Cir. Ct., 7th Div. Ky., April 21, 1976).
23. Castleman B: *Asbestos: Medical and Legal Aspects*, 2nd. ed. New York: Harcourt, Brace and Jovanovich, 1986, pp. 164–179.
24. Memorandum from W. B. Hofferth to J. E. Zeller, Jan. 17, 1962.
25. Compare *Roehling* v. *National Gypsum Co.*, 786 F.2d 1225 (4th Cir. 1986 with *Blackston* v. *Shook & Fletcher Insulation Co.*, 764 F.2d 480 (11th Cir. 1985).
26. Ad Hoc Committee of the Scientific Assembly on Environmental and Occupational Health: The diagnosis of nonmalignant diseases related to asbestos. *Am Rev Respir Dis* 134:363, 367, 1986.
27. Guidelines for the use of the ILO international classification of radiographs of pneumoconiosis. In: *Occupational Safety & Health Series No. 22* (rev.), Geneva: International Labour Office, 1980.
28. Compare Jones JSP: Pleural Plaques, In: *The Biological Effects of Asbestos* (Bogovski, ed.), Lyon: IARC Scientific Publication No. 8, 1972, pp. 243–248, with Schwartz DA: Determinants of restrictive lung function in asbestos-induced pleural fibrosis, *J Appl Physiol* 68:1932–1937, 1990; Bourbeau J: The relationship between respiratory impairment and asbestos-related pleural abnormality in an active work force, *Amer Rev Respir Dis* 142:837–842, 1990. Recent studies on the significance of pleural disease indicate that pleural thickening and plaques are not as benign as previously thought. They are associated with an impairment of lung function and they may predict future cancers. See Selikoff IJ: Predictive significance of parenchymal and/or pleural fibrosis for subsequent death of asbestos-associated diseases (submitted for publication, 1990).

29. Churg A: *Pathology of Occupational Lung Disease.* New York: Igaku-Shoin, 1988, pp. 251–253.
30. Andrion A: Pleural plaques at autopsy, smoking habits, and asbestos exposure. *Eur J Respir Dis* 65:125–130, 1984.
31. Weiss W: Cigarette smoke, asbestos, and small irregular opacities. *Am Rev Respir Dis* 130:293–301, 1984.
32. Surgeon General, *The Health Consequences of Smoking: Cancer and Chronic Lung Disease in the Workplace.* U.S. Department of Health and Human Services, 1985, pp. 241–254.
33. Ibid., p. 241.
34. See cross-examination of Dr. Edwin Holstein in *Kulzer* v. *Owens-Corning Fiberglas,* No. 87–386T, p. 351 (W.D.N.Y., Rochester Div., Apr. 24, 1990).
35. Although plaintiff may not be able to admit corporate documents in the medical phase of a consolidated trial to demonstrate suppression of scientific data, corporate memoranda are certainly admissible to prove that the manufacturers recognize that asbestos is a highly dangerous material. For instance, although the asbestos companies deny in a personal injury trial that asbestosis occurs prior to the development of clinical criteria, they take a quite contrary position in litigation against their insurance carriers. In order to prove an "occurrence" for purposes of product liability insurance policies, the manufacturers have argued in insurance litigation that asbestosis occurs on the inhalation of the fiber, and that one-third of the alveolar sacs must be affected before asbestosis is clinically diagnosable. Policyholders' Proposed Medical Findings of Fact, *In Re* Asbestos Insurance Coverage Cases, No. 1072, pp. 8, 12 (Cal. Super. Ct., S.F. County, Jan. 26, 1987). Although the defendants minimize the hazards of asbestos exposure, internal corporate documents reveal their true concerns when litigation is not a factor. As stated by Dr. Jon Konzen on September 20, 1972: "Irreversible and progressive lung scarring will . . . occur in over-exposed [asbestos] workers before it is apparent to the man or on medical examination. Likewise, occupational exposure to asbestos is known to be causally related to carcinoma of the lung and malignant mesothelioma of the covering or pleura of the lung." J. Konzen to S. Mayer, Sept. 20, 1972. Finally, even though the defendants dispute that asbestos-containing construction materials are hazardous to building occupants, many of them are removing asbestos from their corporate offices.
36. Pneumoconiosis Committee of the College of American Pathologists and the National Institute for Occupational Safety and Health: The pathology of asbestos-associated diseases of the lungs and pleural cavities: Diagnostic criteria and proposed grading schema. *Arch Pathol Lab Med* 106:544, 559, 1982.
37. Churg: supra note 29, p. 260.
38. Ibid.
39. Ibid., pp. 262–263.
40. Ibid., p. 262.
41. Ibid., p. 262.
42. Ibid., p. 285.
43. Doll R, Peto J: *Asbestos: Effects on Health of Exposure to Asbestos.* London: Her Majesty's Stationery Office, 1985, p. 32:

The idea that . . . asbestos-induced cancers occur only secondary to the fibrosis of asbestosis has sometimes been expressed. The idea originated in the days before the discovery of DNA, when cancers were not thought to result from genetic variation in somatic cells, but from the repair of tissue damage that was macroscopically visible. In light of modern knowledge of carcinogenesis, such an idea does not seem plausible. No threshold for the carcinogenic effect of asbestos has been demonstrated in humans or in laboratory animals and, in the absence of positive evidence for a threshold, we have followed standard scientific practice and assume that none exists. One possible reason for thinking that asbestos-induced cancers might be secondary to asbestosis is the high incidence of cancer in the similar condition of cryptogenic fibrosing alveolitis. As, however, the aetiology of this disease is unknown, the argument by analogy does not carry much weight and we have ignored it.

44. Warnock ML, Isenberg W: Asbestos burden and the pathology of lung cancer. *Chest* 89:20, 26, 1986.
45. Selikoff I, Hammond E, Seidman H: *Cancer Risk of Insulation Workers in the United States.* Lyon: IARC Scientific Publication No. 8, 1972.
46. Hendry NW: The geology, occurrences, and major uses of asbestos, In: Biological Effects of Asbestos, *Ann NY Acad Sci* 132:12, 19, 1965.
47. Doll and Peto, supra note 43, p. 17.
48. Report by Dr. Ronald Dodson, Dept. of Cell Biology and Environmental Sciences, University of Texas Health Center at Tyler, May 27, 1988.
49. Report by Dr. Fred Pooley, Dept. of Mining and Minerals Engineering, University College, Cardiff, Wales, June 23, 1988.
50. Report by Dr. Victor Roggli, Dept. of Pathology, Duke University Medical Center, Dec. 4, 1987.
51. Dr. Dodson identified 3,025,082 chrysotile fibers per gram of dry lung tissue; Dr. Pooley identified 7,900,000 chrysotile fibers, 660,000 tremolite fibers, 64,000 crocidolite fibers, and 9000 amosite fibers per gram of dry lung tissue; and Dr. Roggli found 6120 fibers per gram of wet lung tissue. Dr. Roggli counted only those fibers whose length exceeded five microns, whereas Dr. Dodson and Dr. Pooley included all fibers in their counts.
52. Fed. R. Civ. P. 26(b)(4)(B). The rule states: "A party may discover facts known or opinions held by an expert who has been retained or specially employed by another party in anticipation of litigation or preparation for trial and who is not expected to be called as a witness at trial, only as provided in rule 35(b) or upon a showing of exceptional circumstances under which it is inpracticable for the parties seeking discovery to obtain facts or opinions on the same subject by other means."
53. Unfortunately, the defendants consistently rely on one or two pathologists, who, in the face of overwhelming evidence favoring the diagnosis, will testify that the tumor is not a mesothelioma.
54. In one case tried in Virginia federal court, the diagnosis of mesothelioma was confirmed by all pathologists except one who was retained by the defendants. This defense expert contended that the tumor was a metastasis from the thyroid, and the body was exhumed for further analysis. On exhumation, the thyroid gland was found to be free of tumor.
55. In approximately 20% of cases, the history of asbestos exposure was not taken in the occupational history. However, on further investigation, asbestos exposure can almost always be elicited when preparing the mesothelioma case for trial.
56. Pelnar PV: Further evidence of nonasbestos-related mesothelioma. *Scand J Work Environ Health* 14:141–144, 1988. The author is affiliated with the Asbestos Institute.
57. Churg, supra note 29, p. 289.
58. Berry G, Newhouse M: Mortality of workers manufacturing friction materials using asbestos, *Brit J Indus Med* 40:1–7, 1983; McDonald JC, Fry JS: Mesothelioma and fiber type in three American asbestos factories. *Scand J Work Environ Health* 8: 53–58, 1982.
59. As stated by Doll and Peto: "It is not practicable to remove tremolite from chrysotile for commercial purposes and any distinction between the

effects of chrysotile and tremolite may, therefore, be considered academic, unless supplies of chrysotile can be obtained in which little or no tremolite is present." Supra note 43, p. 17.

60. Wagner JC: The complexities in the evaluation of epidemiologic data of fiber-exposed populations. In: *Dusts and Disease* (Lemen R, Dement J, eds.), Park Forest South, IL: Pathotox, 1979, pp. 37–39.
61. In answers to interrogatories, all defendants maintain that they did not use crocidolite in their asbestos-containing pipe insulation.
62. Churg: supra note 29, p. 267.
63. McDonald, JC: Asbestos and lung cancer: Has the case been proven? *Chest* 78:374–376, 1980.
64. Surgeon General: supra note 32, pp. 217–218.
65. Selikoff IJ: Asbestos-associated disease. In: *Public Health and Preventive Medicine*, 12th ed. (Maxcy-Rosenau, ed.), East Norwalk, CT: Appleton-Century-Crofts, 1986, pp. 523–534.
66. 51 Fed. Reg. 22615 (June 20, 1986).
67. 54 Fed. Reg. 29461 (July 17, 1989).
68. Selikoff: supra 65.
69. Ibid.

13. Medicolegal Aspects of Asbestos-Related Diseases: Defendant's Attorney's Perspective

HENRY G. GARRARD, III, IVAN A. GUSTAFSON, AND MERRY REETZ STOVALL

The American courtroom is a forum in which the decision-making process is far removed from the rational discourse that characterizes disputes in the medical/scientific field. In the courtroom, advocates present medical and scientific evidence to a panel of lay jurors. As advocates, the attorneys for both sides will present evidence on pathologic issues without acknowledging the existence of contrary opinion, nor admitting to any doubt as to the validity of the scientific statements involved.

Trial rules allow plaintiffs to present their picture of pathology first. The defense may expose weakness or flaws through cross-examination of plaintiff's experts, or may wait until its case in chief to present its perspective on the medical aspects of the case. Opinions of plaintiff's experts can be shown to be based on untested theory, or to be opposed by the majority of published studies on the subject.

Pathology constitutes powerfully persuasive evidence, for what can be seen is more easily believed. The pathologist has a unique part to play in litigation because physicians of that discipline present for the jury view actual tissue, staining results, digestion analysis, and other information that can be compared objectively to an indisputably normal sample or to a standard by which a process or result can be gauged. The pathologist's slide of tissue from the lung showing emphysema, idiopathic interstitial fibrosis, rheumatoid lung disease, the lack of asbestos bodies, or countless other sorts of information may form the basis of the jury's decision. Available technology such as the direct projection of slides onto television screens, multiple view microscopes, and other types of visual media allow jurors to look at slides concurrently with the expert.

Often in cases dealing with asbestos there are pathologic questions that involve diagnosis, etiology, and the degree to which multiple processes in the same individual can contribute to that individual's problems. From an etiologic standpoint, the presence of asbestos bodies in conjunction with the appropriate type of interstitial fibrosis should be necessary and crucial to the diagnosis. Either the lack of bodies or a count of fibers less than that generally seen in asbestosis could make a difference in what a jury determines an individual's injury to be. For example, a finding of fewer fibers than are generally associated with asbestosis in a lung cancer case or a lack of demonstrable asbestosis as shown by a competent pathologist is strong evidence that the lung cancer is not related to asbestos exposure.

In dealing with both the diagnosis of mesothelioma and questions of etiology, the assistance of a pathologist is crucial. The various sophisticated stains, both histochemical and mucin (if positive for intracellular mucin, the malignancy is something other than a mesothelioma)[1,2] require pathologic performance and interpretation. For example, a slide showing mucin positivity compared to an acknowledged control positive should be very compelling evidence to a jury. Similarly, when an acknowledged mesothelioma can be disputed on etiologic grounds, the pathologist should be called on to show that the number of asbestos fibers from digestion analysis neither exceeds that found in the general population nor equals that seen in mesothelioma cases where the etiology is thought to be asbestos. There is substantial evidence that a significant percentage of mesotheliomas in humans are not asbestos related, and the pathologist should be asked to make that point, as well as to show the physical plausibility of other causes.

Another area where the defense must employ pathologists is in interpreting animal research. Much new research is under way on rats and other animals to look at cellular-level reactions to asbestos exposure. This work is providing new theories on cancer causation and on issues that relate to progression. The pathologist can show that such research does not necessarily apply to processes in humans, or provide information on cancer risk and progression that contradicts epidemiologic experience.[3] The pathologist can tell the jury how experiments are conducted to ensure positive results, how many other substances at the molecular level can produce the same effects, how the animal model grossly is not the same as the human model, and what difference that may make in results.

The pathologist can also be important in regard to the question of the meaning of pleural change, which is often hotly debated at trial. Currently some scientists are attempting to support a proposition that pleural plaques cause impairment of lung function either because of some inhibition of chest wall movement or because of some claimed underlying parenchymal fibrosis associated with pleural plaques. The pathologist is important in helping to show that pleural plaques are located on the parietal pleura (which covers the chest wall) as distinguished from the visceral pleura that actually covers the lungs, to show plaques in general are not expected to inhibit chest wall movement and that when lungs are examined in individuals with plaques there is no general or usual finding that those lungs also have underlying parenchymal fibrosis.

It may also be important to show pathologically how infections, trauma, blood in the chest, empyemas, and other things can cause pleural plaques or changes. Pleural plaques have a typical avascular, basket-weave appearance, and a pathologic exam may show a lack of such findings.

In cases where a death is alleged to have been caused by exposure to asbestos, legitimate questions may exist as to disease, etiology of disease, and the effect of non-asbestos-caused health problems on the individual. A competent pathologist can participate in an autopsy in such cases (it may be appropriate and important to request one if the plaintiffs were not going to have one done). The pathologist should be asked to analyze *all* autopsy material if the pathologist cannot or has not participated in the autopsy. The examination at autopsy or of autopsy material should not be restricted to the malignancy or the lungs, but should cover all parts of the body that may have affected the individual in life or the individual's life expectancy. All too often a pathologist will simply look at slides prepared by someone else when blocks and even formalin-preserved tissue may be available. When ample tissue is available, it can be utilized for fiber burden analysis, adequate sampling for fibrosis, and adequate analysis for other problems that may affect the case.

If a case is a purported mesothelioma, then a thorough examination of multiple parts of the body is essential to prove that the malignancy did not arise from some other part of the body and metastasize to the pleura or peritoneum. One of the possible ways to defend a mesothelioma claim is to show that the tumor did not arise in the mesothelial lining of the pleura or peritoneum but is instead a metastasis from another place and consequently not a mesothelioma at all. Likewise it is important for the pathologist to observe grossly the appearance of the claimed mesothelioma because a true mesothelioma should present grossly in a certain manner. If, for example, the malignancy presents as a number of discrete nodules at autopsy, that should make a diagnosis of malignant mesothelioma very suspect.

The pathologist should be called on more often to show how non-asbestos-related problems actually affect the human being. Such things as the effects of significant diabetes, arteriosclerotic heart disease, emphysema, rheumatoid disease, and liver or kidney disease may cause clinical symptoms similar to those from asbestos-related diseases or may otherwise significantly affect the quality and length of life of the individual. As people in general live to an older age, this is more important. An explanation pathologically of how these various problems affect the body is often overlooked and can have a significant impact on both causation and damages at trial.

Some physicians attempt to relate asbestos to malignancies other than lung cancer and mesothelioma. For example, it may be important in refuting a colon cancer claim to have the pathologist show how a colon section had multiple polyps or a lack of asbestos bodies or fibers, which would cast doubt on the physical plausibility of asbestos' being a cause of such cancer. The pathologist can also show how other agents and body processes make more physiologic and pathologic sense as causes of cancer outside the lung than does asbestos.

An often overlooked important area to cover through the pathologist is that malignancy can be caused without exposure to an external substance. Pathologically it can be shown that cancers often happen in human beings for unexplained reasons, because cells simply began to wildly mutate or because of some genetic predisposition. All this becomes more important today, because for a considerable period of time asbestos exposures experienced by workers have been truly negligible or nonexistent.

PATHOLOGIC DIAGNOSIS OF ASBESTOSIS

While some experts presented at trial have their own personal criteria for diagnosing asbestosis, the published standard diagnostic criteria of medical/scientific organizations such as the American Thoracic Society and the College of American Pathologists make such diagnoses vulnerable to attack. However, the rigid application of diagnostic criteria, without due consideration of other factors, can be misleading. An examination of the current literature illustrates this problem.

Pathology is often helpful to respond to and counter plaintiff's clinical diagnoses. While most cases are resolved through negotiation following clinical examination, most of the more complex cases have some pathologic involvement. Pathology is most useful in these more challenging cases because the clinical diagnosis relies on symptoms that are often shared with other illnesses. The American Thoracic Society has noted a major problem in differential diagnosis when more than one disease is present. There are diseases, unrelated to asbestos exposure, that have symptoms similar to asbestosis that may occur in persons with asbestos exposure.[4] Published studies of clinically diagnosed individuals with asbestos-related disease are often difficult to compare because clinical criteria may vary depending on the purpose of the study: early detection, epidemiologic studies of workers, or establishment of diagnosis in an individual.[5] From the clinical perspective, certainty in diagnosis increases with numbers of positive criteria, keeping in mind the possibility of confounding variables.[4]

Pathologic diagnosis, when available, can be used to refute a weak or an unsupported clinical diagnosis, or to establish the effect of a confounding illness. But pathology may not provide a definitive diagnosis by itself. Pathologic diagnosis of asbestosis requires, at a minimum, the presence of at least two asbestos bodies and the identification of fibrosis, according to the Pneumoconiosis Committee of the College of American Pathologists.[6] These criteria may seem relatively straightforward, but in application overzealous experts may not consider all necessary factors.

Asbestos bodies are considered by some to be nothing more than a marker of asbestos exposure. By themselves, they are not necessarily a manifestation of disease.[6,7] The wide range of reported ratios of uncoated to coated fibers [4:1 to 136,000:1] suggests asbestos bodies are a poor indicator of fiber burden.[8] Recent studies demonstrate that several factors affect the number of asbestos bodies found, such as areas of lung examined and degree of distention of the lung tissue.[8,9,10] Tissue sections frequently show irregular distribution of both asbestos bodies and fibrosis.[11,12] Further problems may be caused by the sample, for it is sometimes impossible to detect asbestos bodies within debris or to distinguish them morphologically from another mineral.[13] It can be seen that a restricted site selection may present a skewed picture of average asbestos burden. It is the task of the defense to expose such circumstances to the jury. This can be done most effectively through the pathologist. In dealing with tissue analysis it is important to have the pathologist examine multiple tissue sites, for an opinion on fiber burden can be attacked if it is based on limited sampling.

The demonstrated presence of asbestos fibers in a lung does not necessarily mean fibrosis will be present. The pathologist should be challenged to find not only bodies or fibers but also appropriate fibrosis in conjunction with the bodies or fibers. Fibrosis may be difficult to evaluate microscopically in the presence of tumor, pneumonia, bleeding, or atelectasis. Indeed the formation of fibrosis may be largely dependent on factors other than fiber burden.[8] Fibrosis near a tumor may be as a consequence of reaction to the natural processes of the tumor. A pathologic examination of fibrosis is most convincing on causation issues where careful consideration is also given to the total clinical picture. Asbestosis can clinically, functionally, radiographically, and, to a great extent, pathologically resemble idiopathic interstitial fibrosis, usual interstitial pneumonia, or fibrosing alveolitis.[7] All this suggests that care must be taken in evaluating pathologic data, both from plaintiff's witnesses and defense experts.

Ultimately any lawsuit for personal injury will focus on the individual plaintiff. In cases involving claimed asbestosis, the seemingly infinite variations of an individual's physiologic response to asbestos exposure comes into play. Host tissues respond variably, and lead to differences in individual immune reaction and susceptibility.[11,14] The uniqueness of an individual's risk for asbestosis is a consistent and well-recognized finding in the majority of epidemiologic, clinical, and pathologic investigations of asbestos workers.[15] There is still no definite explanation of the frequently experienced phenomenon where one asbestos-exposed worker will develop asbestosis while his similarly exposed co-worker will not. Individuals respond differently to the same asbestos exposure. Some of this difference may be accounted for by lifestyle, for it has been observed that radiographic parenchymal abnormalities increase and occur more frequently in smokers than in nonsmokers.[16] Because it is not completely clear why one exposed worker will get asbestosis while a workmate will not, projections as to who will develop asbestosis can rarely be made.

Closely related to the issue of who will get asbestosis is the question of progression. Much time is devoted to this issue at trial, for if the jury is persuaded a plaintiff's asbestosis will progress, the level of damages may increase if the plaintiff prevails. Mild cases of asbestosis, where no lung dysfunction is measurable, are increasingly before the courts. Such cases have added significance if plaintiffs can convince the jury that the injury will progress to the point of dysfunction, impairment, and possible or inevitable premature death. Until recently, there has been little published clinical data on mortality among cases of asbestosis, and even less data about the progression of intrapulmonary fibrosis.[17] Progression can occur and may shorten the lifespan of some patients with established diagnoses, but this is increasingly becoming a feature of "old" asbestosis.[18] The question presented in each individual's case is whether this plaintiff will progress. But what constitutes a predictor of progression remains in dispute.[19] Recent studies, however, suggest that progression is not inevitable.[20,21,22,23,24,25] Parkes observed that, as a general rule, once asbestos has been diagnosed clinically, it tends to progress slowly if at all. Furthermore, progression may cease at any stage.[26] Gaensler et al. studied workers of shipyards, paper mills, and asbestos product plants and concluded that asbestosis is getting rarer; that the great majority (80%) of workers failed to show signs of progression over the course of 11 years; that those who did progress, progressed slowly; and that there was no statistical evidence that progression was more rapid or severe in those with more advanced disease.[27] Jones et al. concluded that, as exposure to asbestos continues to decline, those recently diagnosed with asbestosis will less and less resemble the disease severity shown in former disability claimants.[25]

The importance of cigarette smoking in cases of this type is shown by the more rapid progression of disease in smokers, together with a more severe degree of fibrosis. The evidence from epidemiologic and radiologic studies indicates that, the individual that does not smoke is less likely to get asbestosis than a smoker.[12,16] Chest x-rays and pulmonary function are also generally less affected in the nonsmoker. The pathologist is uniquely situated to show how smoking affects the body's defense mechanisms and is detrimental to the individual in the asbestosis as well as the malignancy context.

PATHOLOGICAL DIAGNOSIS AND LUNG CANCER ATTRIBUTABILITY

The compensation of lung cancer cases that are allegedly attributable to asbestos exposure continues to be one of the major areas of controversy. This dispute focuses particularly on the determination of compensation for the cigarette-smoking asbestos worker with lung cancer.

The relationship between asbestosis and bronchial cancer is not straightforward. It has been observed that asbestos bronchial cancers invariably occur in lungs that are the seat of fibrosis. The site distribution and presence of premalignant changes in the areas of fibrosis in men and animals suggest that lung cancer is a complication of asbestosis, not merely of asbestos exposure.[28]

The evidence to date has not established that asbestos exposure causes carcinoma of the lung in the absence of antecedent asbestosis.[26] In the United Kingdom, compensation for cancer is ascribed to asbestos only if the attending fibrosis is similar to that seen in asbestosis.[29] Modern thought suggests fibrogenesis and carcinogenesis are linked.[30,31] Investigators have shown that the numbers of asbestos bodies in the lungs of the American urban population did not correlate with the presence of bronchial carcinoma.[32] These findings suggest pathologically that asbestos alone is not the cause of lung cancer.

Evidence exists that the risk of lung cancer is raised only among workers exposed to asbestos who also have parenchymal asbestosis.[30,33,34,35] The evidence is also quite strong that, if asbestos-exposed individuals do not smoke, the risk of lung cancer is quite small, if it exists at all.[36,37,38] The conclusion of one recent necropsy study of asbestosis and bronchial cancer in amphibole asbestos miners suggested that asbestos-caused bronchial cancer is almost always associated with some degree of histologically demonstrable asbestosis. Further, that in the absence of asbestosis at necropsy, a bronchial cancer in a person exposed to asbestos is unlikely to be due to asbestos.[35]

Of crucial importance for the defense in the case of the smoking asbestos worker with lung cancer, but without asbestosis, is that there is no method of pathologic examination that can determine that asbestos definitely (more probably than not in the legal arena) was the cause of the tumor. The pathologist should be called in to show that the appearance, cell type, location, clinical presentation, and course of the cancer is exactly what would be expected in a cigarette-related cancer. Further, the presence of asbestos bodies or pleural disease indicates only that exposure has occurred but is not proof of asbestos causation.[2]

THE INFLUENCE OF CIGARETTE SMOKING

The scientific literature continues to support the notion that the greatest contributor to causation of lung cancer is cigarette smoking. The latest information from the American Cancer Society indicates that, among male smokers, the lung cancer relative risk has doubled from 11.35 to 22.36 during Cancer Prevention Study II, which started in September 1982. The findings from this new American Cancer Society prospective study of 1.2 million men and women indicate that mortality risks among smokers have increased substantially for most of the eight major cancer sites causally associated with cigarette smoking.[39] Lung tumors are rare among asbestos workers who do not smoke. While early epidemiologic studies indicated that the effects of asbestos and smoking combine in a multiplicative synergistic fashion to produce lung cancer,[40] several recent surveys have suggested that this model is inapplicable in some cohorts.[41]

The issue of smoking presents several problems in determining causation of lung cancer. The inaccurate classification of smokers as nonsmokers may disproportionately inflate the calculated risk of lung cancer among nonsmokers. Workers' estimates of their own cigarette smoking may be questionable and are not always verifiable. Further, a high incidence of passive smoking in the presence of other workers whose smoking rates were higher than the general population could enhance a risk among nonsmokers.

Some authors remain uncertain whether any type of asbestos acting alone can cause lung cancer in nonsmokers.[41] The majority of epidemiologic and experimental information does not support the hypothesis that asbestos alone is a complete carcinogen in the respiratory tract or an initiator of bronchogenic carcinoma. It is thought that the number of lung tumors that develop in the nonsmoking asbestos worker are few and could be attributable to other occupational or environmental influences.[42]

The carcinogenic potential of cigarette smoke and asbestos in an occupational setting is difficult to assess, because neoplastic disease can be influenced by such agents as smoking habits, exposure to asbestos, contaminating metals, ionizing radiation, and other chemicals that may increase a person's risk of developing lung cancer. Individual variations of smoking and breathing patterns, lung function clearance, and pulmonary infection may also be confounding factors.[42]

The role of cigarette smoking as the leading known preventable cause of cancer cannot be ignored, and should be told to the jury. In fact, tobacco use in the United States is currently responsible for more than 30% of all cancer deaths, including cancers of the lung, larynx, oral cavity, pharynx, pancreas, kidney, bladder, and cervix. The epidemiologic and other evidence supporting a causal relation between smoking and cancer is extensive. Conservative estimates indicate that smoking accounts for 85% of lung cancer cases.[43] Reports from the Surgeon General reveal that smoking is responsible for one of every six deaths in the United States and remains the single most important preventable cause of death in our society.[39,44]

Surveys of the smoking habits of asbestos-exposed insulators, factory workers, and miners and millers have consistently shown that bronchogenic carcinoma is uncommon in those who do not smoke. Whereas there is only a slight increase in the prevalence of lung cancer among nonsmokers, heavy users of cigarettes have an 80- to 90-fold greater predisposition to cancer of the lung.[37,38,45] In the original insulator study done by Dr. Selikoff, only four cases of lung cancer were shown by death certificate to have occurred in those classified as never having smoked regularly.[46] And in the most recent data published on the insulator cohort, the standard mortality rate for lung cancer based on death certificates has declined from 4.6 in 1967–72 to 3.2 in 1980–86.[47]

A study of amosite asbestos factory workers concluded that, had it not been for cigarette smoking, many of the excess lung cancer deaths would have been avoided. The combination of cigarette smoking and asbestos exposure among those studied was calculated to have increased their risk of lung cancer death about 80 times as compared with like men of the same age who neither smoked cigarettes nor worked with asbestos.[38]

To date the contributing evidence that involuntary smoking causes lung cancer and other diseases in healthy nonsmokers also cannot be ignored.[48] Since cancer risk associated with involuntary smoking has focused on household members rather than on exposures in the workplace, the strong possibility exists that there has been an underestimation of the extent of nonsmokers' exposure to tobacco smoke.[43]

The effects of smoking cessation in asbestos workers was evident as early as 1979. Lung cancer mortalities of one group studied were approximately 1:3 for those who stopped compared with those who had continued to smoke. Cessation of smoking is followed by notable reversal of risk.[49] In particular, asbestos workers who stop smoking dramatically decrease their risk of dying of lung cancer.[18] This result further bolsters the proposition that asbestos alone is not the factor in causation of lung cancer that some would suggest.

The health consequences of smoking are apparent. For the majority of American workers who smoke, cigarette smoking represents a far greater cause of death and disability than their workplace environment.[44]

CANCER RISK

Another currently debated and unresolved issue is whether the asbestos-exposed plaintiff is at increased risk for cancer from the exposure alone. Traditionally, plaintiff experts refer to epidemiologic and animal studies in order to estimate the probable cancer risk. These risk estimates are then extrapolated to the individual plaintiff's case. The inaccuracies in such extrapolation as well as the problems in risk assessment are many and have been well documented.[50,51,52,53,54,55] While the process of risk assessment has become increasingly accepted as necessary for decision making, estimation of cancer risk at lower levels of asbestos exposure is uncertain and has limitations. Cancer risk studies must be looked at more critically if they are to be relied on by pathologists and other experts in the courtroom. It is quite simply misleading for a pathologist to use the *old* Selikoff data from the insulator cohort and indicate that the risk numbers or mortality estimates apply to asbestos-exposed individuals irrespective of the nature of exposure.

It has been 13 years since Dr. Selikoff projected that 20% of all asbestos-related deaths were due to lung cancer.[56] Since that time, there has been criticism concerning the projected risks based on the 1978 extrapolated data of American shipyard workers.[50,57,58] The problems have emphasized the lack of agreement on the methods as well as the results of the extrapolated data. In fact even the most recent Selikoff data themselves do not support his earlier projections.[47] A pathologist should be challenged if trying to use the old Selikoff data to make current projections.[47] The pathologist presented by the defense should be armed with current studies, which are more job or workplace specific, and which present more realistic data on which cancer risk estimates can be based.[59,60,61,62,63,64,65]

The 1978 Selikoff projections grossly overestimate the number of future asbestos-related deaths. One review of the prior estimates of the upper and lower limits of ranges determined by Nicholson, Peto, and McDonald estimated that about 76,700 deaths will occur from asbestos-associated lung cancer between the years 1985 and 2009, inclusive.[58] Doll and Peto took issue with the 1978 Selikoff projection and the conclusion that over 10% of all cancers are occupationally related to exposure to asbestos. They noted that most other studies reach the conclusion that many fewer deaths are related to asbestos and that the OSHA and Selikoff projections may be a 10-fold exaggeration.[66]

From the defense standpoint, it is unfair and wrong to tell a jury that asbestos exposure alone carries with it a five-fold increased risk for lung cancer, as many plaintiff counsel and medical experts try to do. An analysis of the statistical risks must look at the circumstances of exposure to determine if there is in fact increased risk, and if so, what the increase may be.

The rate at which lung cancer risk rises with increased cumulative asbestos exposure appears to vary with industrial process.[53] One study found the relative risks for lung cancer ranged from 1 (no increased risk) to 17, with the lowest values in miners and millers and the highest in pipe coverers and insulation workers with old long-term exposures. Such great variability, according to Gaensler et al.,[67] can be attributed to different types of exposure, differences among the groups at risk with respect to age, length of exposure and follow-ups, and the type of control in a reference group. Furthermore, the number of deaths is small in most studies, so the relative risks could be altered substantially by the addition of a single individual.[53,67]

Pronounced disagreement exists as to the magnitude of the range of relative risks. In many of the studies an inappropriate population was used to estimate numbers of deaths; in some surveys death certificates for the at-risk populations were adjusted from data in other medical records. The comparison was made with expected deaths derived from uncorrected death certificates. In the majority of studies the level and duration of exposure are unknown. The standardization of smoking habits is rarely possible. The most important weakness of many studies, in spite of the large numbers of subjects involved, is the very few necropsies conducted to confirm the diagnosis of primary carcinoma of the lung in the absence of evidence of asbestosis both macroscopically and microscopically.[26] The pathologist should serve to explain the effects of all these problems on calculating relative risk.

Pathologically these results are attributable to the dose–response phenomenon and cellular reactions in general. Experts indicate that, while epidemiologic studies in humans can attempt to measure risk directly, their capacity to do so becomes increasingly unreliable as the level of exposure falls. Partly this is due to deficiencies in exposure data, but mainly it is because no referenced population is ever more than roughly comparable with the exposed study group. Valid though the results of well-designed observational surveys are, the components of duration and intensity of exposure have not yet been separately assessed. Estimates of risk carry a wide margin of error.[68] At present, most studies, regardless of index of exposure, still suggest a dose–response relationship. Lung cancers are markedly more common in the groups that were most heavily exposed to asbestos.[69]

PATHOLOGICAL DIAGNOSIS OF MESOTHELIOMA

DIFFERENTIAL DIAGNOSIS

For mesothelioma, the primary problem surrounds the establishment of the pathologic diagnosis.[7] It is accepted that the differential diagnosis between mesothelioma and adenocarcinoma is an area of difficulty. The histologic and cytologic features of epithelial mesotheliomas, pulmonary adenocarcinomas, and other carcinomas may be exceedingly similar.[70]

The differentiation of carcinoma from mesothelioma remains a matter of judgment, despite advances in diagnostic techniques.[71] The presence of a known apparent second independent primary tumor in a case of mesothelioma requires more than the usual rigor in evaluation. In an individual case there may be great differences in lung sections from various areas, and these characteristics may result in a not-insignificant observer variation, even at a high level of expertise.[72]

Additionally, the usefulness of various diagnostic techniques remains an area of considerable controversy. The distinction from other neoplastic processes can be confusing.[73] It is agreed that generous sampling of tissue is required for an unequivocal premortem pathologic diagnosis.[73,74,75]

While the majority of tumors can be diagnosed as mesothelioma or carcinoma, still a small number remain for which a definite opinion one way or the other is not possible.[2] Inflammatory or reactive processes and other malignant tumors may mimic mesothelioma. Metastatic adenocarcinoma to the pleura is not only considerably more common than mesothelioma, but is often extremely difficult to distinguish from the epithelial variant of mesothelioma cytologically and histologically. Adenocarcinomas that frequently metastasize to the pleura include the lung, breast, stomach, ovary, colon, pancreas, kidney, and prostate.[76]

Malignant mesothelioma is still considered a difficult disease to diagnose, despite the fact that the criteria for the pathologic diagnosis of malignant mesothelioma have been described in detail and a standard set of reference slides is available from the Armed Forces Institute of Pathology.[77, 78]

A pathology review of recent United States mesothelioma cases indicates that important differences of opinion still exist in the diagnosis of mesothelioma, even among pathologists with expertise in this disease. In fact, even among experienced pathologists, the diagnosis of mesothelioma is highly subjective.[78,79]

ETIOLOGY

Mesotheliomas are not associated exclusively with asbestos exposure.[2,41,70,80] It is estimated that a significant percentage of men with malignant mesothelioma have no history of exposure to asbestos, and there is usually no excess of mineral fibers in their lungs.[41] While the most common cause of diffuse malignant mesothelioma is asbestos, the cause of a substantial proportion of cases cannot be stated to be asbestos.

Studies exist that enumerate the various nonasbestos agents and other occupational associations that are implicated in the causation of mesothelioma.[80,81,82] Further etiologic agents implicated with mesothelioma in humans include scarring of the pleura, chronic inflammation, chemical carcinogens, viruses, and hereditary predisposition,[82] as well as chronic empyema or therapeutic pneumothorax.[83] The possibility of an association between asbestos and certain chemical carcinogens and mesothelioma as well as unidentified environmental factors has also been discussed.[84] Genetic factors have additionally been implicated.[85] Therapeutic irradiation has been documented as a potential causative agent in mesothelioma.[86,87,88]

Because of the occurrence of large numbers of apparently nonasbestos-related malignant mesotheliomas in humans, and the recent substantiation for a background incidence of mesotheliomas in humans and animals,[80,82] there remains a need for more data concerning the role of nonasbestos exposures that may be associated with malignant mesothelioma. Therefore, exposure to other agents in and outside of the workplace should always be thoroughly explored with the pathology expert. The pathologist should not make the assumption that because a mesothelioma has been diagnosed asbestos was the cause.

UTILIZATION OF THE PATHOLOGIST

A major reason for using the pathologist in litigation when defending an asbestos case is to show where an individual's claim of asbestos causation is ill founded. Despite the eloquent rhetoric of plaintiff's counsel in courtrooms, most ills of the human race are not caused by asbestos. The pathologist is important to show all important health problems suffered by an individual. The pathologist can also show when it is most likely that asbestos is not the cause of a claimed problem. After all, the goal of the justice system is not to make rich people of litigants (or their lawyers) but to give reasonable compensation where it is due.

When utilizing the pathologist, it is important to get all available tissue. If tissue blocks are available, the pathologist should have access to them. If it can be avoided, do not restrict the pathologist only to the slides cut by the other side's expert. If gross tissue is available, the pathologist should examine that also.

The pathologist should always be furnished all available relevant medical records. Even though the desire of many busy pathologists is only to look at tissue slides along with a brief synopsis of the history of the case, the attorney should not succumb to that desire. The pathologist has a unique expertise that allows him or her to gather from records matters that may unravel an entire case. For example, if a pleural effusion is said to be caused by asbestos exposure, the pathologist is uniquely situated to determine from records if the fluid was sterile (if not, asbestos was probably not involved), whether the fluid fits the general published descriptions of asbestos-related fluid, if the occurrence is past the typical latency (20 years or less), and if there are other apparent reasons to explain the effusion.

Much has been written in this chapter about risk estimates, particularly in regard to lung cancer. In putting those risk estimates in perspective regarding an individual case, the pathologist can be quite helpful. The plaintiffs typically desire to take the now-outdated and generally inflated five-fold increased risk that Selikoff et al.[46] reported in long-term insulators with exposures starting decades ago and to apply that risk to the plaintiff in the case. Similar use is attempted to be made for inapplicable British death reports.[89] The pathologist should be called on to show how dose response works in relation to an individual and to compare pathologically the degree of asbestosis generally seen in individuals today to the degree seen in older studies and cases. The point to be shown graphically by the pathologist is that today's disease is not the same as the disease that occurred from exposures of decades ago. The pathologist should be questioned about "old" asbestosis as compared to "new" or "current" asbestosis that is generally being diagnosed today.

Pictorially and graphically, the pathologist, by presenting examples of what is generally seen today and comparing with cases from decades ago, can show from a practical standpoint a disease of "new" asbestosis with the same name as "old" asbestosis but that is quite different, relative to an increased cancer risk and progression. This can be done both macroscopically and microscopically. It can be shown with the aid of the pathologist that asbestosis is not inevitably progressive, does not generally lead to death and disability, and is not usually a harbinger of bad things to come.

REFERENCES

1. Kittle CF: *Mesothelioma: Diagnosis and Management.* Chicago: Year Book, 1987, pp. 1–36.
2. Churg A: Neoplastic asbestos-induced diseases. Ch. 8 In: *Pathology of Occupational Lung Disease* (Churg A, Green F, eds.), New York: Igaku-Shoin, 1989, p. 308.
3. Browne K: Asbestos-related malignancy and the Cairns hypothesis. *Brit J Ind Med* 48:73–76, 1991.
4. American Thoracic Society: The diagnosis of non-malignant diseases related to asbestos. *Am Rev Resp Dis* 134:363–368, 1986.
5. Canadian Thoracic Society: Report of task force on occupational respiratory disease (pneumoconiosis). Department of National Health and Welfare, 1979, pp. 44–45.
6. Craighead JE et al. The pathology of asbestos-associated diseases of the lungs and pleural cavities: Diagnostic criteria and proposed grading schema. *Arch Path Lab Med* 106(11):541–596, 1982.
7. Churg A: Current issues in the pathologic and mineralogic diagnosis of asbestos-induced disease. *Chest* 87(3):275–280, 1984.
8. Warnock ML, Isenburg W: Asbestos burden and the pathology of lung cancer. *Chest* 89(1):20–26, 1986.
9. Churg A: The distribution of amosite asbestos in the periphery of the normal human lung. *Brit J Ind Med* 47:677–681, 1990.
10. Roggli VL, Pratt PC: Number of asbestos bodies on iron-stained tissue sections in relation to asbestos body counts in lung tissue digests. *Hum Path* 14(4):355–361, 1983.
11. Greenberg SD: Asbestos. Ch. 22 In: *Pulmonary Pathology* (Dail DH, Hammar SP, eds.), New York: Springer-Verlag, 1988, pp. 619–623.
12. Roggli VL: Human disease consequences of fiber exposures: A review of human lung pathology and fiber burden data. *Env Health Perspectives* 88:295–303, 1990.
13. Warnock ML, Kuwahara TJ, Wolery G: The relation of asbestos burden to asbestosis and lung cancer. *Pathol Annu* 18:109–45, 1983.
14. Roggli VL, Johnston WW, Kaminsky DB: Asbestos bodies in fine needle aspirates of the lung. *Acta Cytotol* 28:403–408, 1984.
15. Begin R, Menard II, Decarie F, et al. Immunogenic factors as determinants of asbestosis. *Lung* 165:159–163, 1987.
16. Weiss W: Cigarette smoke, asbestos, and small irregular opacities. *Am Rev Respir Dis* 130:293–301, 1984.
17. Coutts I, Turner-Warwick M: *Factors Predicting Outcome in Intrapulmonary Fibrosis Associated with Asbestos Exposure.* London: Cardiothoracic Institute, 1980.
18. Selikoff IJ: Asbestos-associated disease. Ch. 14 In: *Public Health and Preventive Medicine,* 12th ed. (Maxcy-Rosenau, ed.), East Norwalk, CT: Appleton-Century-Crofts, 1986.
19. Gaensler EA, Tederlinic PJ, McLoud TC: Radiographic progression of asbestosis with and without continued exposure. VII International Pneumoconiosis Conference Proceedings, Part I, NIOSH-ILO USDHHS, 1988, pp. 386–392.
20. Becklake MR, Liddell FCK, Mantreda J, McDonald JC: Radiological changes after withdrawal from asbestos exposure. *Brit J Ind Med* 36:23–28, 1979.
21. Gregor A, Parkes RW, Dubois R, Turner-Warwick M: Radiographic progression of asbestosis: Preliminary report. *Ann NY Acad Sci* 338:147–156, 1979.
22. Rossiter CE, Health JR, Harries PG: Royal naval dockyards asbestosis research project: Nine-year follow-up study of men exposed to asbestos in Davenport dockyard. *J R Soc Med* 73:337–344, 1980.

23. Suoranta H, Huesbonen MS, Zitting A, Juentunen Jr: Radiographic progression of asbestosis. *Am J Ind Med* 3:67–74, 1982.
24. Villat JR, Boutin C, Pietri JF: Late progression of radiographic changes in Canari chrysotile mine and mill ex-workers. *Arch Env Health* 38:54–58, 1983.
25. Jones RN, Diem JE, Hughes JM, et al: Progression of asbestos effects: A prospective longitudinal study of chest radiographs and lung function. *Brit J Ind Med* 46:96–105, 1989.
26. Parkes R: Silicates and Lung Disease. Ch. 9 In: *Occupational Lung Disorders*, 2nd ed. Boston: Butterworths, 1982, pp. 268–294.
27. Gaensler E et al.: Third international conference on environmental lung disease. *Chest* 91(2):305, 1987.
28. Sluis-Cremer GK: The relationship between asbestosis and bronchial cancer. *Chest* 78:380–381, 1980.
29. Seal RME: Current views on pathological aspects of asbestosis. In: *Biol Effects of Mineral Fibers* (Wagner JC, ed.), Lyon: IARC Scientific Publications, 1980, 1:217–235.
30. Hughes JM, Weill H: Asbestosis as a precursor of asbestos-related lung cancer: Results of a prospective mortality study. *Brit J Ind Med* 48:229–233, 1991.
31. Rom WN, Travis D, Brody A: State of the art, cellular and molecular basis of the asbestos-related diseases. *Am Rev Respir Dis* 143:408–422, 1991.
32. Churg A, Warnock ML: Number of asbestos bodies in urban patients with lung cancer and gastrointestinal cancer and in matched controls. *Chest* 79:143–149, 1976.
33. Browne K: Is asbestos or asbestosis the cause of increased risk of lung cancer in asbestos workers? *Brit J Ind Med* 43:145–149, 1986.
34. Weiss W: Correspondence—Pulmonary fibrosis in asbestos insulation workers with lung cancer. *Brit J Ind Med* 46:430–432, 1989.
35. Sluis-Cremer GK, Bezuidenhout BN: Relation between asbestosis and bronchial cancer in amphibole asbestos miners. *Brit J Ind Med*, 46:537–540, 1989.
36. Doll R, Peto R: The causes of cancer: Quantitative estimates of available risks of cancer in the United States today. *JNCI* 66:1220, 1981.
37. Craighead JE, Mossman BT: Pathogenesis of asbestos-associated diseases, NEJM 306(24):1446–1455, 1982.
38. Selikoff I, Seidman H, Hammond E: Mortality effects of cigarette smoking among amosite asbestos factory workers. *JNCI* 60(3):507–513, 1980.
39. Shopland DR, Eyre HJ, Pechacek TF: Smoking-attributable cancer mortality in 1991: Is lung cancer now the leading cause of death among smokers in the United States? *JNCI* 83(16):1142–1148, 1991.
40. Saracci R: Asbestos and lung cancer: An analysis of the epidemiological evidence on the asbestos–smoking interaction. *Int J Cancer* 20:323–331, 1977.
41. Mossman BT, Gee JB: Asbestos-related diseases. *NEJM* 320(26):1724–1730, 1989.
42. Mossman BT, Craighead JE: Mechanisms in asbestos-associated bronchogenic carcinoma. Ch. 6 In: *Asbestos-Related Malignancy* (Antman K, Aisner J, eds.), Orlando, FL: Harcourt, Brace, Jovanovich, 1986, pp. 137–150.
43. Ernester V: Trends in smoking, cancer risks and cigarette promotion. *Cancer* 62(8) (supplement):1702–1712, 1988.
44. U.S. Dept. of Health and Human Services. Reducing the health consequences of smoking: 25 years of progress. A report of the surgeon general. DHHS Publication No. (CDC) 89-8411, 1989; p. 11.
45. Selikoff IJ, Hammond EC, Churg J: Asbestos exposure, smoking and neoplasia. *JAMA* 204:104–110, 1968.

46. Hammond EC, Selikoff IJ, Seidman H: Asbestos Exposure, Cigarette Smoking and Death Rates. *Ann NY Acad Sci* 330:473–490, 1979.
47. Seidman H, Selikoff IJ: Decline in death rates among asbestos insulation workers 1967–86 associated with diminution of work exposure to asbestos. *Ann NY Acad Sci* 341:308, 1990.
48. U.S. Public Health Service: The health consequences of involuntary smoking: A report of the Surgeon General; National Research Council Environmental tobacco smoke: Measuring exposures in assessing health defects. Washington DC: National Academy Press, 1986.
49. Selikoff I: Asbestos and smoking. *JAMA* 242(5):458, 1979.
50. Gough M: Sources and interpretation of asbestos exposure data. *J Toxicol Clin Toxicol* 21:211–235, 1983–84.
51. Enterline PE: Estimating health risks in studies of the health effects of asbestos. *Am Rev Resp Dis* 113:175–180, 1976.
52. Brown S: Quantitative risk assessment of environmental hazards. *Am Rev Public Health* 6:247–267, 1985.
53. Weill H, Hughes J: Asbestos as public health risk: Disease and policy. *Am Rev Public Health* 7:171–192, 1986.
54. Crump K: Time-related factors in quantitative risk assessment. *J Chron Dis Vol* 40 (Suppl.)(2):1015–1115, 1987.
55. Hughes J, Weill H: Asbestos exposure—quantitative assessment of risk. *Am Rev Respir Dis* 133:5–13, 1986.
56. Selikoff IJ, Hammond EC: Asbestos-associated disease in United States shipyards. *Cancer J Clinicians.* 78(2):87–89, 1978.
57. Lee P: Assessing the risk of cancer. *Cancer and Detection* 4:15–23, 1978.
58. Lilienfeld DE et al: Projection of asbestos-related diseases in the United States, 1985–2009. *Brit J Ind Med* 45:283–291, 1985.
59. Selikoff IJ: *Disability Compensation for Asbestos-Associated Disease in the United States.* Report to the U.S. Department of Labor, Environmental Sciences Laboratory, 1981, p. 124.
60. Kolonel LN et al: Cancer occurrence in shipyard workers exposed to asbestos in Hawaii. *Cancer Res* 45:3924–3928, 1985.
61. Hanis NM et al: A retrospective mortality study of workers in three major U.S. refineries and chemical plants. *J Occup Med* 27(4):283–292, 1985.
62. Hanis NM et al: A retrospective mortality study of workers in three major U.S. refineries and chemical plants, *J Occup Med.* 27(4):361–364, 1985.
63. Divine B et al: Texaco mortality study. *J Occup Med* 27(6):445–447, 1985.
64. Kaplan SD: Update of a mortality study of workers in petroleum refineries. *J Occup Med* 28(7):514–516, 1986.
65. Cantor KP: Patterns of mortality among plumbers and pipefitters. *Am J Ind Med* 10:73–89, 1986.
66. Doll, Peto: supra note 36, pp. 1305–1308.
67. Gaensler E et al: Thoracic surgical problems in asbestos-related disorders. *Ann Thorac Surg* 40(1):82–85, 1985.
68. Davis JMG, McDonald JC: Low-level exposure to asbestos: Is there a cancer risk? *Brit J Ind Med* 45:505–508, 1988.
69. Newhouse M: Epidemiology of asbestos-related tumors. *Sem Onc* 8(3):250–257, 1981.
70. Hammar SP, Bolen JW: Pleural neoplasms. Ch. 30 In: *Pulmonary Pathology* (Dail DH, Hammar SP, eds.), New York: Springer-Verlag, 1988, pp. 973–1028.
71. Warnock ML et al: Differentiation of adenocarcinoma of the lung from mesothelioma. *Am J Path,* 133:(1)30–37, 1988.
72. Kannerstein M, McCaughey WTE, Churg J, Selikoff IJ: A critique of the criteria for the diagnosis of diffuse malignant mesothelioma. *Mt. Sinai J Med* 44:445–494, 1977.

73. Roggli VL, Kolbeck J, et al: Pathology of human mesothelioma: Etiologic and diagnostic considerations. In: *Pathology Annual*, vol. 22 (Rosen PP, Fechner RE, eds.), Norwalk, CT: Appleton & Lange, 1987:91–93.
74. Hillerdal G: Malignant mesothelioma, 1982: Review of 4710 published cases. *Br J Dis Chest* 77:321–343, 1983.
75. McCaughey WTE: Criteria for the diagnosis of diffuse mesothelioma tumors. *Ann NY Acad Sci* 132:603–613, 1965.
76. Antman KH: Asbestos-related malignancy. *CRC Crit Rev Oncol/Hematol* 6(3):287–306, 1987.
77. Hochholzer L, Johnson FB, Kannerstein M: *Syllabus: Asbestos-related Disease*. Armed Forces Institute of Pathology Publication L00679, 1979.
78. Spirtas R, Keehn R, Beebe GW, Wagner JC et al: Results of a pathology review of recent U.S. mesothelioma cases. *Accomp Oncol* 1: 144–152, 1986.
79. McCaughey WTE, Oldham PD: Diffuse mesotheliomas: Observer variation in histological diagnosis. IARC Sci. Pub. 1973, 8:58–61.
80. Ilgren EB, Wagner JC: Background incidence of mesothelioma: Animal and human evidence. *Reg Tox Pharmacol* 13:1–17, 1991.
81. Malker HSR, McLaughlin JK, Malker BK et al: Occupational risks for pleural mesothelioma in Sweden, 1961–1979. *J Natl Cancer Inst* 74:61, 1985.
82. Peterson JT Jr, Greenberg SD, Buffler PA: Non-asbestos-related malignant mesothelioma: A review. *Cancer* 54:951–960, 1984.
83. Hillerdal G, Berg J: Malignant mesothelioma secondary to chronic inflammation in old scars: Two new cases and review of the literature. *Cancer* 55:1968–1972, 1985.
84. Roggli VL, McGavran MH, Subach J et al: Pulmonary asbestos body counts and electron probe analysis of asbestos body cores in patients with mesothelioma: A Study of 25 cases. *Cancer* 50:2423–2432, 1982.
85. Lynch HT, Cats D, Markricka SE: Familial mesothelioma: Review in family study. *Cancer Genet-Cytogenet* 15:25, 1985.
86. Stock RJ et al: Malignant peritoneal mesothelioma following radiotherapy for seminoma of the testes. *Cancer* 44:914, 1979.
87. Anderson KA, Hurley WC, Hurley BT, Ohrt DW: Malignant pleural mesothelioma following radiotherapy in a 16-year-old boy. *Cancer* 56:273–276, 1985.
88. Maurer R et al: Malignant peritoneal mesothelioma after cholangiography with thorotrast. *Cancer* 36:1381, 1975.
89. Berry G: Mortality of workers certified by pneumoconiosis medical panels as having asbestosis. *Brit J Ind Med* 38:130–137, 1981.

Appendix
Tissue Digestion Techniques
Victor L. Roggli

METHOD A

The digestion procedure used by the author[1] is a modification of the sodium hypochlorite digestion technique described by Williams et al.[2] The details of the procedure follow.

MATERIALS
  0.4-µm pore-size, 25-mm-diameter Nuclepore® filters
  Nuclepore® filtering apparatus, including cylindrical funnel (10 cc), fritted-glass filter support, and 250-cc side-arm flask
  Vacuum source, vacuum tubing, trap
  20-cc plastic-screw-top scintillation-counter glass vials
  Aliquot mixer for blood tubes (Miles Laboratories)
  Two-sided sticky tape
  Scalpel handle, clean scalpel blades
  Forceps (coarse and fine tip)
  25-mm-diameter rubber "O"-rings for filters
  Pasteur pipettes with rubber bulbs
  Rectangular plastic weighing dishes
  Analytical balance

REAGENTS
  All reagents to be prefiltered through 0.4-µm-pore-size filter.
  5.25% sodium hypochlorite solution (commercial bleach)
  8.0% oxalic acid solution
  Absolute ethanol
  Deionized water
  Chloroform (CAUTION: Do not filter through Nuclepore® filter, for it will dissolve the filter!)

PROCEDURE
  Step 1 Weigh the selected specimen (up to about 0.3 gm) wet in a plastic dish on an analytical balance after gently blotting excess fluid with a paper towel.

  Step 2 Mince the tissue into 1- or 2-mm cubes within the plastic dish using fresh scalpel blade and coarse-tip forceps.

  Step 3 Add two Pasteur-pipettefuls of filtered sodium hypochlorite solution to the plastic dish, and carefully transfer the minced tissue in hypochlorite solution into a 20-cc plastic-screw-top scintillation-counter vial.

  Step 4 Rinse the weighing dish with an additional aliquot of hypochlorite solution from a Pasteur pipette, and add this solution to the vial.

Then add two more aliquots (total of 10 cc) of hypochlorite solution directly to the vial.

Step 5   Label the vial for identification, and place it on an aliquot mixer with double-sided tape (Fig. A-1). Allow digestion to proceed until tissue fragments are no longer visible to the naked eye (usually 20–25 minutes for a 0.3-gm sample; however, more time may be required for severely fibrotic or deparaffinized specimens).

Step 6   Transfer the digested suspension into the glass cylinder of the assembled filtration apparatus (see Fig. A-1). It is best to add no more than about 25% of the suspension to the filter at any one time.

Step 7   As the filtration slows, you may add aliquots of 8.0% oxalic acid, absolute ethanol, and fresh hypochlorite solution to the filter surface with a Pasteur pipette to reduce buildup of any organic residues. Add an aliquot of deionized water between additions of oxalic acid, ethanol, or hypochlorite solution to prevent crystal deposition on the filter surface.

Step 8   After the final portion of the suspension has passed through the filter and a final rinse with oxalic acid, ethanol, and hypochlorite solution has been effected, wash a final aliquot of absolute ethanol through the filter.

Step 9   Transfer the filter from the filtering apparatus onto the surface of a glass slide using fine-tip forceps. Attach the periphery of the filter to the surface of the slide with small, torn portions of white, lightly adhesive tape (to prevent folding and buckling of the filter when chloroform is added).

Step 10   After the filter has completely dried, add chloroform dropwise to the filter surface with a Pasteur pipette until the filter is covered and cleared. The tape securing the edges of the filter can then be removed with fine-tip forceps before the chloroform dries.

Step 11   After the chloroform dries, add a coverslip to the slide in a suitable mounting medium (e.g., Permount). The slide is ready for viewing by light microscopy.

Step 9a   If you wish to examine the filter by scanning electron microscopy (SEM) rather that light microscopy, mount the filter on a 25-mm carbon disc with colloidal graphite and sputter-coat with gold, carbon, or other suitable conducting coating (see Fig. A-1).[3] If you wish to employ transmission electron microscopy, then cut out a small portion of the filter and transfer it onto a TEM grid, removing the filter material with chloroform using the Jaffé wick technique.[4,5]

NOTES REGARDING DIGESTION PROCEDURE

In selecting tissue for digestion, avoid areas of tumor, congestion, or consolidation as much as possible. These would affect the denominator in calculations of asbestos-fiber or -body concentrations, and thus would tend to falsely lower the calculated value. Formalin-fixed tissue is preferred by the author, although fresh lung tissue works just as well. An adequate sample is, at minimum, an open lung

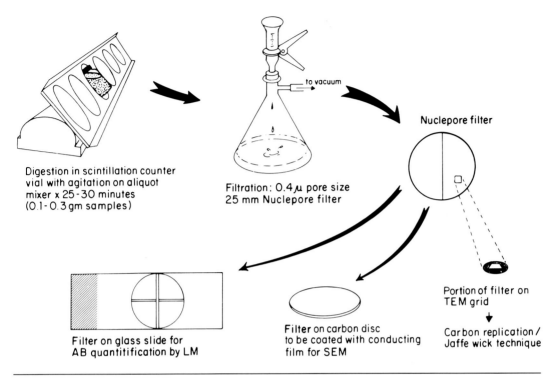

Digestion in scintillation counter
vial with agitation on aliquot
mixer x 25-30 minutes
(0.1-0.3 gm samples)

to vacuum

Filtration: 0.4 μ pore size
25 mm Nuclepore filter

Nuclepore filter

Filter on glass slide for
AB quantitification by LM

Filter on carbon disc
to be coated with conducting
film for SEM

Portion of filter on
TEM grid
↓
Carbon replication /
Jaffe wick technique

FIGURE A-1. *Method A:* Technique for extracting mineral fibers and other inorganic particulates from lung tissue. Tissue is first digested in sodium hypochlorite solution (commercial bleach) and the residue collected on a Nuclepore® filter. The filter may be mounted for light, scanning electron, or transmission electron microscopy. See text for details.

biopsy; lobectomy, pneumonectomy, or autopsy tissue is even better. Transbronchial biopsies are inadequate to give meaningful results.[6] If a lobectomy or pneumonectomy specimen is available, the author generally prepares two or three filters, and for autopsy cases, four filters (one from the upper and lower lobes of each lung). At least one filter is examined by SEM for asbestos bodies and uncoated fibers; the rest are examined by light microscopy for asbestos-body content.

Sometimes, only paraffin-embedded lung tissue is available. In such cases, a portion is selected from the block, deparaffinized in xylene, and rehydrated through absolute and 95% ethanol. The usual times for deparaffinizing tissue are doubled to maximize paraffin removal, since residual paraffin clogs the pores of the filter, obscuring fibers and bodies. The wet weight is obtained from the specimen in 95% ethanol. A correction factor has to be applied to deparaffinized specimens because of lipids removed at the time the tissue was originally processed[6] (see last paragraph of upcoming section on "Counting Rules and Calculations").

There may be some variability in Steps 6 and 7 (filtration), depending on the individual sample. Some samples pass readily through the filter and require little rinsing with oxalic acid, ethanol, or hypochlorite solution to remove residues. Other cases may sharply decrease their rate of filtration and require considerable effort to remove organic residues. Sometimes ethanol most readily restores the filtration rate, while in other cases oxalic acid is more effective. Occasionally it is necessary to add a drop of Tween 80 or some other detergent to the suspension to facilitate filtration.

METHOD B

In some cases, the asbestos-body content is too low to obtain an accurate estimate from a 0.3-gm sample. If accurate quantification is desirable in such cases, then the procedure of Smith and Naylor[7] employing a larger sample size may be preferable. The details of the procedure follow.

MATERIALS
0.4-μm-pore-size, 25-mm-diameter Nuclepore® filters
Nuclepore® filtering apparatus, including cylindrical funnel (10 cc), fritted-glass filter support, and 250-cc side-arm flask
Vacuum source, vacuum tubing, trap
300-cc glass jar with lid
Scalpel handle, clean scalpel blades
Forceps (course and fine tip)
25-mm-diameter rubber "O"-rings for filters
Pasteur pipettes with rubber bulbs
50-cc screw-cap conical centrifuge tubes
Rectangular plastic weighing dishes
Analytical balance
Tabletop centrifuge

REAGENTS
Filtration is optional.
5.25% sodium hypochlorite solution (commercial bleach)
Chloroform
95% ethanol
50% ethanol

PROCEDURE
Step 1   Weigh the selected specimen (approximately 5 gm) wet in a plastic dish on an analytical balance after gently blotting excess fluid with a paper towel.

Step 2   Mince the tissue into 2- or 3-mm cubes within the plastic dish using fresh scalpel blade and coarse-tip forceps.

Step 3   With a scalpel blade, transfer the tissue from the dish into the glass jar. Rinse the dish with a 2-cc aliquot (one Pasteur-pipetteful) of sodium hypochlorite solution, and add this solution to the jar. Then add about 250 cc of hypochlorite solution to the jar (approximately 50 cc hypochlorite solution per gram of tissue).

Step 4 Let the glass jar sit for several days to allow time for the tissue to digest and for the asbestos bodies to settle to the bottom (Fig. A-2).[8]

Step 5 Remove the supernatant by gentle aspiration using a Pasteur-pipette attached to the vacuum system, being careful not to disturb the sediment at the bottom of the jar.

Step 6 Add a 20-cc aliquot of chloroform to the jar to suspend the asbestos bodies embedded in the sticky layer on the bottom of the jar. Swirl the chloroform to dissolve these residues, then add a 20-cc aliquot of 50% ethanol to the chloroform suspension. Transfer the ethanol-chloroform mixture to a 50-cc screw-cap conical centrifuge tube.

Step 7 Label the centrifuge tube for identification, and place it in the tabletop centrifuge. Use a tube from another sample or a tube filled with water for balance. Centrifuge the specimen at 200 G for 10–15 minutes.

Step 8 Remove the supernatant by gentle aspiration using a Pasteur-pipette attached to the vacuum system, being careful to remove pigment and lipid residues at the chloroform-ethanol interface and leaving approximately 5 cc of chloroform and sediment at the bottom of the tube (chloroform is heavier than ethanol and settles to the bottom).

Step 9 If the sediment remaining after Step 8 is black, then you may add an additional 20-cc aliquot of chloroform and 20 cc of 50% ethanol to the centrifuge tube and repeat Steps 7 and 8. Otherwise, add about 15 cc of 95% ethanol to the sediment and residual chloroform.

Step 10 Suspend the sediment in the 95% ethanol using vigorous shaking or a vortex mixer if necessary. Then transfer this suspension into the glass cylinder of the assembled filtration apparatus (see Fig. A-2), and collect the sediment on the filter surface.

Step 11 Transfer the filter from the filtering apparatus onto the surface of a glass slide using the fine-tip forceps. Then prepare the slide for examination by light microscopy as described earlier in Steps 9–11 of Method A.

NOTES REGARDING DIGESTION PROCEDURE

Tissue selection guidelines are similar to those outlined earlier for Method A. Generally, a lower lobe sample abutting the pleura is used. The values obtained for asbestos bodies per gram of wet lung using Method B are generally quite comparable to those obtained with Method A. In a study of 10 cases in which both methods were used to quantitate the asbestos-body content, the average ratio of the results obtained by Method B to those obtained by Method A was 1.1 (range 0.3–3.5).[9] Although filters prepared by Method B can also be examined by analytical electron microscopy, the author does not recommend this because there is evidence of a significant uncoated-fiber

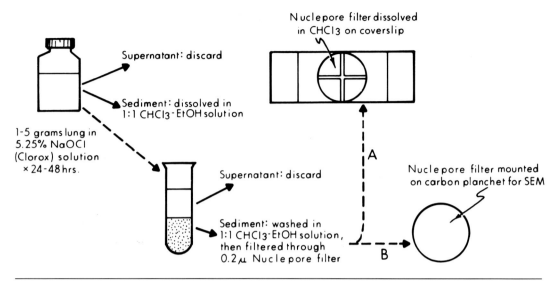

FIGURE A-2. *Method B:* Technique for extracting asbestos bodies from lung tissue. Tissue is first digested in sodium hypochlorite solution (commercial bleach), followed by a centrifugation step to separate the inorganic particulates from inorganic carbon and undigested lipid residues, the latter remaining at the chloroform-ethanol interface. The residue is recovered on a Nuclepore® filter, which may then be mounted on a glass slide for examination by light microscopy. See text for details. Reprinted from Ref. 8, with permission.

loss at the chloroform-ethanol interface during the centrifugation step (unpublished observations). Others have also reported fiber losses with each sequential centrifugation step.[10]

It is extremely important to maintain scrupulously clean glassware. Studies have shown that asbestos bodies and fibers adhere to glassware surfaces and may be removed with difficulty.[11,12] Such loss of fibers or bodies may give a falsely low count. Of greater concern, however, is the contamination of glassware with carryover of bodies or fibers from a case with a heavy burden to a case with very low tissue asbestos content.[13] A new scalpel blade, centrifuge tube, or glass vial should be used for each case. The cylindrical glass funnel and the glass jars should be carefully cleaned with warm soapy water and a scrub brush between cases, rinsing with copious amounts of deionized water.

Filtration of reagents is optional for Method B because asbestos bodies derive only from biological systems and do not contaminate these reagents. (Uncoated fibers, on the other hand, may contaminate many different reagents and give falsely elevated fiber counts by electron microscopy. This is especially problematic for small chrysotile fibers, which are ubiquitous. Reagent blanks should be prepared and examined to control for this possibility whenever electron microscopic techniques are employed for asbestos fiber quantitation.)

COUNTING RULES AND CALCULATIONS

The morphologic features of asbestos bodies are described and illustrated in detail in Chap. 3. Asbestos bodies, which have thin translucent cores, are to be distinguished from pseudoasbestos bodies, which have broad, yellow sheet-silicate or black cores. The author enumerates the true asbestos bodies and pseudoasbestos (nonasbestos ferruginous) bodies separately. Except in rare cases, true asbestos bodies are more numerous than pseudoasbestos bodies. Indeed, asbestos bodies are identified in more than 90% of cases, whereas pseudoasbestos bodies are observed, in the author's experience, in about 25% of cases. Identification of asbestos bodies by scanning electron microscopy is dependent on morphologic features alone, since one cannot appreciate the additional information regarding the color of the core fiber that is available from light microscopic observations. However, EDXA studies of the core fiber allow for precise identification of fiber type (see Chap. 11).

Fibers are defined as particles with a length-to-diameter (aspect) ratio of at least 3:1 and with roughly parallel sides. The author does not count particles with aspect ratio less that 3:1 or with sides that are nonparallel or excessively irregular. Clumps of fibers are seldom encountered with the digestion procedures just described. Both asbestos and nonasbestos fibers are counted together (total uncoated-fiber count). Although there is considerable morphologic overlap, most of the fibers that are 10 μm or greater in length with aspect ratio greater that 10:1 are asbestos, whereas nonasbestos mineral fibers tend to be shorter than 10μm in length and have aspect ratios less than 10:1. Asbestos fibers are distinguished from nonasbestos mineral fibers on the basis of their morphology and chemical composition as determined by energy-dispersive spectrometry (see Chap. 11). Asbestos fibers must also be distinguished from crystals that may form on the filter surface, which often have pointed ends. Such crystals are *not* included in the total fiber count.

Quantification of the asbestos-body content of a lung tissue sample requires a determination of the numbers of bodies per unit area of filter surface. This can usually be accomplished by counting the number of bodies in a portion of the filter of known area, and multiplying this value by the total effective surface area. The author usually counts the number of bodies in two perpendicular strips at a magnification of 400× (see Fig. A-1 and A-2). In cases with a low asbestos-body burden, the entire filter surface may need to be counted to obtain accurate results. In quantifying the asbestos-body and uncoated-fiber burdens by scanning electron microscopy, the author counts 200 fibers or 100 consecutive 1000× fields, whichever comes first. The latter amounts to approximately 1% of the surface area of the filter. The total numbers of bodies or fibers on the filter can then be determined by multiplying the number of bodies or fibers per square millimeter of surface area by the total effective surface area of the filter. Determination of asbestos-body or fiber concentration can then be accomplished by dividing the numbers per filter by the amount of wet tissue digested in preparing that particular filter.

For paraffin blocks, the value must be multiplied by 0.7 for the results to be comparable to wet fixed lung tissue[9] (see earlier). Some investigators prefer to report their results in terms of bodies or fibers per gram of dried lung. In this circumstance, a portion of lung adjacent to the one actually digested should be weighed wet and then dried to constant weight in a 60–70°C oven. Then the asbestos-body or fiber concentration per gram of wet lung can be multiplied by the wet-to-dry weight ratio, yielding an asbestos-body or fiber concentration per gram of dried lung (see also Chaps. 3 and 11).

SAMPLE CALCULATION
Sample weight = 0.308 gm
Total effective filter area = $\pi r^2 = \pi (10.5 \text{ mm})^2 = 346 \text{ mm}^2$
Asbestos bodies counted in two perpendicular strips of filter
  (see Figs. A-1 and A-2) = 423
Empirically determined diameter of one 400 × field = 0.42 mm
Area of two perpendicular strips = $2 \times 21 \text{ mm} \times 0.42 \text{ mm} = 17.6 \text{ mm}^2$
Asbestos bodies (AB) per mm^2 = 24

Therefore,

$$\frac{AB}{gm} = \frac{(24/mm^2)(346 \text{ mm}^2)}{0.308 \text{ gm}}$$

$$= 27,000$$

REFERENCES

1. Roggli VL, Brody AR: Changes in numbers and dimensions of chrysotile asbestos fibers in lungs of rats following short-term exposure. *Expl Lung Res* 7:133–147, 1984.
2. Williams MG, Dodson RF, Corn C, Hurst GA: A procedure for the isolation of amosite asbestos and ferruginous bodies from lung tissue and sputum. *J Toxicol Environ Health* 10:627–638, 1982.
3. Roggli VL: Scanning electron microscopic analysis of mineral fibers in human lungs. Ch. 5 In: *Microprobe Analysis in Medicine* (Ingram P, Shelburne JD, Roggli VL, eds.), Washington, DC: Hemisphere Pub., 1989, pp. 97–110.
4. Churg A: Quantitative methods for analysis of disease induced by asbestos and other mineral particles using the transmission electron microscope. Ch. 4 In: *Microprobe Analysis in Medicine* (Ingram P, Shelburne JD, Roggli VL, eds.), Washington DC: Hemisphere Pub., 1989, pp. 79–95.
5. Churg A, Sakoda N, Warnock ML: A simple method for preparing ferruginous bodies for electron microscopic examination. *Am J Clin Pathol* 68:513–517, 1977.
6. Roggli VL: Preparatory techniques for the quantitative analysis of asbestos in tissues. *Proceedings of the 46th Annual Meeting of the Electron Micros-*

copy Society of America (Bailey GW, ed.), San Francisco: San Francisco Press, 1988, pp. 84–85.

7. Smith MJ, Naylor B: A method for extracting ferruginous bodies from sputum and pulmonary tissues. *Am J Clin Pathol* 58:250–254, 1972.

8. Roggli VL, Shelburne JD: New concepts in the diagnosis of mineral pneumoconioses. *Sem Respir Med* 4:138–148, 1982.

9. Roggli VL, Pratt PC, Brody AR: Asbestos content of lung tissue in asbestos-associated diseases: A study of 110 cases. *Br J Ind Med* 43:18–28, 1986.

10. Ashcroft T, Heppleston AG: The optical and electron microscopic determination of pulmonary asbestos fibre concentration and its relation to the human pathological reaction. *J Clin Pathol* 26:224–234, 1973.

11. Corn CJ, Williams MG, Jr., Dodson RF: Electron microscopic analysis of residual asbestos remaining in preparative vials following bleach digestion. *J Electron Microsc Tech* 6:1–6, 1987.

12. Gylseth B, Baunan RH, Overaae L: Analysis of fibres in human lung tissue. *Br J Ind Med* 39:191–195, 1982.

13. Roggli VL, Piantadosi CA, Bell DY: Asbestos bodies in bronchoalveolar lavage fluid: A study of 20 asbestos-exposed individuals and comparison to patients with other chronic interstitial lung disease. *Acta Cytol* 30:460–467, 1986.

INDEX

Squamous metaplasia, 229–230
Staining. *See also specific stains*
  dispersion, polarizing microscopy
    with, 8–10, 11
Standardized mortality ratio (SMR)
  for gastrointestinal cancer, 212
  for laryngeal cancer, 215
Stanton hypothesis, 280
Superficial parenchymal invasion,
    in pleural mesothelioma,
    114, 115
Superoxide anions, production of,
    asbestos fibers and, 272
Surgery
  in mesothelioma treatment, 153
  in peritoneal mesothelioma diag-
    nosis, 147
Synergism
  between polycyclic aromatic hy-
    drocarbons and asbestos
    exposure, 283, 284, 285
  between smoking and asbestos
    exposure, 284
    in lung cancer production,
    192–194
Systemic disease, asbestosis-
    related, 98
Systemic sclerosis, silica exposure
    and, 98

T-cells, in pleural mesothelioma, 237
Talc, 338, 339. *See also* Serpentines
  ovarian cancer and, 218
  parietal pleural plaques and, 167,
    175
  in sheet silicate pseudoasbestos
    bodies, 61
Talcosis, 167
TEM. *See* Transmission electron
    microscopy
Textiles, manufacture of, 21
  exposure measurement and, 28
  lung cancer and, 194
Thoracotomy, tumor sampling at,
    pleural mesothelioma diag-
    nosis and, 117
Thorium dioxide (Thorotrast), me-
    sothelioma and, 113
Threshold limit value (TLV), medi-
    colegal issues and, 351

Thymidine kinase, in pleural
    mesothelioma, carcinoma
    vs., 128
Tissue ashing, 301
Tissue burden
  analysis of. *See* Tissue mineral
    fiber content analysis
  asbestos bodies in sputum and,
    239, 242
  proportion of coated fibers and,
    41, 46
Tissue digests. *See* Digestion studies
Tissue mineral fiber content analy-
    sis, 299–339. *See also* Histo-
    logic sections
  in asbestosis, 307–314
  in benign asbestos-related pleural
    diseases, 318–321
  digestion techniques in, 301. *See
    also* Digestion studies
  exposure category and,
    329–336
  for fiber identification and quanti-
    fication, 301–305, 336–339
  historical background of,
    299–300
  interlaboratory variations in, 306
    medicolegal aspects of, 356
  intralaboratory variations in, 306–
    307, 308
  in lung cancer, 322–326
  in mesothelioma, 314–318
  methods for, 300–307, 308
  in neoplasia other than lung,
    326, 327
  in normal lungs, 326, 328–329
  results of, variability of, 306–
    307, 308
  in testimony, for plaintiff, 354
  tissue selection for, 300–301
Tissue sections. *See* Histologic
    sections
Tissue selection, for mineral fiber
    content analysis, 300–301,
    384–385, 387
Titanium, in pseudoasbestos bod-
    ies, 62
Titanium dioxide, 339
TLC (total lung capacity), in asbes-
    tosis, 81–82
TLV (threshold limit value), medi-
    colegal issues and, 351

125.00
112.50